Mental Health Practice with the Elderly

MARK A. EDINBERG

Center for the Study of Aging,
University of Bridgeport

Prentice-Hall, Inc., Englewood Cliffs, New Jersey 07632

Library of Congress Cataloging in Publication Data

Edinberg, Mark A., 1947-
    Mental health practice with the elderly.

    Bibliography: p.
    Includes index.
    1. Aged—Mental health services.   I. Title.
RC451.4.A5E35   1985   618.97'689   84-15877
ISBN 0-13-5759 94-3

Editorial/production supervision and
   interior design: Virginia McCarthy
Cover design: 20/20 Services, Inc.
Manufacturing buyer: John Hall

Printed in the United States of America

10 9 8 7 6 5 4 3 2 1

ISBN 01 0-13-575994-3

Prentice-Hall International, Inc., *London*
Prentice-Hall of Australia Pty. Limited, *Sydney*
Editora Prentice-Hall do Brasil, Ltda., *Rio de Janeiro*
Prentice-Hall Canada Inc., *Toronto*
Prentice-Hall of India Private Limited, *New Delhi*
Prentice-Hall of Japan, Inc., *Tokyo*
Prentice-Hall of Southeast Asia Pte. Ltd., *Singapore*
Whitehall Books Limited, *Wellington, New Zealand*

FOR JOEL

Contents

Section III
Interventions with the Aged

Section IV
Delivery of Mental Health Services

Preface

This text, while focusing on emotional and mental health of the aged, is designed to be of value to people of several professions. We are at a historical point at which the numbers and types of disciplines called upon to give "mental health" to older adults is extremely varied, including (but not limited to) clergy, counseling, medicine, nursing, occupational therapy, psychology, psychiatry, recreation, and social work. However, there is often a lack of a common knowledge base and language when the multi-faceted problems of the aged are handled in any interdisciplinary setting. *Mental Health Practice With the Elderly* grew out of my concern that there be a text that pulls together information to introduce professionals to literature, knowledge, issues, and skills used in treating the mental health problems of older adults. It is designed so that a person unfamiliar with the field of aging or with a given treatment modality can understand relevant background and how varied approaches may be used in practice with the older adult.

Although many types of treatment approaches are reviewed, I have avoided making a "final" judgment on any approach but have focused more on the potential utility of most methods. While others may disagree with this decision, I think the professional should make her or his own judgments as to the "correct" method or most effective combination of approaches. We know that psychotherapeutic methods work. We do not know, with certainty, which are the "best" for the range of mental health problems and adaptive situations faced by the aged.

This text is divided into four sections: I—Processes of Aging; II—Psychopathology and Assessment; III—Interventions with the Aged; and IV—Delivery of Mental Health Services. The four chapters in Section I address Myths and Theories of Aging (Chapter 1), Aging and the Individual (Chapter 2), The Social Context of Aging (Chapter 3), and Death, Dying, and Bereavement (Chapter 4). Theories, research, and data on aging are related to mental health care of older adults in four ways: discussion of implications for the mental health care of the elderly, delineation of areas in which mental health intervention can benefit older persons in adapting to changes related to aging, suggestions of roles and functions for the mental health practitioner, and suggestions of stylistic and strategic approaches as they have been presented in the literature.

Section II is presented in three chapters: Functional Disorders (Chapter 5), Organic Brain Disorders (Chapter 6), and Assessment of the Elderly (Chapter 7). Each of the first two chapters reviews major psychiatric disorders found in the Diagnostic and Statistical Manual of the American Psychiatric Association (DSM-III). Disorders are then discussed in terms of their occurrence, symptomology, and how they are commonly treated in the aged, including major drugs used to control symptoms. Chapter 7 has three purposes: to introduce the reader to issues in assessment, to present methods and instruments used in screening the elderly, and to provide a decision-making framework (presented as a list of questions) to aid in determining how to use assessment procedures. The review of instruments excludes those requiring significant clinical training to administer or interpret.

Both the guides to treatment and description of drug regimens are introductory. The reader wishing more advanced information on interventions can refer to the chapters in Section III of this text, and the reader wishing more information on drug interventions should refer to cited references in medicine and nursing.

Section III starts with a chapter on General Considerations in Mental Health Practice with the Elderly (Chapter 8). This chapter focuses on areas of practitioner and client interaction that affect the therapeutic process regardless of type of therapeutic approach: How interventions with the aged differ from those with the young, the nature of helping relationships with the aged, professional ethics, and how the contact between client and practitioner is structured.

Chapters 9 to 14 review several types of approaches to intervention with the aged: Psychodynamic Approaches (Chapter 9), Behavioral and Cognitive Approaches (Chapter 10), Humanistic and Creative-Expressive Approaches (Chapter 11), Group Approaches (Chapter 12), Family Approaches (Chapter 13), and Indirect Approaches: Pets, Plants, and Environmental Manipulation (Chapter 14). Each chapter presents some introductory information about the approach and then provides examples of techniques and methods used with the elderly. Each approach is also evaluated using the following framework: *goals* (cure, adaptation, enrichment, prevention), *focus* (physical health, attitude/values, cognition, emotions, behavior, socialization), *targeted population* (types of clients most likely to benefit), and *strengths and weaknesses* (including scientific validity of the approach, flexibility of the approach, clarity of the approach, and the degree to which the approach can be integrated into the multi-dimensional and multi-system problems of the aged). The framework is based on work by Huyck and Hoyer (1982).

Section IV is designed to introduce readers to the mental health delivery system as it pertains to the aged. A short history of mental health legislation is given, followed by a description of existing institutional and community structures, some assessment of their relative strengths and weaknesses, and some considerations about organizational issues and dynamics that influence mental health care of the older client. Three current trends, outreach, peer counseling, and support groups, are also described. In part due to space limitations, all of this material is contained in one chapter: Delivering Mental Health Services to the Elderly (Chapter 15).

There are many people who deserve mention in helping create this text. Allison Bailey, Barbara Demmerle, Margaret Kane, and Lynn Hodgson all read sections of the text and made helpful suggestions. Frank Benito and Judith Sugarman added certain clinical observations. Marsel A. Heisel, Michael A. Patchner, Ron Toseland, Ramón Valle, and Patricia Wisocki were reviewers. Their interest and astute criticism is appreciated. My colleagues at the Center for the Study of Aging, David Carboni, Judith Naden, and Donna Wagner, provided emotional support through two years of writing. Joseph Nechasek, Dean of the College of Health Sciences, also provided important input in specific areas.

If there is ever an award for patience and deciphering, it should go to Lorry Goorevich, our secretary, who typed this manuscript. Mary Chaco, Regina Kliczewski, Siobhan Kelly, Barbara Hunter, Marie Prezioso, Dorothy Stanewich, Mary Winfield, and Lori Piazzola also helped in preparing parts of the text and references.

There is a group of people without whom this text would not exist. They are the people involved in its production. To all of you at Prentice-Hall, including Bill Webber and Susan Taylor (editors), Barbara DeVries (assistant), and Virginia McCarthy (production editor), heartfelt thanks for a job well done.

Finally, there is my family. To my parents, Ruth and Harold Edinberg, and my grandmother, Selma Cohen, thank you for your love and support. To my wife, Barbara, and my children, Daniel and Joel, you are the most important people in my life.

M.A.E.

Acknowledgments

Materials in Chapter 2 adapted from Butler, R.L. & Lewis, M.I., *Sex After Sixty.* New York, Harper & Row, 1976, with permission.

Materials in Chapter 3 adapted from Kart et. al., *Aging and Health: Biologic and Social Perspectives.* Menlo Park, Ca.: Addison-Wesley Publishing Co., 1978, with permission.

Materials in Chapter 5 adapted from Libow, L.S.: Senile Dementia and "Pseudo-senility": Clinical Diagnosis, In C. Eisdorfer & R. O. Friedel (Eds.) *Cognitive and emotional disturbance in the elderly: Clinical Issues.* Copyright © 1977 by Year Book Medical Publishers, Inc., Chicago, with permission.

Materials in Table 6-1 adapted from the following sources with permission of publishers:

Mental Status Questionnaire from Kahn, R.L., Goldfarb, A.I., Pollack, M., & Peck, A. (1960) Brief objective measures for the determination of mental status of the aged. *American Journal of Psychiatry, 117,* 326-328, with permission of American Psychiatric Association.

Short Portable Mental Status Questionnaire from Pfeiffer, E. (1975). A short portable mental status questionnaire for the assessment of organic brain deficit in elderly patients. *Journal of the American Geriatrics Society, 23,* 433-441, with permission of W.B. Saunders, publisher.

Materials in Chapter 8 adapted from Kane, R.A. & Kane, R.L., *Assessing the Elderly*. Lexington, Mass.: Lexington Books, with permission of the publisher. Copyright 1981, the Rand Corporation.

Materials in Chapter 13 adapted from Herr, J.H. & Weakland, J.H., *Counseling Elders and Their Families*. New York: Springer Publishing Company, 1979, with permission.

Myths and Theories of Aging

INTRODUCTION

Being "old" means different things to different people: Mrs. O., a seventy-eight-year-old widow, lives alone in an apartment and is dependent on public transportation and a senior center for her connections to the outside world. While she has good health and adequate income, being "old" for Mrs. O. means being dependent on others when she used to depend on her husband.

Mr. and Mrs. Y. are a married couple in their sixties who have just moved into a retirement community. Mr. Y. has retired from an executive position, Mrs. Y. raised a family and worked part-time. For Mr. and Mrs. Y., being "old" may mean relaxing and enjoying life.

Dr. B. is a seventy-four-year-old dentist recovering from a heart attack. He is married, but his wife is arthritic and cannot care for him. He also does not have substantial savings or investments and must work part-time. For Dr. B., being old may mean being concerned about health, sexuality, ability to work, or living in a nursing home.

Mrs. Q. is an eighty-two-year-old widow who goes out and publicly speaks for the rights of the elderly. She is self-sufficient and independent. For Mrs. O., being "old" means having the opportunity to correct some of society's mistakes.

Bob Hope, George Burns, justices of the Supreme Court, many elected officials, and other elderly are living at the peak of professional or personal lives. For them, being old may mean doing the same things that they have been doing in the past.

We are living in a time when conventional views and expectations of aging are changing. There is even disagreement about how to define *old*. Should age be defined chronologically (how many years one has lived), functionally (what one is capable of doing in a specific area of functioning), or socially (one's roles, activities, and use of supports)? For our purposes, the chronological definition will be used to limit the focus of this text to people sixty-five years and older.

Even with an arbitrary definition of who is old, the question still remains: Who are the elderly? As a starting point, consider the four following generalizations:

1.   The aged are quite varied on almost any dimension. Some are at the peak of their professional and personal lives; others are not. Most manage quite independently on their own; others are in desperate need of health care or in need of varying degrees of support to maintain themselves, including institutional care. The aged represent every cultural, racial, religious, and socioeconomic class.

2.   At its best, aging can represent opportunities for continuing or developing satisfying roles, relationships, and activities. At its worst, aging can represent painful losses of one's intimates, health, and roles.

3.   Individuals vary considerably in their reactions and abilities to adapt to losses and age-related changes. Some reach deepened self-understanding and integration even in the face of death; others may have trouble adapting to role changes rising from retirement. How an individual has coped with change throughout life is a good indicator of how she or he is likely to "adapt" to aging.

4.   While "age" does not directly cause most of the conditions associated with being older, there are certain changes in aging and specific conditions (such as senile dementia of the Alzheimer's type) that are primarily found in the elderly. However, it is frequently difficult in an individual case to determine the degree to which a person is suffering from a physical, mental, or socially created problem.

These generalizations have three common themes: Aging has the potential to be a positive part of life, individuals are quite varied in how they live and adapt in old age, and aging-related issues and changes will affect individuals to varying degrees. Unfortunately, most people do not share this view of both the possibilities and variations in aging; rather, they have some vague or overgeneralized negative stereotypes about how the elderly live, feel, and adapt to their situation. A closer examination of these commonly held beliefs is useful as a way to begin uncovering the realities of aging.

STEREOTYPES OF AGING

Negative attitudes and stereotypes of the elderly have been described as evidence of "agism," a general prejudice against the elderly (Butler, 1968). Agism is expressed in some commonly believed myths about the elderly, all of which are untrue as stated, although some elderly individuals may act in such a manner or may even believe the myths themselves.

Some Common Myths About the Elderly

Unproductivity   It is commonly believed that older adults do not lead productive lives, that they cannot contribute to society (Butler, 1975). In fact, 25 percent of older people are gainfully employed. Older workers have fewer accidents and better attendance than younger workers and are equally productive. In terms of responsibility, older persons have held proportionately more public offices (including justice of the Supreme Court and presidency of the United States) than younger persons (Palmore, 1981).

Inflation and legislated changes that raise the age of retirement and eligibility for social security benefits are likely to create an even greater interest and need for the aged to work in the future. The myth of unproductivity can make obtaining work unnecessarily difficult for the older worker since many employers still mistakenly believe that any older worker is inherently less able than a younger one.

Senility   The myth of senility implies that confusion and loss of mental facilities is inevitable in old age, cannot be helped, and leads to death. According to this belief, it is only a matter of time until each of us starts to forget where we are, who we are, and what we are doing.

In fact, while many elderly may have some minor memory loss, only 15 percent are likely to show signs of disorientation, that is, confusion as to where they are, who they are, and what day it is. When disorientation occurs, it is due to specific conditions such as overmedication, depression, or brain diseases; it is not a sign of "old age" (Jarvik, 1980).

Minor memory loss, such as misplacing the keys or forgetting a newly learned set of directions, is not a sign that death is imminent or that all mental faculties will soon fail. Moreover, some memory loss can be recovered or aided, as is discussed in Chapters 2 and 5 of this text.

The senility myth can cause substantial harm to the elderly. Both older people and professionals may pay no attention to changes in functioning that signal onset of a specific problem because they attribute the changes to age and think they are inevitable. At another level, the input of older adults may be discounted by families, courts, or neighbors as the ramblings of "senile" old people, particu- larly if there is a disagreement or an emotional confrontation. Finally, older people themselves may not take appropriate risks in social situations, such as being assertive or asking someone to repeat a statement, for fear of being labeled senile.

Sexlessness   The major stereotypes of sexuality in old age are that the elderly are sexless, that sexual interest should stop in the forties, fifties, or at retirement, and that any sexual interest by the elderly is abnormal—or at best humorous.

These attitudes are reflected in jokes about "dirty old men," cartoons about "sex-starved" older women in magazines such as *Playboy*, and numerous television "comedy" sketches. In fact, many elderly are interested in sexual activity and are sexually involved when a partner is available (Ludeman, 1981).

Unfortunately, these stereotyped beliefs reinforce any tendency by older persons and caregivers to avoid discussing matters of sexual functioning. Many professionals feel uncomfortable with this topic as it relates to the elderly; as a colleague once said, "We're pretty sure our parents didn't do it, but we *know* our grandparents didn't."

Rigidity   Another myth about the elderly is that they are rigid in behavior and thinking, that they cannot change their ways. While psychological research has shown that there are several types of rigidity, some of which are associated with age (cf. Botwinick, 1978), it is more likely that "rigid" elderly people were rigid in their youth and have only become more so through the years. One could even argue that today's "successful" older adult requires a greater ability to cope with change (in roles, attitudes, and status) than a person from any other age group.

Emotional Fragility   There are a series of misconceptions about the aged regarding their emotionality. These include stereotypes such as the aged are too passive, feel miserable and unhappy, or conversely, are easily upset, cranky, or chronic complainers. Actually, a person's emotional style remains similar through-out the life cycle, although there may be a heightened sense of turning inward or a magnification of existing traits in old age (Botwinick, 1978). A quiet, polite older person was likely to have been quiet and polite in earlier years; a cantankerous, assertive older person was probably quite the same way when younger.

Incompetence   The myth of incompetence implies that older persons are sick and cannot take care of themselves, their households, and their affairs. A related misconception is that most older persons end up in nursing homes.

The facts are somewhat different. Approximately 90 percent of the elderly manage their own affairs. Although 43 percent of the nation's more than 25 million elderly have chronic conditions that limit activity and 86 percent have a chronic condition requiring medical care, only 5 percent live in institutions at any moment in time (Butler & Lewis, 1983; Kastenbaum & Candy, 1973). Furthermore, most chronic impairment is not completely debilitating. Conditions such as arthritis, hypertension, and diabetes can be controlled. With appropriate physical, social, and psychological supports, the individual having these conditions can continue to lead a full and productive life in his or her community. Too often, the need for a specific support (e.g., a wheelchair or home-delivered meals) is overgeneralized to mean that the older individual is incompetent in all areas of functioning.

Homogeneity   This myth reflects the idea that "they are all alike." In fact, the variation in abilities, interests, needs, and health and mental health status among the aged is greater than in any younger population group. Each older person needs to be considered first and foremost as an individual, with beliefs, feelings, behavior, and a specific set of social and cultural supports and needs rather than simply being considered "old."

Portrayal of the Elderly

Negative views of old age are continuously expressed in media, especially on television (Kubey, 1980). Older people, though occasionally portrayed as wise, are usually presented as weak, eccentric, dependent on others, and incompetent. In advertising, much of the fashion and cosmetic industries have focused on and emphasized "looking young." Looking "old"—or even one's age—is, by implication, unattractive.

Similarly, many common expressions in America carry with them a negative view of age and the elderly as well as reflecting common stereotypes and myths. A few examples include:

Oh-oh, I must be getting old (when something is forgotten).
You're too old to be doing that.
You're as young as you feel (implying that feeling "old" is feeling bad).
He's a dirty old man.
She's a little old lady in tennis sneakers.

Stereotypes of the elderly are often conveyed in public settings by a look, body language, or comment. The older adult who is a little slow counting out change because of arthritis might hear comments from people in a grocery store checkout line. In other situations, people might be oversolicitous or patronizing.

Families may also treat older members in stereotyped ways. Their assumptions that an older person will not understand, will be angry, cannot hear, or should not make his or her own decisions are as often as not a reflection of their own anxiety, discomfort, or misperceptions rather than an accurate assessment of the older person's condition.

Implications for Mental Health Practice

The myths and stereotypes about the elderly affect how older persons view themselves and how others act toward the elderly. Inasmuch as an older person believes he or she is becoming senile or is incompetent because of age, he or she will have an attitudinal set that works against solving problems, creating a positive self-image, taking responsibility for his or her life and living life to its potential. These misconceptions should be identified and challenged when they arise as part of therapeutic intervention.

At the same time, the mental health practitioner should acknowledge and change his or her own stereotypic beliefs about the elderly. The practitioner should also consider how to decrease the impact of negative stereotypes on the older client's self-image and functioning. Educating family members and others about the realities of a client's condition may be useful in this regard. Also, direct confrontation may be used, with the goal of helping the support system identify and challenge inappropriate beliefs about aging and the older client. In the latter case, use of the cognitive methods presented in Chapter 10 of this text is a recommended approach.

A final focus of concern is preventive; that is, the mental health practitioner can serve as an educator or advocate for conveying accurate views of aging in school curricula, in media, and to the general public. The purpose of such efforts is to decrease the likelihood that others will perpetuate the myths and related behaviors that in turn create or reinforce psychological distress in the aged.

THEORIES OF AGING

Even armed with all of the facts about the aged, we are still left without answers to questions such as "What is the purpose of aging?" or "How can we conceptualize human development in the later years?" Theories of aging attempt to answer these questions and define the "purpose" of aging, although they vary in their scope, specificity, and focus. While it is beyond the scope of this text to review all theories of aging, several of the most prominant that have implications for mental health care are summarized below. They represent major psychological, sociological, and social-psychological approaches to aging.

Theories of Human Development

A Developmental Stage Perspective: Erikson's Stages of Man

Developmental stage theories, starting with the work of Freud, attempt to describe human development as a sequence of steps or stages. Each stage is different from all others, with specific tasks, problems, and outcomes, the preferred outcomes usually being the development of traits or characteristics such as trust, autonomy, or capacity to love. The concept of stages is fluid; that is, they may overlap or flow into each other without an obvious onset or termination at a specific age.

One of the earliest developmental stage theories with direct application to aging is that of Erik Erikson (1963). Erikson's theory proposes eight stages of development, each consisting of a basic conflict with two possible solutions, one adaptive (e.g., attaining trust in others), one unadaptive (e.g., mistrust of others). If an early stage is resolved with a low degree of adaptation, resolution of later conflicts will be made more difficult. A raft negotiating a river provides a useful metaphor for understanding the stages. If the raft is damaged in an early turning point (conflict resolved with poor degree of adaptation), it will be more difficult to navigate the rest of the river (later stages), although the later turning points can still be negotiated (Kimmel, 1980).

The conflict in each of Erikson's stages is between two naturally occuring opposite states or tendencies. The conflicts are viewed as inevitable and important processes in the individual's development.

The first six stages (characterized by outcomes of basic trust versus mistrust, autonomy versus shame and doubt, initiative versus guilt, industry versus inferiority, identity versus role confusion, intimacy versus isolation) focus on development up to early adulthood. Only two stages (adulthood and maturity) focus on adulthood and old age, even though these stages may encompass as many as fifty years of a person's life.

Adulthood: Generativity Versus Stagnation   In Erikson's seventh stage, adulthood, generativity refers to "concern in establishing and guiding the next generation" (Erikson, 1963, p. 267). There is a creative impetus in generativity, often expressed in raising children or in job-related activities, such as being a mentor to younger workers (Levinson, 1978).

Stagnation, however, implies a tendency to remain static in a manner characterized by concern only with oneself or by lack of interest (boredom). A successfully resolved struggle will result in satisfaction with one's creative productivity at work and an interest in the growth of younger family members. An unsuccessful resolution of the struggle may result in boredom, disinterest in work and family, and a sense of "biding one's time."

Maturity: Ego Integrity Versus Despair   Ego integrity is the culmination of all adaptive resolutions of earlier conflicts. It is the state in which a person is wise, mature, and has an integration of self and outer world realities. Ideally, the adult who has successfully resolved earlier conflicts has the capacity to achieve ego integrity and appreciate her or his life for what it is has been.

Despair reflects disgust, anger, fear of death, or other feelings that suggest one's life was a waste. Despair reflects failure to resolve earlier conflicts successfully. The depressed older person or the one who continually "starts over" to find meaning in life reflects despair.

A Continuation of the Stages Proposed by Erkison

The stages proposed by Erikson are broad both in their scope of concerns and the number of years they encompass. An extension of both stages has been proposed by Peck (1955). For old age, he proposed three essential conflicts:

Ego Differentiation Versus Work-Role Preoccupation   In successfully resolving this conflict the individual must have varied sources of interaction and satisfaction from the world, not just from a single work-role, in part so that retirement or children leaving home will not be a catastrophic blow to self-esteem.

Body Transcendence Versus Body Preoccupation   This conflict revolves around how the person copes with the increased likelihood of illness, pain, or infirmity. While most older people have a chronic illness, some manage to live full lives in spite of the pain or infirmity. Some even grow by coping with the illness. These individuals show evidence of body transcendence. Individuals who "live" through their illnesses, be it by continually discussing the illness, being overdependent on medication, or inappropriately going from doctor to doctor, can be considered to show signs of body preoccupation.

Ego Transcendence Versus Ego Preoccupation   Ego transcendence refers to any tendency to interact with the world as if it will continue after one's own death. The need to leave a legacy and the need to share the knowledge one has gained through the years are two examples of ego transcendence. A graphic example of ego transcendence is the story of a traveler who watched an old man planting fig trees. The traveler asked the old man why he was doing this, since the trees would bear no fruit while the man was alive. "I am doing this so my grandchildren will have the fruit," the old man replied.

Ego preoccupation is, conversely, the tendency to treat the world as if everything ends with the individual's demise. There is little evidence that plans are made for the parts of life that will continue after the individual is deceased. One can wonder if reticence to make a will and plan for one's own funeral are, at some level, a reflection of ego preoccupation.

Research Evidence Supporting Erikson's Approach

There is some evidence that socialization patterns in aging reflect early experiences considered important in Erikson's framework (Lowenthal, 1968). For example, different patterns have been found for persons who had little contact with family and for those who had an "excessively harsh, punitive, or deserting parent" (Lowenthal, 1968, p. 195), compared to those who did not report this type of background. Perhaps even more important is the proven relationship between having a confidant (one with whom the older adult feels intimate) and decreased emotional impact of losses, lessened likelihood of psychiatric problems, and increased likelihood of satisfaction with current social interactions (Lowenthal & Haven, 1968). The related ability to trust others is a cornerstone of Erikson's first stage of development.

Implications for Mental Health Practice

Developmental stage theory raises several important considerations for mental health practice. First is that early experience influences many aspects of current behavior in the elderly. This in turn reflects what is called *continuity theory*, that older persons have a range of coping styles and approaches to life's problems that they have developed over many decades. Some styles and approaches that are currently ineffective were effective at another point in time. In terms of mental health practice, a client who appears to be showing "resistance" could, from his or her perspective, merely be holding on to what has been a useful way of coping in the past. This means not that change is impossible, but rather than an appreciation of a client's social and personal history is important in implementing "new" ways of approaching problems or coping with sources of emotional turmoil.

A second consideration is that having a confidant seems to be an effective preventative measure against likelihood of psychiatric illness and/or institutionalization. This suggests that actively finding ways to enable older persons to develop meaningful relationships is an appropriate endeavor for the mental health practitioner.

A third consideration is that developmental stage theory helps conceptualize aging as a phase of life in which certain conflicts are to be expected and need to be resolved. For example, consider the struggles of the older person who will not make out a will but who worries at the same time how a spouse will carry on after his or her death. It may make more sense to conceptualize this as an attempt to resolve the issue of ego transcendence versus ego preoccupation, an understandable conflict, rather than simply as the irrational rambling of a demented older person.

Finally, developmental stage theory provides several goals and a focus for mental health intervention with the aged. One goal may be the resolution of current age-related struggles. Another may be the resolving of conflicts arising out of the past. A third may be more adaptive, that is, teaching the client how to use successful strategies from the past in lieu of currently unadaptive strategies rather than examining why the client is using the unadaptive strategies. A final goal is to consider the quest to make meaning out of one's life an appropriate issue in mental health treatment of the elderly.

Sociological Perspectives: Disengagement and Activity Theories

A sociological perspective is one in which the individual's status and relationship to society are considered crucial in examining adaptation to aging. The most noteworthy sociological theories of aging are the theories of disengagement and activity. These two theories are viewed as contradictory in that each predicts different patterns of social behavior in the elderly who age "successfully." Successful aging in this case is frequently defined as being satisfied with one's life or having a high degree of "life satisfaction."

Disengagement Theory

The theory of disengagement is based on studies of older men in Kansas City showing that there were consistent declines in role activities, social interaction, and involvement with current roles as individuals aged (Cumming & Henry, 1961). The basic tenet of disengagement theory is that there is a mutual (and desirable) separation between older persons and society as the elderly prepare for death.

Disengagement has four characteristics: It happens slowly and continually;

it is universal; it is mutual and satisfying for the individual and society; and it is sanctioned by society through mechanisms such as retirement (Crandall, 1980).

Subsequent research has not shown disengagement to be either inevitable or desirable, although some individuals are quite content with less social and role activity in old age (e.g., Maddox, 1964; Carp, 1968). A competing set of concepts, called activity theory, has been proposed as a more accurate conceptualization of successful aging.

Activity Theory

Activity theory, which was actually developed prior to disengagement theory, argues that while there are age-related physical changes, the psychological and social needs of elderly are similar to those of the middle-aged adult. Therefore, the successfully aged individual remains involved in activities in which she or he was engaged in middle age (cf. Havighurst & Albrecht, 1953; Tobin & Neugarten, 1961), resisting the tendency of the social environment to withdraw support or status. If there are losses in roles or relationships with others (such as death of spouse), these losses should be replaced with appropriate substitutes (e.g., friendship or volunteering) to achieve maximum life satisfaction.

Activity theory underlies the development of senior citizen centers in the United States as well as services such as the meals program of the Older Americans Act of 1965. The philosophical assumption that older adults should remain active as a way of promoting life satisfaction and "successful" aging has hit a responsive chord in the delivery of social services to the aged.

Implications of Disengagement and Activity Theories for Mental Health Practice

Both disengagement and activity theories focus on activity as a critical variable in determining happiness in old age. Furthermore, both theories attempt to describe normal and desirable aging. Although they represent opposite viewpoints, these theories suggest strategies to prevent emotional problems in old age. Disengagement theory suggests working through one's decreasing interaction with society. Activity theory suggests staying active. Engaging in meaningful activities may also be an effective preventive measure and source of satisfaction to compensate for the losses in status and role that accompany aging.

Although most research supports activity theory, it is important to consider that for some individuals a degree of disengagement may be quite satisfactory. Some older adults seem to enjoy relinquishing current responsibilities; also, some older adults prefer to observe activities in institutional settings, even though at one point they were participants.

Conversely, many adults blossom in old age, finding new relationships and activities that provide a high degree of satisfaction. For the mental health provider, the question of which is the correct theory may not be as important as paying attention to how individual clients derive satisfaction in their lives and knowing that there are many ways in which individuals can have a "successful" old age. The latter point is particularly important in making sure the mental health practitioner does not force her or his values of "successful aging" on the older client.

A Social Psychological Perspective: The Social Reconstruction Model

A somewhat different perspective on aging is presented by Kuypers and Bengtson (1973). It is particularly applicable for any professional working with older people on issues of self-esteem.

Although not a theory of adult development per se, Kuypers and Bengtson's approach draws from several backgrounds, including systems theory and "labeling theory." Kuypers and Bengtson are concerned with the impact of "being old" on the individual, which can take place in the following manner. First the older person is susceptible to a "psychological breakdown." Then, others label the individual as incompetent or deficient (stereotype of aging). The individual assumes a sick and dependent role and loses previously held coping skills. Finally, the individual identifies with the role and subsequently labels himself or herself as deficient (Bengtson, 1973).

FIGURE 1-1   The Social Reconstruction Syndrome

From Vern L. Bengtson, *The social psychology of aging.* Copyright © 1973 by Bobbs-Merrill, Inc., reprinted by permission.

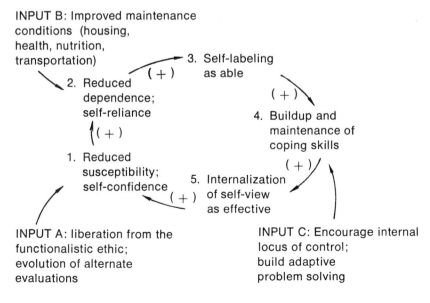

INPUT B: Improved maintenance conditions (housing, health, nutrition, transportation)

2. Reduced dependence; self-reliance

3. Self-labeling as able

4. Buildup and maintenance of coping skills

1. Reduced susceptibility; self-confidence

5. Internalization of self-view as effective

INPUT A: liberation from the functionalistic ethic; evolution of alternate evaluations

INPUT C: Encourage internal locus of control; build adaptive problem solving

Kuypers and Bengtson then argue that the elderly are likely to be victims of social labeling because of their loss of roles and status. Also, their loss of identity as workers or parents makes them even more vulnerable. If an individual accepts a negative label as the basis of his or her identity, he or she will become dependent, losing previous skills. Finally, accepting the negative label means the person is self-defined as inadequate, which allows the cycle to repeat itself.

The social reconstruction syndrome seeks to prevent or stop the breakdown syndrome for the elderly. It is one of the few models or theoretical perspectives that suggests types of intervention to improve competency and well-being as well as prevent the onset of emotional distress. It also presents a model of how the individual interacts with social systems.

The five steps of the model are:

1. *Reducing susceptability and promoting self-confidence.* Because there are few roles that can give older adults a positive self-identity, they are vulnerable to externally determined self-labeling. However, an older adult who has self-confidence is, by definition, less likely to experience the beginnings of social breakdown. Interventions at this point need to focus on freeing the individual from the work ethic (i.e., that one's self-esteem should be based solely on how well one works). This also fits Peck's ego differentation versus work-role preoccupation stage.

2. *Reducing dependence and increasing self-reliance.* In a social breakdown, the individual falls prey to others' labeling him or her as feeble, sick, helpless, or "senile." The goal of the social reconstruction model is to encourage independence and the capacity to rely on oneself as the source of one's own identity. Interventions that improve access to the environment (see Chapter 14), nutrition programs, housing, or health maintenance programs are suggested at this point. However, these programs should be designed so that participation in them does not cause lowered self-esteem.

3. *Self-labeling as being capable or able.* Interventions that address issues of self-labeling include cognitive and client-centered therapies (reviewed in Chapters 10 and 11). Also, group interventions (Chapter 12) are recommended, as they provide cohesion and a sense of positive identity.

4. *Building and maintaining coping skills.* Kuypers and Bengtson suggest that older adults can be encouraged to develop an internal locus of control and learn adaptive problem-solving skills. This is also the point at which cognitive problem solving and application of behavioral/learning approaches would be helpful.

5. *Internalizing the new view of oneself as an effective human being.* The role of mental health interventions at this point should be to provide mechanisms for peer support and continued mastery over new situations. These in turn should enable the older adult to internalize his or her "new" self-image. Although the individual with an internal locus of control theoretically needs little outside validation, there is enough theory and research to indicate that while new learnings are being integrated, continued outside support makes the process much easier. One interesting implication for mental health practice is that the "helper-helpee" relationship would not be beneficial at this point. The older client now needs a more equal relationship with a helper, one similar to that psychoanalysts discuss at the "reeducation" phase of analysis.

Implications of the Social Reconstruction Model
for Mental Health Practice

The social reconstruction model presented above includes specific types of interventions for the mental health practitioner at various points. In order to carry these out, the practitioner needs to be well versed in therapeutic skills and knowledge about other social and supportive services. Ideally, the practitioner can choose to be an advocate for better housing or nutrition programs, a developer of plans for meaningful activities in senior centers, or even a "storefront philosopher" to challenge our societal norms embodied in the work ethic. Rather than taking the traditional low status position given to professionals who work with the elderly, effective mental health professionals in gerontological settings may need more sophisticated skills, knowledge, and approaches to client problems than those in more traditional mental health settings.

Beside implying an expanded knowledge and skill base for mental health providers, the social reconstruction model suggests that the role relationship between worker and client varies at different points in the relationship. Sargent (1980) has begun the discussion of how therapy can be provided in indirect and nonthreatening ways to the elderly. What may be even more important is a rethinking of the role of the helper. Do the labels "counselor" or "therapist" imply that the client has to be dependent? Is it possible to be a helper without making the client feel dependent? How can we, as mental health professionals, do our work in ways that promote social reconstruction as opposed to social breakdown from the onset of the relationship? These questions are not easily answered. The social reconstruction model raises them in a direct and useful manner.

SUMMARY AND CONCLUSIONS

Aging has the potential to be a positive part of life. Individuals are quite varied in how they live and adapt in old age, and there are aging related issues and changes that differentially affect older people. Several common myths about aging are the myths of unproductivity, senility, sexlessness, rigidity, emotional fragility, incompetence, and homogeneity. Although reality is quite different, the elderly are frequently portrayed as incompetent and in other negative ways in media. Stereotypes of the aged can affect how the older person acts as well as how others act toward the older person. Both education and direct intervention are needed to counter the effects of stereotypes about the elderly.

Theories of aging, including Erikson's stages of man, activity and disengagement theories, and the social reconstruction model, attempt to explain expected tasks and problems of aging. Each has implications for conceptualizing and designing mental health interventions for the aged in terms of the goals and focus of mental health interventions.

2

Aging and the Individual

INTRODUCTION

Mrs. G. is a ninety-two-year-old widow. She lives in an apartment, does her own shopping, and generally takes care of herself. She appreciates a visitor and calls her sixty-seven-year-old daughter regularly. She knows she is not as strong as she used to be, she wears glasses for reading, she has trouble hearing, and her "memory isn't as good as it used to be." Other than some arthritis and mild hypertension, her health is good.

Mr. C., however, is seventy-nine and is in a nursing home. He was finally institutionalized by his family after several small strokes and loss of memory as to his address and the date. Mr. C. cannot cook for himself, uses a walker to get around the institution, and has to have someone light his cigarettes as he is "careless" with matches. He also needs help dressing and bathing.

Mr. H. is in his mid-sixties. As he begins to think about aging, he seems to be concerned. When he forgets anything, he wonders if he will turn out like his uncle, who died of "Alzheimer's disease." He wonders what the next ten years will bring. Will he be healthy (like Mrs. G.) or will he deteriorate (like Mr. C.)?

What happens to individuals as they age? What changes should be expected? Which are signs of specific problems rather than the "aging process"? What impact will expected changes and/or impairment have on the individual and how can the mental health practitioner intervene in these areas?

These questions provide the framework for this chapter. It will focus on individual change in areas of psychological functioning, sexuality, and health. In each area, likely changes and consistencies are described. Also, abnormal or pathological conditions found in the aged are noted. At the end of each section, age related changes are discussed in light of their implications for the mental health of the aged. Finally, roles of the practitioner as well as goals and strategies for mental health intervention in the various areas are presented.

PSYCHOLOGICAL CHANGES IN AGING

Personality Changes

Personality is an individual's patterns of organizing his or her beliefs, perceptions, and behavior. As was mentioned in Chapter 1, older adults are quite diverse on many dimensions, personality being one of them. However, most aspects of personality remain stable throughout adulthood. Certain ones, such as degree of extroversion, may have different meanings, serve different purposes, or be expressed differently in old age (Costa & McCrae, 1977).

One noteworthy change in aging is that older people have a tendency to turn inward. That is, they have less energy and emotionality in relating to the world. This change certainly seems related to cautiousness in responding to the environment, more introversion, and the general slowing down of sensory and physical systems (Botwinick, 1978).

Yet this turning inward does not mean increased mental health problems. Nor does it mean that older adults dramatically change with age. Many of the changes are subtle (Neugarten, 1977). The "turning inward" is perhaps more a question of how the individual thinks and feels than how he or she acts.

A second expected personality change is towards less stereotyped differences between men and women. Generally, men may become "more expressive and women more instrumental" (Huyck & Hoyer, 1982, p. 238) in late life. Other changes may be improved ego functioning and less impulsiveness.

These expectations—that is, stability of most traits but a general turning inward and changes in traditional sex-role orientation—are offered cautiously. Even with our current tentative knowledge, one implication for mental health practice is that dramatic changes "for the worse" are not to be expected and are likely to be due to specific problems, either psychological, physical, or some combination of the two.

Changes in Cognitive Functioning

One of the most commonly accepted beliefs about age is that intelligence declines in the later years. Related beliefs include a sense that older people are rigid and cannot learn as well as younger people and that, in general, cognitive functioning can be expected to diminish with age.

The difficulty with these beliefs is that they are at best partially true. It turns out that while age may have a slight impact on cognitive functioning, other factors such as health and education say more about an older adult's intelligence or cognitive functioning than his or her age.

Intelligence

Intelligence is commonly measured by performance on intelligence tests such as the Wechsler Adult Intelligence Scale (WAIS). The WAIS has been tested on large numbers of elderly so that normative (average) scores exist for the aged. The WAIS is subdivided into two areas, each having five or six subtests: verbal (information, vocabulary, comprehension, similarities, arithmetic, and digit span) and performance (object assembly, digit symbol, block design, picture arrangement, and picture completion).

Early studies indicated that when young and old people were given the WAIS, younger people scored higher, leading to the conclusion that there is a decline in intelligence with age. These studies were cross-sectional; that is, they measured two different age groups at one moment in time.

These studies, however, did not take into account that intelligence test scores are affected by familiarity with testing and education. While their results were accurate (that is, older people scored lower than younger), the differences may not have been solely due to age. Later longitudinal studies have attempted to follow a group of individuals over time to see how their intelligence test scores change. These results can be summed up as a "classic aging pattern," specifically that verbal abilities show little change, but performance or psychomotor skills show a decline with age (Botwinick, 1978).

Even more important than a report of general decline in one area is the question of "So what?" What does the decline mean? To what can it be attributed? What are the implications for the individual client?

Various causes for the decline have been proposed, including disease, health, low motivation, unfamiliarity with testing and resulting cautiousness, expectations of failure, age bias in the tests, changes in capacity, and physiological changes (Crandall, 1980). Part of the problem in determining causes stems from the fact that intelligence, as measured by tests, is not a single or simple concept. There is a wide range of individual differences among the elderly in terms of knowledge and ability to learn (Willis & Baltes, 1980).

A more important consideration is what "intelligence" means in terms of adaptation, coping, and learning new ways of handling the "real world" the older person faces. No existing intelligence test measures capacity or ability in these areas for the elderly (Botwinick, 1978). One of the dangers of overreliance on intelligence tests with the elderly is that results from a test can inappropriately be transformed to a prediction about how the older person will either peform or adapt to new surroundings. From a practical viewpoint, it is more important to ask "Does the older adult have the (intellectual) ability to maintain him or herself or adapt to new circumstances?" than "What is her or his IQ?" It has also been argued that the environment (personal, social, and cultural) in which older persons live is not conducive to maintaining or developing intelligence in old age (Willis & Baltes, 1980). While the research results suggest a decline with age in certain abilities, we still do not know how much is innate and how much is due to physiological changes or environmentally induced conditioning.

Learning and Memory

Learning and memory are closely related, although they are considered somewhat separately in psychological research. They are related in that problems in one area will affect the other. Without memory, there is no evidence of learning; similarly, without learning or with faulty learning there is no memory. Craik (1977) separated the two processes by suggesting that learning is represented by acquiring skills or knowledge whereas memory reflects both retaining and being able to retrieve the skills or knowledge. That is, learning focuses on how the new content gets into the person; memory focuses more on filing and retrieving the content (Botwinick, 1978).

Learning   In discussing learning, a further distinction must be made. There is a difference between learning (or the ability/capacity to learn) and performance (the ability to put forth what has been learned). At the same time, learning is usually measured in terms of performance on a task or test. Older people show some decline in performance of newly learned tasks compared to younger people 1978). The unanswered question is "Is this due to changes in ability or changes that only (primarily) affect performance?"

Only certain conclusions can be drawn about this issue. For example, when older people have limited time exposure to new verbal tasks (such as learning new sets of paired words) they do less well than the young. Also, older people perform poorly when there is less time to respond with what they have learned (Canestrari, 1963; Monge & Hultsch, 1971).

Furthermore, other factors seem to affect learning and performance. Botwinick (1978) had identified *motivation, cautiousness,* and *meaningfulness of task* as three such factors. It can be argued that older people are less motivated than younger people to learn new material or that they are less motivated in laboratory settings. In fact, it seems that older adults are highly motivated in these settings, at times to the point where their anxiety actually works against effective learning and performance (Eisdorfer, Norolin, & Wilkie, 1970).

It has been demonstrated that the elderly make more errors of omission than commission in learning/performance tasks. That is, they are more likely not to respond than to make a guess when they are unsure of answers. This tendency may be considered a sign of cautiousness. However, in one instance when older adults were rewarded for each response, the hesitancy to guess disappeared and learning rates improved (Leech & Witte, 1974).

Finally, the question of task meaningfulness has been raised. That is, do older persons learn meaningful tasks at a different rate than less meaningful tasks? How does this compare to younger people? Although there is little research in this area, it is reasonable to expect that motivation and learning will be higher when the task has meaning to the older adults (e.g., Botwinick & Storandt, 1974). At the same time, "meaningfulness" is a complicated concept and may refer to familiarity of material, value to the learner, or even type of task (Botwinick, 1978).

Memory   As was mentioned earlier, memory can be considered the retention and retrieval of new material. There are two general theories of memory that are used in psychological research. The first distinguishes between *short-term* and *long-term* memory; short-term being used to describe periods of time from a few seconds to several weeks, long-term being used to describe memory of events in the more distant past. The second theory, which is more accepted, again distinguishes two types of memory, *primary memory*—a temporary memory of immediate nature with no processing taking place; and *secondary* memory—any memory that is longer than a few seconds or requires "processing" (integration, organization or abstraction) (Waugh & Norman, 1965). Botwinick (1978) also suggests there may be two other types of memory—sensory memory, an almost perceptual process, and very long-term memory.

Traditionally, researchers have shown that the elderly have poorer short-term and long-term memory than younger people (e.g., Bahrick, Bahrick, & Wittlinger, 1975). While some experts conclude that there is no primary memory decline and that secondary memory decline is expected with age (e.g., Botwinick & Storandt, 1974), others are finding that if conditions are "demanding" or if a cognitive ordering of material is immediately needed, primary memory of the elderly is not as effective as that of younger people (Craik & Simon, 1980). It also should be noted that the age differences are not dramatic; in fact, when very bright elderly are compared to very bright younger people, there are few memory differences (Botwinick, 1978).

Even with general age differences, other factors have been found that improve older people's performance on memory tasks even to the point of virtually "catching up" to younger people. The key factors seem to be:

Slowing "presentation" or pacing of materials to be learned
Instructing older people to organize material as it is presented
Rehearsing material once it has been learned
Providing techniques for memorization

Creativity

Although not usually considered a traditional aspect of cognitive functioning, creativity is an area of functioning that can be used to enhance the quality of older persons' lives. While early work (e.g., Lehman, 1958) shows that highly creative people do their best work before the age of forty, this work has been challenged (e.g., Dennis, 1966; Bullough, Bullough, & Mauro, 1978). There are numerous examples of individuals who have remained creative in their later years, such as

Picasso and Will Durante, as well as those who become "more" creative with age, such as Grandma Moses, who began painting after the age of sixty.

A more relevant question for the mental health practitioner is how to enable older persons to be creative or develop creativity. Rather than measuring creative accomplishments against Picasso—a measure by which virtually all of us would fail, old or young—or even measuring creative output, qualitative or quantitative, against what the individual "used" to do, the focus of creative work with the aged may be best focused on what can take place in the present.

Implications for Mental Health Practice

A word of caution must be given before examining implications of cognitive age changes for mental health practice. Virtually all of the work in cognition and aging is based on the study of groups of elderly. Individual older adults, by they clients, friends, or family, will vary considerably in both cognitive capacities and deficits.

The mental health practitioner may assume a role of instructor to help older persons compensate for memory loss or changes in ability to learn new information. The goal of such intervention is to help the individual adapt to current levels of ability rather than cure the memory loss or loss of ability.

A first point of intervention is to appreciate the impact of anxiety on cognitive functioning in the elderly. It may well be that some poor memory, inability to learn new information, and even cautiousness in responding are related to high levels of anxiety that have a detrimental impact on cognitive functioning. The older client who has cognitive (learning, memory) impairment may be anxious, have a serious underlying condition, or have a combination of the two.

Several specific steps can be taken to improve memory, learning, and performance difficulties.

Slowing the Pace of Learning   Older clients may need more time than younger persons to receive, store, and practice new knowledge, concepts and skills. For example, two situations in which new learning is necessary are relocation to a new house or apartment and moving into an institution. Given anxiety about the move, anyone working with an older client should appreciate that it may take the person a while to become acclimated and learn how to negotiate a new neighborhood or adapt to institutional procedures. Older clients should be encouraged to respond, ask questions, venture forth in the new environment, and, at the same time, take their time in responding.

Reducing Autonomic Arousal   Autonomic arousal (anxiety) can be decreased in several ways:

Ensuring a sense of privacy in sessions (perhaps by finding a quiet room or "corner" in a nursing home)

Having the client sit in a comfortable chair or, if bedridden, be as comfortable as possible

Establishing personal contact, rapport, and trust before delving into the "work" at hand

Using relaxation techniques such as successive relaxation (see Chapter 10) before moving to cognitive material

Reassuring the client that other activities (meals, visitors, etc.) will be tended to—that the counseling session will not interfere with other activities

Decreasing background noise and stimulation (visitors, television)

Utilizing Specific Strategies to Increase Ability to Learn, Retain, and Use New Knowledge and Skills   Very often, a poor memory or difficulites in learning can be helped by simple structural arrangements, such as having pertinent information written down in an easily seen place in the client's room or apartment. It is also helpful to have the client be involved in writing information and planning the design or placement of a noteboard of phone numbers or instructions for medication.

In addition, several techniques and strategies have been suggested that can improve learning and/or memory with the elderly. They include:

1.   Having the mental health professional encourage and support the older client responding to (trying out) the new information or skill to overcome cautiousness (errors of omission).

2.   Having the client use a "thinking-aloud" process (Giambra & Arenberg, 1980). This is seen as particularly useful with problem solving.

3.   Using group intervention. Older people can see that others have similar problems, receive peer support, and address self-worth issues that may make memory problems seem more severe than they are (Zarit, 1980; Zarit, Gallagher & Kramer, 1981).

As Botwinick (1978) has pointed out, however, older people do not spontaneously use mediators and may have more difficulty with them than younger people. Some possible reasons include lack of motivation, inability to use the device, a negative reaction to having to learn or use a "crutch," and a related loss of independence and self-worth.

4.   Encouraging step-by-step learning. The older client will generally do better if one task is well learned before another is undertaken (Botwinick, 1978).

SEXUALITY AND AGING

There has been growing interest in how aging affects sexuality and sexual expression. We know that one's sense of personal identity is strongly related to one's sexual identity. Sexuality is also one area in which psychological concerns are closely interrelated with physical functioning.

The Importance of Sex and Sexuality
for the Elderly

While *sex* usually refers to intercourse, being *sexual* more appropriately encompasses a range of behavior between people (including persons of the same sex) such as smiling, flirting, holding, touching, kissing, or feeling attachment to another human being. The sharp barriers that we create to separate "sex" from the rest of the continuum of emotional expression are inappropriate in understanding sexuality.

Dailey (1981) discusses five aspects of sexuality that provide a useful way to think about the topic: sensuality, intimacy, identity, reproduction, and sexualization.

Sensuality refers to physiological or psychological reactions to one's body or that of another—the "joy of sex," including "skin hunger," the need to be touched. Sensuality does not have to be genital, although genital arousal is a part of sensuality. Being held, massaged, or touched by another is an important part of sensuality. Unfortunately, many women have been brought up to believe that they have few rights to sensual pleasure. There may be an attitudinal set against sensual pleasure in the current aged cohort.

Intimacy is the emotional counterpart to sensuality. There is closeness, openness, and emotional exchange when there is intimacy. Widows and widowers experience a double loss of sexual and personal intimacy. Many also "give up" opportunities for personal intimacy by ignoring or denying their own feelings and interests in other personal relationships.

Identity is one's sense of gender, being male or female. Concerns such as one's sex role, changes in male and female identities in the last twenty years, and flexibility in defining oneself as an elderly man or woman are important questions in considering sexuality and identity.

Although *reproduction* is usually not a direct concern in aging, one's sense of success or failure in having or having raised children can influence identity and self-worth in old age.

Sexualization is the use of sexuality to influence others through power and control. Sexualization can reflect other aspects of a relationship. One can also argue that society puts older people "in their place" through sexualization by perpetuating the myths of the dirty old man and the asexual female, as well as the notion that old people "can't" and "shouldn't" have sex.

Physiological Changes in Sexual Functioning

There are four phases to sexual response—excitement, plateau, orgasm, and resolution. For older men, the following changes can be expected with age (cf. Masters & Johnson, 1966, 1970):

1. The excitement phase takes longer than for younger men. Achievement of erection may take several minutes.

2.   The plateau phase, a phase in which sexual tension is considered "enjoyable," may be comfortably maintained for a considerable period of time. Younger men are prone to desire ejaculation sooner than their older counterparts.

3.   Unlike the expected two-stage orgasmic process in younger men (the feeling that ejaculation is inevitable and actual ejaculation of seminal fluid), older men vary considerably in type of orgasms. The first stage may blend with the second. In the second stage, there is likely to be less seminal fluid. These natural changes may cause anxiety in the older male.

4.   In the resolution phase, the refractory period (the time before the male is able to respond again to sexual stimulation) is often considerably longer than for younger men. It can take hours for the older male to respond sexually after ejaculation. Also, after ejaculation, the erection may be lost quite rapidly.

None of these changes mean that satisfaction from the sexual experience is lessened for the elderly male. In fact, there are distinct advantages to the decreased demand for ejaculation in that partners can receive pleasure and sex can be reciprocal. However, several of these changes may lead older men to believe they are rapidly losing the capacity to perform or achieve erection. This, in turn, can lead to increased anxiety, impotence, or cessation of sexual activity.

For older women, expected physiological changes with age related to sexual functioning (by stages) include (Masters & Johnson, 1966, 1970):

1.   Onset of lubrication in the vagina is not as rapid as for younger women. It may take several minutes of stimulation before lubrication takes place. While the vagina does not have the expansive capacity of that of younger women, it is usually elastic enough to accommodate sexual intercourse. Intercourse can be painful due to changes in the vagina and/or abstinence from sex over a period of time. There may also be related bladder or urethra inflammation.

2.   In the plateau stage, there is less voluntary elevation of the uterus than in younger women. Both the color and position of labia are different, and the size of the cliotris may be smaller.

3.   In orgasm, uterine contractions may be fewer or even spastic in nature. The spastic pattern may be painful. Steroid therapy is helpful for some of the unpleasant aspects, although there is considerable concern about side effects, including the incidence of cancer and bleeding.

4.   Perhaps surprisingly, resolution in the older woman is quicker than for younger women. Both the uterus and pelvic viscera return to an unstimulated state quickly.

Again, as is true for the aged male, none of these changes mean that sexual activity must cease, although sexual activity may be painful. Also, some changes such as more extensive foreplay may be needed. Close consultation with medical personnel is suggested whenever pain is involved.

The Effects of Medical and Emotional Problems on Sexuality in Old Age

Some of the most debilitating myths about sexual functioning have to do with the impact of disability and illness on it. Misinformation and lack of client education has led to undue caution and unncessary cessation of sexual activity by older adults (Butler & Lewis, 1976).

One of the most common illnesses in the elderly is *heart disease*. Although many older people stop sexual relationships after a heart attack, it is often due more to fears about exertion than to actual dangers. While abstinence is generally recommended for a short period of time, the amount of energy needed to have intercourse is only that required for climbing a flight of stairs. Masturbation and variations in position (e.g., side by side) are suggested aids.

Other major diseases that may affect sexual functioning are *strokes, arthritis, prostatitus* (inflamation of the prostrate gland) and *diabetes. Diabetes* (diabetes mellitus) is somewhat different than the preceding conditions in that it can cause impotence in men, which is also an early sign of the disease. Although impotence may not be reversible if it occurs in a severe or long-standing case, in other instances it often can be (Butler & Lewis, 1976). In all of these conditions, attention needs to be paid to self-image and communication between partners.

An additional consideration is the impact of *surgery* on sexual functioning. In this regard, the most traumatic forms of surgery are hysterectomy (removal of the womb), mastectomy (removal of a breast), prostatectomy (removal of the prostate gland), and colostomy and ileostomy (removal of sections of the intestine). None of these causes a decrease in either desire or functioning after appropriate recovery time. However, the reactions to the loss of a breast or womb or the reaction to the smells and appearance of a bag attached to the ostomy opening are likely to create apprehensions about self-concept and capacity for intimacy, two major aspects of sexuality. Adjustment to these operations is complex. It may take considerable time and much counseling to help the older person and his or her partner work through their reactions so that they may reinstate sexual activity (Butler & Lewis, 1976).

Homosexuality

Although not considered a formal psychiatric disorder, homosexuality is not fully accepted in our culture. While the stereotype of the older homosexual is one of poor coping and isolation (Corby & Solnick, 1980), it may well be that being gay is less of a problem than its stigma in society (Kelly, 1977). There is no evidence that homosexual elderly are any less adapted to aging than heterosexual elderly.

Implications for Mental Health Practice

Some older persons have a history of sexual difficulties that have occurred throughout their lives. Cultural norms (e.g., the idea that women should only serve their husbands) may have influenced inhibited patterns of sexual expression throughout life. Belief in stereotypes about decreased sexual interest in aging will also inhibit self-expression in the aged. Fear and anxiety may arise from a lack of knowledge about either the significance of expected physical changes or a specific health problem. The ability to communicate about one's sexual concerns and problems with a partner is also a major source of difficulty. Finally, the lack of an acceptable partner is a major barrier to sexual expression, especially for older women. Sexual problems may be expressed in several ways.

One of the major symptoms of sexual dysfunction is male impotence, the inability to have an erection. Impotence is not "normal" for the elderly. It is even possible for males who have been impotent most of their lives to gain potency in old age with appropriate treatment (Masters & Johnson, 1970).

Other forms of dysfunction include lack of interest, lack of energy, and obviously, lack of sexual activity. Although intercourse may occur with less frequency than in earlier years, long periods of abstinence may be a sign of sexual problems.

The role of the mental health practitioner in sexual problems of the aged will vary depending on the specific problems and their underlying causes. One role is that of educator, giving clients accurate information about aging changes and implications of specific health conditions. Another is that of counselor, working with clients to uncover beliefs and feelings about themselves or aging that interfere with sexual expression and helping them change these beliefs, feelings, and related self-esteem. A third role is that of facilitator, helping a client and his or her partner learn how to communicate with each other about feelings, concerns, and specific sexual needs.

Similarly, the goals of mental health intervention vary. One goal is to "cure" a specific problem, such as impotence. Another may be to encourage more adaptive patterns of coping with physical changes or conditions and their implications. A third is to provide what can be called "enrichment," helping clients expand their options for physical pleasure (e.g., having massage "courses" in nursing homes and senior centers or developing activities that increase physical contact and intimacy in both community and institutional settings). A fourth is preventive, designing educational and group interventions to dispel inaccurate information and beliefs about sexuality and aging, encourage communication about sexual concerns between couples, and encourage options such as older women dating younger men.

A range of specific techniques and approaches have been developed for working with sexual prolems (cf. Masters & Johnson, 1970; LoPiccolo & LoPiccolo, 1978). They often combine instruction (including step-by-step approaches to create a better awareness of one's sexual response), counseling, facilitating communication between partners, and having clients explore many aspects of sexuality. The mental health practitioner who wishes to treat sexual problems of older clients directly is encouraged to take formal certification in this area.

Several other considerations are important in intervention in the area of sexuality and aging:

1.   Mental health practitioners should feel comfortable discussing their own sexuality as well as listening to and counseling others.
2.   The life style, personal values, and generational values of the older client need to be appreciated and respected.

3.   The ability to listen and be nonjudgmental (see Chapter 11) is a cornerstone of any intervention, be it curative, adaptive, enrichment, or preventive.

4.   If problems are identified, careful assessment should be made to determine the extent to which physical problems, anxiety, fear, misinformation, and difficulties in partner relationships contribute to the problem. The type and scope of intervention should be planned only with adequate understanding of the client's total situation.

HEALTH AND AGING

Traditionally, health and health care focus on diagnosing and curing single disease entities (Kart, Metress, & Metress, 1978). However, most of the physical discomfort faced by the elderly is chronic, influenced by aging-related changes, and is likely to involve several body systems. Many health problems of the elderly are overlooked because symptoms are similar, complaints can be incorrectly thought of as signs of aging, and older persons may be reticent to discuss their problems (Brody & Kleban, 1981).

At the same time, how older people view their health and health status may be as important as their actual physical conditions in determining well-being, adaptation to illness, and ability to function independently. This is, of course, one of the contentions of Peck (1955), that how a person handles illness and pain is a developmental task in old age. The person who lives through his or her illnesses by considering himself or herself "sick" or a "patient" will have a different outlook on life than another person with the same impairment who considers himself or herself "basically well."

Most elderly consider themselves in good or excellent health compared to others of their age (Harris and associates, 1975), in spite of the fact that the vast majority of them have at least one chronic impairment. The rest of this section outlines the major age-related changes that contribute to the impairments experienced by the elderly.

Physical Changes in the Elderly

If a general statement could be made about bodily changes and the elderly, it would be that "there is a gradual decline in capacity for all physiological systems; however, the decline does not affect most day-to-day activities." Most of the changes are so gradual that the individual is unaware of them except in times of exertion or stress.

Musculoskeletal System

The musculoskeletal system refers to those parts of the body (bones, muscles) whose function is both to support other organs and provide movement. With age, a person's physical strength, agility, and capacity to endure strenuous effort gradually decline. Muscles in the skeletal system atrophy (i.e., decrease in size) because muscle cells do not replicate. Also, there is a decrease in bone density called osteoporosis, which may make bones more fragile and susceptible to fracturing or breaking (Grob, 1971).

Changes are also reflected in the older person's posture, which can be hunched forward, with wrists bent and a slight flexing at the knees or hips. These changes are due to changes in the spinal column, including "compression fractures" (Grob, 1971). Despite these changes, however, there is little sense of weakness in the individual.

The changes noted do not, in and of themselves, cause death or even lower life expectancy. However, they can cause considerable discomfort and decrease mobility, which in turn can lead to dramatic changes in socialization, relationships, and quality of life. Unfortunately, people mistakenly assume that joint and muscle pain is natural and expected; therefore, they do nothing about it. Consistently recurring pain is not part of old age and should be examined.

The major symptoms of musculoskeletal disorders are stiffness, aching, and muscle cramps. Specific diseases associated with these symptoms are arthritis (characterized by swelling and pain in joints) and gout (characterized by high levels of ureic acid in the blood stream).

The Skin (Integument)

The skin serves several purposes, including sensation, protection, and regulation of temperature. With age, several types of changes can be expected. Generally, the skin becomes drier and more prone to wrinkling and itching, and there is a decrease in functioning of sweat glands (Tindall, 1971). Although these changes in and of themselves are not serious threats to health, they do make the individual susceptable to several diseases or disorders. Individuals who have been exposed to extensive sunlight through the years are more likely to contract circulatory, metabolic, or hormonal problems and skin cancer (Magnussen, 1980).

Besides senile pruritus (itching), the most common skin problem of the elderly, specific diseases or conditions related to the skin are *decubitus ulcers* (frequently caused by patients being left unmoved in beds or chairs), *keratoses* (thickening of the skin in areas exposed to sunlight), and *skin cancer.* The most common form of skin cancer is *basel cell carcinoma*, which does not spread (is nonmalignant) and is easily detectable. The other forms of skin cancer *(squamous cell carcinoma, malignant melanoma,* and *secondary skin cancer)* are more serious. They can spread (metastasize) and, at least in the case of malignant melanoma, lead to a lowered life expectancy.

Several sensible procedures can be followed to protect the skin in old age. A humidifier, pots of water on radiators, or filled bathtubs can add moisture to dry air. Sensitivity to sunlight can be avoided by wearing hats or sitting in the shade (Magnussen, 1980).

The Gastrointestinal System

Most chronic problems reported by the elderly are in the gastrointestinal system, which consists of body organs associated with ingesting and digesting food: the mouth, esophagus, stomach, small intestine, gallbladder, liver, pancreas, and large intestine. Many of these problems are caused not by disease but by poor nutrition, eating habits, or overconcern with bodily functioning (Sklar, 1971).

Age changes in the gastrointestinal system are generally not as great as in other systems. There is less stomach acid secretion and a slowing of digestion, which has implications for absorption of medicine and alcohol (both have longer half-lives—the time taken for one-half to be absorbed and metabolized).

While some loss of taste buds may take place, more serious oral problems such as sores or pain may be dismissed as "inevitable," leading to poor oral hygiene. Only one-half of all elderly have any natural teeth. Periodontal disease is also prevalent.

There are some changes in the stomach's walls and motor activity. The colon and rectum show little change in motor activity or capacity to secrete (despite the many complaints about constipation) and changes in other organs such as the pancreas or liver may be neglible in terms of impact on general functioning (Sklar, 1971).

Common Complaints and Illnesses Common gastrointestinal complaints of the elderly include heartburn, diarrhea, gas, and constipation. Common illnesses associated with the gastrointestinal system include *gastritis* (inflammation of the stomach), ulcers (painful irritation of one part of the stomach lining), *stomach cancer* (growth of malignant cells in the stomach), *gall bladder disease, diverticulosis* (a herniation or protrusion of the colon), *hiatus hernia* (where the stomach "slips" out of place, causing pain), *malabsorption,* and *maldigestion.*

Common single-organ symptoms and diseases include *jaundice* (a yellowing of the skin, a symptom that could indicate cirrhosis, hepatitis, drug effects, or cancer), *cirrhosis,* a serious liver condition, considered irreversible and the most drastic stage of liver degeneration (often related to alcoholism), and *cancer* of the various components (liver, bowels, gallbladder) (Kart et al., 1978; Sklar, 1971).

Nutrition In part because practitioners have been influenced by the beliefs that nothing can be done or that older people need less for survival, their nutritional status has generally been ignored. Older adults have similar nutritional needs as middle-aged adults. One exception is caloric intake, which decreases by about 5 percent per decade from age fifty-five. However, a physically active older adult may have the same caloric needs as a younger person (Kart et al., 1978). Common nutritional problems of the elderly include: potassium deficiency, obesity, vitamin C deficiency (many vitamin C foods are costly, the potato being one exception), and certain other vitamin deficiencies, some due to metabolic changes that lower absorption. Many dietary and nutritional problems of the elderly can be accounted for by poor dietary habits, including faulty food preparation and lack of a balanced diet. Many older adults to not have financial resources to buy standard forms of food groups (Berger, 1976) and they may not know cheaper substitutes (e.g., potatoes for vitamin C). Also, grocery store pricing (larger volumes for less money) works against the single older adult, who is cooking for one person. Nutritional assessment is beyond the scope of this text (see Christakis, 1973, for an extensive overview); a nutritionist or specially trained nurse and/or physician should be used for referrals.

Nutrition does not take place in a social or cultural vacuum. For most people, where and with whom food is eaten is of paramount importance. Holidays, special events, and other cultural traditions are closely intertwined with food and eating. The relative social isolation of many elderly (particularly the poor) has had a profound impact not only on mental health but on nutritional intake. For these reasons, meal programs at congregate sites have been developed through Title III (formerly Title VII) legislation of the Older Americans Act. Theoretically, both the nutritional content and socialization offered by sharing a meal with others has a positive effect on physical and emotional well-being, although it is also important to know how often clients attend (Ebert, 1980).

The Cardiopulmonary System

The cardiopulmonary system refers to those organs and systems in the body that serve to move blood to body cells and aid in the removal of waste from the cells.

Age-Related Changes   Like changes in other systems, changes in the cardiopulmonary system are gradual and represent a decline in capacity and performance. However, normal or expected changes are similar to pathological changes, which presents diagnostic problems. Expected changes include less elasticity in the aorta (the major artery from the heart), less cardiac muscle strength, and a resultant decrease in the rate of blood pumped by the heart at rest. Valves in the heart may increase in thickness and be the site of calcium deposits. In addition, changes in blood cell elasticity means that less oxygen can be absorbed from the lungs. Also, the lungs are less able to absorb oxygen due to physiological-related decline of muscle capacity in both the abdomen and chest (Kart et al., 1978). Several common health problems are related to this system.

Hypertension   Hypertension, or what is commonly known as high blood pressure, is the result of either loss of capacity of the heart to pump blood or loss in relative elasticity of the arteries. It has been called the "invisible illness." High blood pressure is not noticeable; however, it is dangerous in that it can lead to severe heart problems and/or strokes. Heredity, diet, exercise, environmental stress, reactions to stress, and obesity are all related to hypertension.

Coronary Artery Disease (Ischemic Heart Disease)   Coronary heart disease is the main cause of heart problems and death in the elderly. In this disease, blood cannot get through to tissues because arteries are either clogged due to a buildup of plaques on their inner walls (atherosclerosis) or lack sufficient elasticity to allow blood through easily (arteriosclerosis).

Heart Failure   Hear failure is the cessation of the heart to function properly. It is not so much a disease but the outcome of one or more several symptoms, including hypertension, atherosclerosis, and arteriosclerosis.

Heart Attack (Myocardial Infarction)   A heart attack is a sudden blockage of part of the coronary artery, either leading to interference with heart functioning and death or to some tissue death and the formation of scar tissue in its place (Brown, 1979).

Stroke (Cardiovascular Accident)   A stroke occurs when there is no blood supplied to a part of the brain, often due to atherosclerosis. Both the number of brain cells affected and their location influence the degree of damage to the individual's functioning. Some elderly suffer "ministrokes," short-lived incidents, which can lead to speech problems, blacking out, and lack of strength (Kart et al., 1978).

A condition where a blood vessel in the brain ruptures is called a cerebral hemorrhage. This is the most dangerous of all strokes in the elderly, often leading to coma and death.

A stroke can lead to paralysis, severe speech problems, and various problems in locomotion and use of limbs, depending on its location in the brain. A stroke on the left side of the brain affects speech, behavior (the client may appear cautious), language use, and movement on the right side of the body, including paralysis. A stroke on the right side of the brain will affect perception of spatial relationships, behavior (the client will appear impulsive or "fast"), and movement on the left side of the body, including paralysis (Kart et al., 1978). Recovery is often possible but requires patience and support from the patient and family.

The Genital and Endocrine Systems

The endocrine system refers to those organs that produce hormones, including the thyroid, adrenal glands, and the pituitary gland. The genital system refers to those organs used in the reproductive process. The functions of both systems are interrelated.

In terms of age-related changes, there are few specific changes in the genital system (most have been discussed earlier in this chapter). The most common diseases in males are inflammation of the prostate gland, inflammation of the testicles (treated by rest and antibiotics) and, occasionally, cancer. For females, cancer of the cervix and uterine cancer are concerns in late middle age.

Diabetes   The major disease associated with the endocrine system is diabetes, a condition in which a lack of insulin in the body and a decreased capacity in the liver to change sugar to more useful substances leads to an increase in glucose (sugar) in the bloodstream (Smith & Germain, 1975).

Diabetics are now referred to as Type I (insulin-dependent) or Type II (non-insulin-dependent, treated by oral hypoglycemics, diet, and restriction of carbohydrate intake). Diabetics are faced with an unending condition. Not only do they have to grapple with the fact that they will never get better or be cured, but they must also be active participants in their own care. Signs of disease progression include numbness, changes in vision (visual impairment is not uncommon), or changes in ambulation. Maintaining a balanced diet is difficult, as it often means changing eating habits established over a lifetime. In addition, social problems (such as how to refuse birthday cake) may need to be confronted so the client can learn how to handle them assertively and with high self-esteem.

Changes in Sense Organs

Although most changes in the sense organs of the elderly do not mean total loss of the sense or dramatic impairment, it can be argued that sensory loss creates as much functional hardship for the elderly as disease. Along with increased difficulty in handling the environment, the individual has to cope with embarrassment over needing physical or social support. Medicare does not cover the cost of sense-correcting devices such as glasses, hearing aids, or corrective shoes; moreover, many older adults are reticent to use them because they symbolize dependency, weakness, or "being old."

Changes in Vision   Most older people have adequate vision. However, the eye lens does become less flexible, leading to difficulty in seeing close. This condition is called *presbyopia* and may necessitate glasses for reading. Also, the lens may become somewhat yellow, making it easier to see oranges, reds, and yellows but more difficult to distinguish greens and blues.

There are three common and debilitating eye conditions found among the aged. One is *cataracts*, a seemingly age-caused clouding of the transparent eye lens. Cataracts cause blurring of vision and may require surgery. A second is *glaucoma*, a serious condition in which there is an increase in pressure of aqueous fluid in the eye, evidenced by loss of peripheral vision, blurring, and "halos" around lights. Fortunately, it is less common than other eye problems, occurring in 1 to 3 percent of the elderly (Kart et al., 1978).

The third condition is *senile macular degeneration*: The cells of the macula, the part of the eye responsible for making fine visual discrimination, begin to die. Ordinarily, there is not a total loss of vision. Magnifying glasses and environmental aids such as large-print books can help compensate for this condition.

Changes in Hearing   Hearing ability decreases with age. Caused by loss of the ear's nerve tissue starting in the mid-twenties, slightly more than one in ten "young" elderly (between sixty-five and seventy-four) and about one in four older elderly (over seventy-five) have noticeable hearing problems (Burnside, 1976).

There are three hearing-related problems for the elderly. First is loss of pitch discrimination—ability to determine how "high" or "low" a sound is. Loss of ability to hear high pitches is the most common hearing problem for the elderly.

The second problem is volume loss. Because most people believe that the "hard of hearing" need increased volume, they may yell at an older person, never realizing that "raising" their voice also raises the pitch. Hearing aids, while important for volume loss, do nothing for pitch problems.

The third problem is that some older people may only understand every third or fourth word spoken. The older person who answers questions incorrectly because he or she does not hear well may seem confused. The older person who has to be told everything twice can seem depressed. In addition, loss of hearing can lead to depression or fear of new settings, both because of the inability to distinguish sounds and the fear of failure, embarrassment, or others' reactions to the older person with a hearing deficit.

Changes in Taste and Smell While many studies have suggested that taste and smell decline with age, there is some controversy as to whether this decline is caused by aging or other factors. Whatever the cause, the decline of these senses has one important drawback. Foods may seem "tasteless," leading to a lessening of food intake. The older client, especially one on a restricted diet, may have to be encouraged to use new or different spices to compensate for his or her taste loss and make meals enjoyable.

Changes in Touch and Mobility Older people are less sensitive to touch stimuli than younger people. Also, reaction time is longer in a variety of ways. One outcome of this change is a tendency for the elderly to be slightly cautious in the physical environment and to respond slowly to physical stimuli, which can include elevator doors, paying at the grocery checkout, and verbal requests. While the changes are not debilitating, they bring expressions of impatience and ridicule from others, which can feel devastating to the older adult.

Medication

Any discussion of health, well-being, and mental health of the aging must at least recognize the importance of medication and its impact on older people.

Use and Misuse Older people use more than twice as much medication as younger people. Three-quarters of the elderly regularly use drugs (Hale, Marks & Stewart, 1979). Medication includes drugs prescribed by physicians as well as those bought "over the counter," (not requiring a prescription).

Older people with chronic diseases are likely to have several prescriptions for their illnesses, some dating back ten or more years. Some will not take recommended dosages or finish the prescription but will save "left-over" pills in case the symptoms recur, not realizing that the effectiveness of the medicine may have dissipated. Others will borrow pills from those with similar conditions or ignore the potential dangers of mixing pills with each other or with alcohol. Other problems arise from not using the medication correctly and using prescriptions from several physicians who are unaware of each other's treatment of the problem.

Aging Changes   Even when medication and regimen are carefully managed, consideration has to be given to the impact of aging on relevant body systems. For example, changes in the liver's ability to metabolize drugs to harmless substances can mean that "normal adult dosages" may have twice the effect of an older person (Ebert, 1980a). Other drugs have "paradoxical effects" on the aged, causing reactions unlike those encountered in younger adults.

Commonality with Other Health Problems   Some of the effects of over-medication, misuse of drugs, drug-drug interaction, and improperly followed regimens include tiredness, constipation, inability to eat, confusion, disorientation, and indigestion (Ebert, 1980a). These signs can indicate other problems, but improper use and side effects of medication should be ruled out as a matter of course in any dramatic change in client functioning.

Implications for Mental Health Care In the Treatment of Illness in the Elderly

The 1980s are witnessing the birth of fields or subspecializations such as behavioral medicine and health psychology. There is also a trend to take a so-called "holistic" view of health care—that is, to consider psychological, spiritual, and medical aspects as being part of a "whole" rather than separate and completely distinct entities. These trends suggest growing interest in mental health aspects of health care.

One potential goal of intervention for a mental health practitioner is to help the elderly person adapt to physical limitations and cope with illness. This may take the form of teaching the older client to comply with a medical regimen, to make changes in diet, activities, and hygiene to improve his or her health status, or to cope and stress. It may mean helping the client accept physical limitations and maintain self-worth in light of significant changes in health status and resulting changes in daily, weekly, or monthly routine.

A related role can be that of an authority figure who instills hope and, by showing concern, provides emotional support (cf. Frank, 1975). Goldfarb's "brief therapy," described in Chapter 9, is an example of how the "healing relationship" can bring benefit to hospitalized elderly.

A second intervention goal is direct control of symptoms. The general techniques use to control symptoms are behavioral, including reconditioning certain responses (e.g., incontinence), relaxation, guided imagery, and biofeedback (which can be defined as using machinery to have the client link "voluntary" actions with "involuntary" responses, such as relaxing to lower blood pressure). Generally, the more the symptom reflects a specific disease entity, the less effective the techniques have been. For example, people have been trained to control high blood pressure through these techniques, but not to cure or alleviate arteriosclerosis.

A final role is in decreasing external sources of induction into dependency (see the social reconstruction model in Chapter 1). Simple procedures such as not leaving the client alone at known critical moments (such as entry into the hospital and awakening from surgery), fully orienting the client to his or her disease and to hospital or nursing home procedures, and being sure staff introduce themselves by name and state the purpose of their visit, interview, or procedures (Bradley & Edinberg, 1982) can help the client's adaptation and progress through the treatment of an illness. In addition, the physical environment can sometimes be altered to improve the patient's independence and mastery, with a resultant positive sense of worth (see Chapter 14 for some specific environmental manipulations).

These roles are being realized in many health settings. The following descriptions of potential mental health interventions in health-related areas (stress management, cancer, pain control, and reversing incontinence) are but a few examples of how mental health interventions can be used in the health care of the elderly.

Mental Health Interventions that Can Benefit the Health Care of the Elderly: Some Examples

Stress and the Elderly

Stress management is a popular topic in the health field. The term *stress* is generally used to describe ineffective physiological and behavioral changes in an individual in response to a perceived threat. Individuals vary in their perceptions of what constitutes a threat, their physiological reactions to it, and their behavioral responses to threatening situations. Common reactions to a stressful situation include feelings of anxiety or dread; increased blood pressure, respiration and pulse rate; a physical readiness to take evasive action; and finally, exhaustion and temporary loss of capacity for positive action (Selye, 1974).

While stress reactions are generally considered short-lived, they can contribute to more chronic problems, such as hypertension (Zarit, 1980). Stress has also been linked to cancer and other illnesses (Simonton, Matthews—Simonton, & Creighton, 1978).

The relationship between events, stress, and disease in the aged is complex. Level of stress has been gauged by the number of stressors an individual encounters over time (Holmes & Rahe, 1967). Older people are generally exposed to more potential stressors than younger persons (Lowenthal, 1975). However, for the most part, older persons seem to adapt well to potential stressors such as retirement and institutionalization (Eisdorfer & Wilkie, 1977), adaptation being related to both an expectation and a psychological sense that these events are on time in the individual life cycle (Neugarten, 1977). Even when there is difficulty in adapting to stressors, the impact on the elderly may not be as long-lasting as we expect (Palmore et al., 1979). Finally, stress can actually be raised by exposing the older person to full knowledge about a condition over which he or she has little control, such as an operation (F. Cohen, 1980).

Personality and Heart Disease   Heart problems have been found three times as often among persons with certain personality characteristics (Type A) as opposed to persons without these characteristics (Type B). Type A individuals are characterized as aggressive, competitive, impatient, trying to do many things at once and having low self-esteem; Type B individuals are characterized in the opposite manner (Suinn, 1981). There is interest in changing Type A behavior (such as anger and impatience, two stress-related states) to decrease likelihood of heart conditions. However, it has also been argued that there may be survival value in exactly these traits and behavior for the elderly and that a more appropriate goal would be teaching older persons how to experience and express these traits rather than eliminating them (Sparacino, 1979).

Again, the relationships between personality, stress, and disease states are only beginning to be understood. The following treatment guidelines should be considered as useful, provided we acknowledge that there is still much to be uncovered about these relationships and that there are considerable individual variations in reaction to stressors, coping skills, and ability to handle stress reactions.

Intervention Guidelines   The role of the mental health practitioner in stress management is that of a guide and teacher. The client is taught how to identify his or her own potential sources of stress, is guided towards uncovering his or her own unadaptive reactions to stressful events, and is then taught one or more methods to change the stressful situations, physiological reactions, self-defeating thoughts, and unadaptive behavior that result from a stress reaction. Guidance may involve exploration of ambivalent reactions to potential stressors (e.g., the client who is both relieved and guilty when her ill husband finally dies, freeing her from burdens of caring), helping the client connect pieces of a stress-related behavioral pattern (e.g., feeling tired and run-down the first six months after retirement), or challenging self-defeating attitudes that prevent the client from attempting to learn more effective ways of handling stressors.

The goals of intervention can include alleviation of specific symptoms (e.g., elevated blood pressure in certain situations), decreasing frequency and duration of physiological and behavioral responses to stress (e.g., feelings of anxiety or helplessness), substituting specific nonstress responses for stressful ones (e.g., becoming relaxed before a confrontation with family members), and adding stress-reducing activities (exercise, proper diet, meditation) to the daily routine as a preventive measure.

The techniques used in stress management are varied. They include problem-solving approaches (one of which is described in Chapter 10) to identify sources and reactions to stress; behavioral and cognitive approaches such as relaxation and use of pleasant images as a substitute for stress-increasing thoughts (see Chapter 10 for a description of several techniques); and using props such as tapes of music or instructions to help a client practice new physical and psychological reactions privately. Before any technique is used, the practitioner should have a good idea of the stress-producing pattern of the individual client and how the client thinks about the stressor (e.g., is it "an act of god" or "something that should be changed"?). A final consideration is to design interventions so that the client has maximum control over the situation and his or her response—that is, to give the client a sense of ownership over parts of the stress-producing situation and his or her subsequent response.

Cancer

Cancer is a term that also means tumor or neoplasm (Hogan, 1979). It refers to a growth caused by abnormal cell reproduction. Probable causes include viruses, health habits (e.g., smoking), heredity, environmental factors (e.g., pollutants), diet, and life style. Cancer can appear in virtually any part or organ of the body. The severity and prognosis varies, depending on its location and the amount of cancer. There is also the possibility that *cancer* is too general a term and that various types of cancers, while being similar, should be considered separate disease entities. Cancer treatments include surgery, radiation of specific body areas, chemotherapy (the use of chemical substances in the entire system), and the use of pain control medication. Arguments have been made that there is a relationship between cancer and personality, thus suggesting adjunctive treatment by psychological methods using imagery and/or hypnosis (Simonton, Matthews-Simonton & Creighton, 1978).

A point should be made here about miracle cures for cancer. A series of substances, diets, and techniques (the most recent being laetrile) have been promoted as "cures" for cancer. Most have no scientific basis. Some, such as laetrile, may cause more problems than they alleviate. "Miracle cures" should be avoided. Other methods, such as imagery, can certainly be recommended in conjunction with medical treatment. However, the decision to forego medical treatment for dietary or psychological intervention is not recommended in light of current knowledge.

Some common emotional reactions to the diagnosis of cancer include: grief and grieving accompanied by denial of the illness, guilt, a sense of isolation, concerns about sexuality, and concerns about dying. Cancer affects both the client and family. Clients sometimes feel that they are unacceptable to others or that others are abandoning them. Family members and others may at some level believe that the client with cancer is contagious and should be avoided (Coping with Cancer, 1980). Other negative family reactions may include pity and overconcern, talking about the client as if he or she were not present or dead, and "mixed" messages about emotional closeness. The client who can clearly discuss his or her feelings may be turned off by others, especially those who cannot handle their feelings about the client (Wortman & Dunkel-Schetter, 1979).

When surgery is imminent, clients may go through grief reactions (loss of appetite, feeling blue, feeling anger, frustration, or denial) before or after the organ or body part is treated or removed. An older women losing a breast may have as many concerns about being attractive as a younger person. The client needs psychological supports starting the day of surgery (Coping with Cancer, 1980).

Implications for Mental Health Practice   The major role and function of the mental health practitioner in working with the cancer patient is to decrease emotional difficulties encountered by both the label of "cancer" and the realities of the condition. The goals of treatment may range from attempting to aid the curing process or pain control through the use of techniques such as guided imagery (imagining one's white blood cells killing cancerous cells or imagining one's body recovering from the side effects of radiation therapy) to helping a family member talk about his or her own fears about catching the disease from a spouse.

The older client who has an emotional reaction to any aspect of the disease (diagnosis, surgery, others' responses) may benefit from an informed and concerned "outsider" who is an active listener (see Chapter 11). The client and family may need to talk through their own reactions with the practitioner or need support to be able to share their concerns with each other. They may also benefit from peer support groups, such as those run by chapters of the American Cancer Society or Make Today Count. A final implication is that the mental health practitioner will be working with other professionals in the care of the older person with cancer. By being the one most concerned with emotional functioning, the mental health practitioner may have an important perspective to add to other aspects of planning a patient's care.

Pain

A common symptom reported by the elderly is pain, be it from a specific illness or from a chronic condition such as arthritis. Pain may also be related to psychological conditions. The physical aching experienced in mourning is one example. Finally, clients can complain of pain when there is no apparent physical cause.

One critical aspect of pain is that it is both subjective and perceptive; that is, the old ideas of pain being sensations translated into direct feeling are over-simplified and incorrect (Smith, Merskey, & Gross, 1980). A complicated series of relationships exist between glandular functioning, brain functioning, and perception of pain, with substances such as endorphin being posted as the body's "pain killer."

Implications for Mental Health Practice   Inasmuch as pain is related to psychological state, the mental health practitioner may be able to design interventions to decrease its effects. Relaxation, suggestion, hypnosis, and behavioral techniques have been used with some success for pain control in all age groups (Merskey, 1980). Also, since pain may represent a response to loss or a reaction to other aspects of an individual's situation, helping the individual in pain decrease sources of tension in other areas of functioning may also serve as indirect pain control.

Incontinence

One of the most embarrassing and socially debilitating health problems for the elderly is urinary or fecal incontinence, the inability to hold urine or bowel movements until they can be voided appropriately. Incontinence may occur in almost one out of ten elderly and is a factor in considering nursing home admission (Yeates, 1976). While there are measures that can be taken to control or even eliminate incontinence, the fear of being incontinent will inhibit many elderly from socializing or participating in social activities, even in structured settings such as nursing homes.

The reactions of others plays an important part in how the incontinent person views himself or herself. It is demeaning for an adult to have to wear a diaper, but it is doubly so if staff or family make disparaging comments or joke about it.

Intervention Guidelines   Before any program of retraining is begun, one should have information as to when and how often urination or defecation take place, how well (long) the client can hold urine, and how much urine is passed. Physical diagnosis for both fecal and urinary blockages or diseases is also suggested (Ebert, 1980b). If there is a physical defect, muscle exercises, medication, or even catherization may be recommended. Some clients may never regain continence.

The physical and social environment should be conducive to toileting. That is, the client should be able to get to a toilet or bed pan, the bed (in the home) should be low enough so that the individual can reach the floor and individual patterns of toileting need to be respected (Willington, 1975; Ebert, 1980b).

Conceptually, the model for regaining continence is fairly simple: desire to defecate/feeling of full bladder (stimulus), leading to defecation/urination in appropriate place (desired response), followed by positive reinforcement (feeling of relief, rewards from staff). Schematically, it can be represented as:

Stimulus - - - - - - - - - Desired response - - - - - - - - Reinforcement

(urge to   (voiding in   (relief,
urinate/   correct place)   reward by
defecate)   staff)

For bowel incontinence, Willington (1975, 1976) suggests medically controlling the timing and urgency of bowel movements through antidiarrheics (to allow fecal buildup) and suppositories (to start bowel movements in a short time). In this manner, the client can be watched, placed on the toilet when the urge comes, and be rewarded. Willington reports that within two or three weeks, the "bowel reflex" usually is reinstituted and suppositories can be eliminated. Clients have to be closely monitored, but eventually fecal continence will be regained.

A related approach for urinary incontinence has successfully been implemented by Hussian (1981). In his approach, nursing home aides did the following: Take the client to the toilet five minutes after awakening (if he or she does not urinate, retoilet every half hour); offer toileting every half-hour with praise for accepting the offer; give praise for success and information if no urination takes place; wait no longer than four hours to toilet again (every half hour if needed);

toilet within fifteen minutes of inappropriate urination ("accidents"); and check clothing one hour after every toileting with praise for dry clothes and a change of clothes if they are wet.

Incontinence will affect many aspects of a person's social functioning. By reversing the condition, a person's self-worth is likely to be raised and he or she will realize new opportunities for satisfying social activities.

SUMMARY AND CONCLUSIONS

The aging individual can be said to undergo some gradual changes in most psychological and physical areas of functioning. None of these changes themselves create insurmountable problems; most are hardly noticed except under conditions requiring greater than average exertion. Many of the cognitive changes reflect a slowing down of functioning rather than a loss of ability. One implication is to decrease levels of anxiety when new learning is to take place. A second implication of psychological changes is to help clients to structure new learning so that they have adequate time to learn tasks, information, or skills.

Sexual functioning in the elderly may reflect the same slowing of response. However, if a normal slowing of response is misinterpreted as a sign of inevitable decline in this area, it may become a self-fulfilling prophecy. Stereotypes about the "sexlessness" of old age and discomfort about discussing sexuality contribute to difficulties in handling problems related to sexuality in the aged.

One result of the changes in aging seems to be increased susceptability of the elderly to illness and disability. The vast majority of the elderly have a chronic impairment, yet most can manage on their own with appropriate supports.

There is growing interest in the emotional component of physical losses and aging. Mental health intervention has focused on direct control of symptoms, using the power of the helping relationship to enhance treatment, and aiding personal adaptation and coping with loss. Managing the environment, while equally important, has historically been less of a concern.

Although some of the intervention approaches noted in this chapter focus on curing or alleviating conditions, much of the assistance we can give to the aged concerns ways of coping with change, an adaptive focus of intervention. The differences between curative and adaptive approaches are discussed in chapter 7 of this text, but one point to remember is that they are qualitatively different. One is not simply an extension of the other. The future should see development of varied mental health approaches to adaptation in aging, an area that can be considered uncharted territory at the present.

3

The Social Context of Aging

INTRODUCTON

Mrs. E. is ninty-two years old. She was married, raised a family, and cared for her husband during a five-year terminal illness. Her family is scattered, although one daughter lives close by and calls daily. Mrs. E. has been a widow for three years. She misses having her husband and a close companion, although her daughter tries to fill the gap.

Mr. F. is a seventy-three-year-old retired tool worker. Upon retirement, he decided to go back to college and received an associate's degree in gerontology from a nearby university. Mr. F. spends much of his time working with local agencies as a volunteer and sits on several boards of community agencies as a representative of the elderly.

Mrs. J. is a black woman in her mid seventies. She has by her own account "never stopped working," having raised a large family and been a salesperson over a fifty-year-span. She has trouble making ends meet but is active in a senior center and the church. She, like Mrs. E., is a widow. Her husband died twenty-five years ago and, while she misses him, other activities and concerns fill up her life.

These three cases typify some of the different ways social changes affect the elderly. The social context of aging refers to the nature of older persons' relationships to others, be it family, friends, the community, or society. Social aspects of aging are broad and have been described through numerous theoretical approaches (Huyck & Hoyer, 1982). For purposes of this text, four major aspects affecting social relationships and behavior of the aged are reviewed: family relationships, minority group membership, retirement, and widowhood. Implications of each area's impact on the elderly in terms of mental health care are discussed, including potential roles of the mental health practitioner, goals, and strategies for intervention.

FAMILY RELATIONSHIPS

Living Arrangements

More than half of all elderly live with their spouses. Another 15 percent live with other family members—a child or other relative. Almost 30 percent live alone. Of the remaining elderly about 5 percent live in institutions and about 2 percent with unrelated persons (Kastenbaum & Candy, 1973; Butler & Lewis, 1982).

Most studies of how the aged prefer to live and how they actually live share the same results. Older adults prefer to live independently in their own houses, condominiums, or apartments as long as possible, although many would like to be near family (Kart, 1981).

A relevant question is: How happy are people with these arrangements? It turns out that older people living with family (not spouses) may actually be less satisfied than those living with spouses or alone (Murray, 1973). Living in an inter-generational setting means that potentially difficult issues such as control, authority, and how chores are handled are encountered on a daily basis (Lopata, 1973).

Marital Status

Most older men are married; most older women are not, primarily due to widowhood. Among the single elderly, the odds are much greater (six times as great) that a widowed man will remarry than that a woman will. The disparity in remarriage rates in part reflects greater numbers of women, the social acceptability of men marrying younger women, and a social norm that women should "honor" the memory of the dead spouse (Treas and Van Hilst, 1976).

Another group is the elderly who never married. This group includes those who took care of their own families in lieu of marriage, those who had mental or physical handicaps that effectively precluded them from considering marriage, or those who simply chose to live as single adults.

Marital status is related to positive life satisfaction, positive mental health, and longevity in the elderly (Crandall, 1980). However, one cannot conclude that the act of marriage brings with it all of these blessings. Individuals who had difficulty maintaining intimate relationships may well be divorced or have never married, making the elderly who are married a more "fit" group by attrition. Also, the individual who never married may be quite capable, despite the relative lack of structured social supports for single persons in our society.

The Married Older Couple

Research on older couples indicates that marital satisfaction in old age is somewhat higher than in child-rearing years. Most older people are satisfied with their marriages, although aspects of the relationship such as conversation topics or sources of satisfaction may change (Treas, 1975).

Men are likely to be more satisfied with marriage in old age than women. The major sources of dissastisfaction in marriage in old age for men are amount of respect they receive and (when ill or disabled) their increased dependency on spouses. For women, the major source of dissatisfaction is the quality of communication in the relationship (Stinnett, Collins & Montgomery, 1970).

The marriage partnership provides an immediate support for any age changes or disabilities. Most couples have long established patterns of coping with stress. These coping patterns are tested by what can be called transitional crises for the older couple (Bengtson & Treas, 1980). There are four such crises: children's leaving home, retirement, death of a spouse, and development of chronic disabilities. Children's leaving home is often referred to as the "empty nest" syndrome. Older couples can expect fifteen years without children. The absence of children can mean the loss of a major role and source of self-worth for parents, especially women. For some, however, the "release" from child rearing is positive.

While most people manage the transition from work to retirement quite well, there are several inherent changes for the marital couple at this time, including mourning or depression over the loss of a job, the retiree getting "underfoot" at home, and conflict over how to share household tasks. Loss of income can also create marital stress.

Both anticipation of and living through the death of a spouse can be expected and are major crises for marital couples in old age (see Chapter 4 for a discussion of grieving).

Older people have a proportionately large percentage of chronic disabilities. The impact of the disability on the marital partner may be quite severe. The healthier spouse, usually a younger wife, must become either a partial or full-time caretaker of the other, a change in terms of traditional role relationships. Caretakers may have feelings of anger, despair, and frustration with limited opportunities to vent them. Social norms do not allow them to express such feelings toward an ill or incapacitated spouse. Concerns about sexuality, "living ones' own life," financial burdens, or structural changes due to medical or transportation needs are also potential sources of stress. The mental health practitioner should be alert to the impact of disability on the spouse and the marital relationship and should appreciate that the realities of the disability may exist for the couple over many years.

Relationships with Other Family Members

There is a substantial amount of interest in how older adults relate to family members. One common belief often expressed is that older people are abandoned by family members, that family dump older people in nursing homes and then forget them.

Is this really the case? It turns out there is usually contact between family and older relatives. Studies have shown that the vast majority of elderly see children on a regular basis; 75 percent have a child living within thirty minutes travel time (Shanas, 1979). Daughters are more likely to keep in close contact than sons; direct descendents more than in-laws, and geographically close children more than those living far away. Also, ill elderly are more likely to have a child living close by than those in good health (Treas, 1975). Finally, even when institutionalization results, positive family ties may be strengthened, as less burden of care is placed on family members (Smith & Bengtson, 1979).

Having people within close geographic proximity does not, of course, mean that family bonds are strong or beneficial to any family members. There are two approaches to assessing the quality of the relationships. One is to determine the dynamics of the relationship—that is, to find the answers to such questions as, "How does it feel to be a member of this family?" or "How does this family provide emotional support?" This approach is a family therapy/systems approach and is extremely important for mental health work. It is explored as a separate topic in Chapter 13.

This second approach, one most commonly used by sociologists, is to examine what are called *exchanges between the generations* (Bengtson & Treas, 1980). The theoretical framework for this approach, called *exchange theory*, examines the types of exchange between individuals and groups. According to this theory, successful exchanges are those that are mutually rewarding. Each side should feel it is getting as well as giving. This sense of mutuality may be felt even though different variables are being exchanged, such as goods, services, "roles," values, or knowledge.

Many older adults prefer to go to their families in time of need as opposed to agencies (Hill et al., 1970). In times of need, it is also likely that family will respond to older family members' problems. The ways in which older family members give assistance include: help with children, gifts, financial assistance, advice on business or other matters, running errands, and taking in grandchildren or other relatives to live with them (Harris and associates, 1975). The ways in which family members give assistance to older family members include: housework, financial assistance, chores, advice and help on insurance, health, or other matters, transportation, and taking an older family member into their home.

Along with these possibilities for exchange between generations, some "new" roles are emerging for both older adults and their children.

Parenting the Parent   One role change in family relationships of the elderly is referred to as "parenting the parent," where a child takes on the care and support of a parent. The support may take many forms, including emotional, economic, or service. Needless to say, this shift in roles can be uncomfortable for the elderly, resulting in loss of self-esteem, increased dependency, and unresolved guilt or ambivalence. From an exchange theory perspective, the problem is one of non-reciprocity—that is, the older person "gets" but has little or nothing to "give." From the family member's point of view, being the "parent of the parent" has similar difficulties, including feelings of guilt or even anger over the loss of one's independence as well as feeling one is giving but getting nothing in return.

The issues in parenting the parent are complex. The older person's physical, psychological, housing, and economic status; availability of social supports; family norms about caring for older relatives; the quality of older person-child relationships; and the child's physical, psychological, economic, and social status all come into play in determining the extent to which the child can parent the parent. Ideally, the family can provide a first line of defense to increased frailty in the elderly, and external support can then be provided for circumstances the family cannot handle. Unfortunately, needed external supports are not always available, and families vary considerably in their willingness and ability (both economic and psychological) to "parent the parent."

One of the unrealized ways in which family members can aid the older person is to be an advocate and broker in obtaining support or services, including those to which the older person is entitled. However, some recent research has indicated that family members are not playing this needed role (Wagner & Keast, 1981).

The Role of Grandparent   The traditional role of older people in families is that of grandparent. Becoming a grandparent can take place at quite an early age. Over 70 percent of the elderly have grandchildren (Brody, 1978). While many grandchildren seem to enjoy the contact they have with grandparents, some grandparents or grandchildren do not enjoy the relationship. There are also varying expectations between members of individual families as well as cultural differences ranging from assumed child care to the grandparents' appearing on major holidays.

It should be noted that the role of grandparent is not usually a full-time job. However, the accomplishments of offspring are a source of satisfaction to the aged, which may lead to older people's thinking there is more closeness between generations than younger family members do (Treas, 1975).

Implications for Mental Health Practice

There are several issues for the mental health practitioner to consider in responding to family concerns of the aged. The first is that family relationships are not stagnant. Both life cycle issues and role changes may create new problems on rekindle dormant ones. Changes in economic conditions and onset of physical disability and ensuing role changes may create difficulties for all members of a family, even if only for a short time. The focus of a mental health provider's interventions may need to focus on helping older marital partners and family members accept the realities of change and adapt to them, rather than only working to cure "unhealthy dynamics."

A second consideration is the family's expectations of care. The ease or difficulty with which families handle the life cycle changes will be in part determined by how the family's needed response fits its expected response. A general knowledge about how many families help elders is a useful reality check for the mental health practitioner in listening and responding to family concerns.

A third consideration for the mental health practitioner has to do with reciprocity of exchange. Self-esteem and sense of independence are promoted through reciprocal or equal exchanges between older persons and other family members. This is not to say that each dollar or hour of time given to an older family member has to be returned on a one-for-one basis. It is the sense of reciprocity that is important. Thus, advice, emotional support, and "wisdom" may be exchanged for financial support, shopping, and house chores between generations. The mental health practitioner can work with families and older members on how to identify sources of exchange in a problem-solving or educational manner. This should lead to a sense that exchanges are not one-way transactions.

One potential role of the mental health practitioner is that of therapist and/or facilitator helping family members learn to communicate their concerns and problems effectively and discover mutually satisfying sources of exchange. A second role is that of arbitrator or educator, focusing on providing ways (e.g., use of a problem-solving approach) to help families find mutually satisfactory solutions to problems. A third potential role is that of resource expert, being an initial link between families, older persons, and needed services or entitlements.

The goals of intervention are likely to be helping the family adapt to change or providing experienced options for families (including developing support groups and services such as day care, friendly visiting, or respite care, as discussed in Chapter 15) rather than "curing" unhealthy dynamics. The nature of expected life cycle events, limits of time, and access to families are reasons for considering adaptive as opposed to curative approaches.

The types of intervention strategies likely to be used with families are a reflection of these roles and goals as well as a recognition that many problems experienced by older persons and families will require specific actions to resolve them. Herr and Weakland (1979) have devised a useful approach to family work that is reviewed in Chapter 13.

MINORITY GROUP STATUS
AND MENTAL HEALTH OF THE ELDERLY

If it can be said that older adults have to cope with physical, economic, and social disadvantages in old age, it can also be claimed minority group elderly suffer from multiple jeopardies of being old and nonwhite (Jackson, 1980). Minority elderly are less likely than whites to receive or seek all types of services for a variety of reasons, including lack of access, racism, perceived racism, and cultural and language barriers.

Definition of Minority Groups

Several characteristics define minority groups: a *shared culture* and cultural traditions; a *common language* (usually not the language of the dominant culture); *common customs*; a particular set of *role relationships* for men, women, children, and families; *a shared history*; and a *psychological sense of belonging to the group*, reinforced by cultural behavior that sets the group apart from the dominant culture (Watson, 1982).

General Status of Minority Elderly

While it has been difficult to determine accurately the status and numbers of minority elderly, certain trends can be identified. A smaller proportion of minority group members are elderly than is the case for whites. Whereas 11 percent of the white population is elderly; only 7 percent of the nonwhite population is elderly. This difference is due to many factors and clearly suggests that minority group members have a more difficult time in all stages of life than whites.

One interesting finding in the research is what has been called the *crossover effect*. This refers to changes of lifespan or life expectancy that actually favor minority group members. For example, as of 1970, minority women born in that years have a slightly higher life expectancy (68.4 years) than white males (68.1 years) (Schwartz & Peterson, 1979). Also, it seems that blacks and other minorities who live to age seventy-five may have a higher life expectancy than white of the same age (Watson, 1982).

At the same time, minority group elderly are worse off than white elderly in most areas (economic, housing, health, mental health, and access to services). This is due to discrimination and economic disadvantages, including not having had high-paying jobs, not being in positions that provide social security eligibility, job discrimination (working for less pay than whites), or not knowing English and lacking the educational or training opportunities to achieve high income during working years (Jackson, 1980). Finally, it seems that these multiple health and social stressors have a differential and greater impact on minority groups, leading to higher mortality rates in earlier years.

Variations Among Minority Elderly

The previously mentioned disadvantages of minority elderly neither mean that "they are all alike" or that a minority background is somehow inferior to that of mainstream American culture.

Minority groups vary considerably in their values, roles, language, history, and customs. These differences are often more pronounced among the elderly, many of whom were born and raised in other countries. Even within a cultural group (e.g., Asian-Americans, Hispanics), there can be subgroups with differences in almost any area of normative behavior. Variations in cultural behavior are a potential source of identity and strength for the elderly as well as the young. Only by appreciating the cultural background and context of minority older persons can we develop effective and meaningful intervention approaches to improve the quality of their lives.

Attributes of several major minority groups are as follows:

Black Aged   The black aged are quite varied in terms of education, income, and life experiences. In 1980, there were 26,495,000 blacks in the U.S., 2,090,000 (eight percent) of whom were over sixty-five (Statistical Abstract of the United States, 1982-83). Eleven percent of the general population is black, 9 percent of the elderly population is black (Hill, 1978). Despite the existence of a distinct middle-class and upper-middle-class black elderly group, older black adults do not do as well as whites in several ways: They have higher rates of poverty (38 percent vs. 13 percent for whites, which actually represents an improvement over prior decades) and chronic health problems; they suffer from less access to health care, nursing home care, adequate housing, and support services (statistical abstract of the United States, 1982-83; Jackson, 1980; Hill, 1978). Blacks have had a history of being promised much but receiving little by apparently trustworthy whites. Many have had to put up with being called "boy" or by their first names while being expected to address whites as "Mr." or "Mrs." It may be more respectful to use formal last names with black older clients to indicate respect rather than to put the relationship on a first-name basis, as is often done in counseling.

Many black elderly have a natural and important support network of kin. The church has also been a strong influence for many, providing a positive sense of identity in a hostile social environment.

Hispanic Elderly   The term *Hispanic* includes many different nationalities, each with its own set of values, roles, and social structures. Hispanics include Mexicans, Puerto Ricans, Cubans, and elderly from every nation in Central and South America. Most Hispanics (primarily of Mexican descent) live in the Southwest, although Puerto Ricans and Cubans live primarily in the East. As of 1980, there were 14,609,000 Hispanics in the U.S., 709,000 of whom were elderly (statistical abstract of the United States, 1982-83). A smaller proportion (4.9 percent) of Hispanics are elderly than whites or blacks, which is an indication of the hardships Hispanics face throughout the life span.

Hispanic elderly are worse off than whites on almost every variable. They have higher mortality rates and poverty rates (30.8 percent poverty rate in 1983); they are much more likely to suffer from poor nutrition, poor health, and inadequate housing conditions than whites (cf. Kobata, Lockery, & Moriwaki, 1981; Dowd & Bengtson, 1978; statistical abstract of the United States, 1982-83).

It is important to realize that one-half of the Hispanic elderly were born in their native countries. Along with substantially higher rates of poverty and illiteracy than whites, many come from rural backgrounds. For all of these reasons, Hispanic elderly may feel that the family should be a primary source of support. However, the family itself may not be able to provide support. Needed support may be beyond the family's abilities (e.g., twenty-four-hour care), leading to intergenerational problems and value conflicts. The lack of trained professionals who speak Spanish is a major roadblock in providing better care to this group.

American Indians In 1980, there were 1,420,000 American Indians in the U.S., five percent of whom were over age sixty-five (U.S. Bureau of the Census, 1983). American Indians are somewhat similar to Hispanics in that many divergent cultures and tribal groups exist. In addition, American Indians are the worst off of all minority groups, with a much lower life expectancy and high rate of poverty prevailing. High rates of alcoholism, lack of adequate nutrition, and high rates of chronic disabilities are also characteristic of older American Indians.

American Indians live in urban, rural, and reservation settings. Each group has its own set of problems and concerns. By living on the reservation in which one is registered, an American Indian is entitled to certain benefits, including health care and housing. However, employment opportunities are quite scarce on most reservations, leading to an "enforced" state of poverty. Also, the land given to Indians historically has been of little agricultural and mineral value. Health care and other supportive services may be minimal or inadequate. Alcoholism, while not universal, is a major concern in health care, as is lack of adequate nutrition. Elderly Indians may be dependent solely on families, although communal sharing is also a norm.

Within this context, it should be mentioned that American Indian elderly have lived through an era in which their status within the tribe has been eroded. Formal decisions on reservations are made by elected councils, not a "council of elders," although the elderly may be consulted.

An additional cultural consideration with American Indians is that theirs is a very different culture from that of the rest of America and one that has maintained itself separately from the rest of society. Values and questions of the role of human beings in nature may be conceived quite differently by the Indian than by the helper. This is not to say helping is impossible. Rather, the helper needs to appreciate and respect cultural differences and the underlying cultural context in which mental health care is understood by the Indian client and not assume that Indians refuse treatment or are too stoic to help themselves (e.g., Baldwin et al., 1981).

Asian-Americans Asian elderly include Chinese, Japanese, Hawaiian, Korean, Filipino, Vietnamese, East Indian, Laotian, Cambodian, and other elderly of Asian descent or born in Asia. Six percent of the 3,259,000 Asian-Americans in the U.S. are over sixty-five (U.S. Bureau of the Census, 1983).

Two of the main myths about Asian-American elderly are that they are homogeneous and that they have successfully assimilated into the culture of the United States. Sue (1977) and others have raised questions about the poverty, health, and mental health of Asian-American groups. It is likely that they suffer from levels of health and income similar to those of other minority groups. Many may be hidden in ghettolike areas, or remain out of contact with needed services in

Chinatowns or "little Tokyos" throughout the United States. The influx of refugees from Vietnam, Laos, and Cambodia in the 1970s has also created an increase in elderly from these groups.

One cultural issue for several Asian-American groups is the question of filial piety. Whereas, in the past, respect and obedience to the parents had been an assumed value, the American focus on nuclear family allegiance leads to some potential problems between generations, which in turn may lead to embarrassment and shame that the older adult will not wish to discuss. This phenomenon is similar to the problem elderly Hispanics face.

Implications: Overcoming Barriers
to Mental Health Services

Major barriers to providing mental health services to minority elderly include traditions of relying on family for support, a sense that mental health care does not fit into cultural traditions, lack of access to service, and overriding needs for food, shelter, and health care. In addition, there is a possibility that service providers hold inappropriate stereotypes of minority elderly, that minority members distrust the service providers, and that language barriers exist.

Stereotypes about Minority Groups   Most mental health practitioners are white. Most have little cross-cultural experience or training. When confronted by a client from a minority group, they are likely to lack knowledge about the group. Despite attempts to focus solely on the individual older client, both the client's cultural identity and the practitioner's potential stereotypes about the cultural group make ethnic issues a critical consideration, as bias or misinformation can only hinder mental health interventions.

For example, one of the myths about several minority groups (blacks, Hispanics, and American Indians) is that the family will always take care of the older adult. While these groups do have a strong history of family support and loyalty (e.g., Billingsley, 1968; Ragan & Simonin, 1977), the economic and social burdens of care may be great for a minority group family, which is likely to have far fewer economic reserves than its white counterpart. Also, even if a family can take care of its older member, certain problems need professional care. In fact, the client and family may need reassurance about the appropriateness of seeking help outside of the family.

A second myth is that certain groups (Asian-American and even Jewish elderly) have no problems. It is likely that the number and severity of economic and mental health problems is underestimated in these groups, especially Asian-Americans (Sue, 1977). Belief in these myths may lead a mental health provider to avoid working with minority clients because "nothing is really wrong" or "someone else should be taking care of the problem."

A third myth is an expectation that the minority group members will not accept any help from an outsider, that minority elderly will not change, or that they are rigid. Certainly, some individuals will not accept help and some may not change. However, the expectation of failure is both a self-fulfilling prophecy and may place the mental health providers' anxiety, fears, or discomfort on the clients.

Low Trust in Mental Health Practitioners (Perceived Racism) Minority elderly may not initially trust mental health practitioners for several reasons. They may believe that treatment was developed for whites or that it does not work. At another level, the way in which help is presented may violate cultural norms about help. In several groups (e.g., American Indians) health providers have traditionally had a personal relationship with the client or have built one during service (primary relationship). The mental health provider who presents herself or himself to members of these groups as a "professional" (objective, scientific, or distant) may be distrusted by older adults because he or she is violating the norms for how to give help, not because the older adults do not want help, do not need it, or that the help will not work.

The difficulty in discovering this problem is that the reaction of the elderly will be conveyed subtly. Many minority elderly have learned from bitter experience not to trust "majority" professionals by being open and sharing concerns. Developing mutual trust takes considerable effort, but it is not impossible.

Language Barriers One of the most frustrating barriers in delivering mental health service to minority elderly is lack of a common language between provider and client. Mental health practitioners may feel that minority members should learn or speak English. Minority group elderly may feel that the language of their culture is important to them, and, besides, why should they be the one to learn two languages? After all, it is the older person who needs help. Why not help him or her in the native tongue?

For many Japanese, Chinese, American Indian, and Hispanic elderly, language will be a barrier for some years to come. Besides encouraging mental health practitioners to learn other languages, several strategies can be employed to overcome language barriers:

1. A bilingual interpreter can be available in any agency or from another agency. A little diligent searching can uncover adults who speak the language in question and who may be willing to volunteer or be paid for their time.

2. Another member of the family can serve an interpreter, although there are certain inherent difficulties with this solution. First, the older adult may not want to discuss personal feelings in front of family members, particularly concerns about sexuality, death or dying, or concerns that make the translator uncomfortable. Second, the family member may selectively perceive and color the older person's statements with his or her own interpretations. Third, if the family member is a child, he or she may not understand certain concepts. Children under the age of twelve do not have a good understanding of body parts and functions, so that if medical information is needed, their translations may be misleading (Smith, 1977). Fourth, the role of translator, when the translator is younger than the client, may

represent a reversal of translation cultural roles where the elder is supposed to be in charge (Solomon, 1979).

3.   Finally, while "verbal" language will need translation, nonverbal aspects, including body language, intonation, eye contact, and use of silence are still available to the practitioner and may have heightened importance to the client.

Other aspects of working with minority elderly are covered in Chapter 8 of this text.

RETIREMENT

Retirement, or the mandated loss of a job, is becoming one of the more controversial life-cycle issues facing the elderly. Questions are being raised about the value of retirement and stability of economic supports, such as social security (which was intended as a supplemental income source in old age). Also, economic conditions are such that many older adults cannot retire. The 1978 raising of the age of mandatory retirement to seventy in many professions reflected these concerns.

For many people, retirement does not lead to poor health, lower life satisfaction, or onset of mental illness (Streib & Schneider, 1971). Retirement can be a pleasant time, especially if one is financially and emotionally prepared. Also, the question of how people use leisure time is becoming more of a concern to social planners.

Within this context, the question of adaptation to both loss of job and related economic and life-style changes becomes important. This is particularly so because few people actively plan for retirement, even though successful adaptation to the retired role can be enhanced by plans made far in advance of retirement (Atchley, 1980).

Adaptation to Retirement

Most retirees view retirement as a positive experience although individuals vary considerably in their reactions and experiences (Foner & Schwab, 1981). Dissatisfaction with retirement can be caused by many factors. Poor health and lessened income are two major sources (Foner & Schwab, 1981). There is not only the loss of income but also loss of status and of relationships with coworkers, a feeling of uselessness, and, at times, the additional stress of spending more time in the home with a spouse. The fact that retirement is mandated rather than chosen can also be detrimental.

Stages of Retirement

Retirement can be viewed as having six phases (Atchley, 1980). Although the onset and duration of each phase will vary among individuals, the phases provide a framework of expected steps in the retirement process. They are:

1. *Preretirement.* This is the time in which people begin to consider the possibility of retirement. Expectations ("fantasies") about retirement will affect the transition to retirement, depending on how well they match reality. Some people seriously consider and plan for retirement; others may deny it or "let it happen."

2. *Honeymoon.* Immediately after retirement, there is likely to be a time of vacationing—either taking trips, sleeping late, traveling, or doing things one always wanted to do. Many people end this phase by establishing a retirement routine, which can be satisfying if it builds on existing interests or represents a desired life change, such as continued participation in community organizations or a move to a better climate.

3. *Disenchantment.* Some people experience a letdown or sense of depression soon after retirement. Although they are only a small percentage, these are the people who can be considered as having difficulties adapting to retirement. Boredom, restlessness, or feelings related to depression may be found in this phase.

4. *Reorientation.* Even without professional help, many disenchanted retirees will "reorient" themselves to available options for socialization, recreation, and identity in the community, such as peer groups, senior citizen centers, or volunteer work. Reorientation should result in a routine that is both satisfactory and manageable within the retiree's economic, health, and social resources.

5. *Stability.* At this stage the daily routine has become consistent and comfortable. The time it takes to reach this point varies considerably. Most people reach it within a year. However, at least one study found over a third of the studied group reported the process took more than twelve months (Glamser, 1981).

6. *Termination.* Atchley also includes a termination phase, a time in which "being retired" is not meaningful role for the older adult. This can happen when the retiree takes on another role (having another job, being a volunteer), becomes disabled or institutionalized (sick role), or even becomes so far removed from work that the idea of being "retired" from a job has little meaning.

Implications for Mental Health Practice

Many of the problems reported by older persons in retirement are related to health and economic difficulties. Others, such as feeling lonely, difficulties in establishing a retirement pattern, or compensating for the loss of the work role, are usually seen as social problems by the persons experiencing them rather than mental health concerns. While mental health interventions can help persons having emotional difficulties to adjust to retirement, the interventions are more likely to succeed as part of a preretirement and followup program or a program designed to help people handle all problems of being retired (including health and economic concerns) than as a separate entity.

Within this context, interventions should be seen as having three potential goals: One is aiding adaptation to the changes and realities of retirement. Another is enriching options for retirement, such as helping people learn the social skills needed to take on new roles and activities, whether leisure or work-related. A third is preventing difficulties in adapting to the changes of retirement through the design and implementation of preretirement programs and group interventions aimed at future retirees.

Preretirement planning is slowly becoming part of the benefit packages offered by business and industry. The range of programs offered include: simple information sessions on retirement benefits, one-day seminars focusing on financial planning, a series of lectures, seminars with several sessions designed to help with adaptation and planning (economic, social, health), and individual counseling. From the mental health perspective, the last two types of programs make the most sense, since they provide the opportunity to discuss personal reactions and expectations about being retired. However, it is not clear that preretirement programs as they now exist significantly improve the retiree's long-term adaptation to retirement (Glamser, 1981). There is a need for better integration of mental health concerns with financial and social planning in most programs currently offered to preretirees.

Because of the diverse needs of the retiree, the mental health practitioner may have to play several roles: counselor, helping the client discuss and resolve reactions to the loss of the work role and challenging any beliefs that unnecessarily inhibit choosing new and/or satisfying activities; resource person, guiding the client to authorities who have expertise in financial planning; and trainer, teaching the client social and problem-solving skills needed to take on new roles and activities. Occasionally, the mental health practitioner will also serve as either therapist or referral source in those rare occasions in which retirement precipitates an abnormal response, such as a major affective reaction (depression). The specific strategies employed will be a function of the goal of intervention and may include listening, cognitive skills, and problem solving.

Other considerations in designing interventions are: respect client values about social, economic, or personal issues; include family members (especially spouses) in retirement planning and counseling; be aware of community resources such as clubs, organizations, and self-help groups; attempt to initiate enrichment and preventive programming before persons become retired; and keep continued contact with retirees past the initial phases of retirement, even if it is only periodic followup on the telephone.

Certain problems of the retiree are best handled before retirement. However, we need better ways of identifying individuals likely to be "at risk" due to retirement and more emphasis on preventive approaches to handle these problems.

WIDOWHOOD

Being a widow or widower brings with it a series of potential problems, including economic, social, and psychological concerns.

By age sixty-five, 36 percent of all women are widowed, and the percentage increases until, for women eighty-five and older, over three quarters are widows. The elderly have a higher rate of death of spouses than any other age group. Current estimates also suggest that older women can expect to live alone for fifteen years after the death of their spouse (Lopata, 1979).

Older widows face many problems, including inability to earn wages, agism, and inadequate educational background due to traditional limitations imposed on women. Their lack of supports for social contact and fear of rejection can lead to less use of social resources. They also face sex imbalance—fewer available men for relationships—as well as dangerous housing, lack of contacts for emergencies, and, when housebound, lack of social contact and of medical and nutritional care (Lopata, 1979).

One of the most serious disadvantages facing widows is their economic status. In all racial and ethnic groups, widows have less money than other people. Most widows are poor; black widows are one of the poorest groups in America.

The reasons for these economic problems are multifaceted: Pensions and social security are biased toward males; women as a group do not have prerequisite skills and education for well-paying jobs, and they have traditionally been paid less for the same job than men with equivalent backgrounds. Elderly minority widows have the added jeopardy of being from a minority group, which substantially adds to the types of discrimination suffered by older widows.

Along with financial difficulties, older widows suffer in several other ways. They have a higher rate of death, suicide, and mental problems requiring treatment than other elderly (Berardo, 1970).

Older widowers also face certain problems, despite relatively high remarriage rates and income levels. Widowers are relatively unlikely to live with children, have extensive interaction with family, receive or give support to others, or even have many friends. The necessities of self-care, which include shopping, preparing meals, and cleaning, are traditionally female tasks that have to be learned. Finally, the family role of grandfather has less value and fewer specific tasks than that of grandmother (Berardo, 1970).

Racial and ethnic differences affect widows. Generally, black widows are worse off than white. They are widowed earlier and more likely to be poor. Widows in many ethnic groups are likely to be foreign born and to hold generational or cultural values about their role that differs from those of their families. These differences in expectations, in which the widow expects to play a more active role than the family wishes, can lead to conflict (Lopata, 1979).

Certainly, some of the difficulties widows face originate in the change from being married to being single. Widows really have no role in today's society. They have to create their own identities knowing there is no one to take the place of a deceased spouse and having limited roles as mothers, grandmothers, or aunts (Block et al., 1978).

Creating a new life as a widow is difficult, in part because a woman's status and identity are traditionally determined by her husband's role. Also, social norms require her to keep her husband's memory alive, not being interested in other men, and confine her to doing things only with other widows (Atchley, 1980).

How widows cope with their new role varies considerably. Somehow the widow has to adapt to others' expectations (such as referring to her as Mrs. X), although they may not reflect her current activities and self-definition as she attempts to create a new life. While it can be expected that some widows will begin to participate in new relationships and roles, some will want to be isolated, participate primarily in family relationships, or have a somewhat restricted sphere of activities (Lopata, 1979).

Implications for Mental Health Practice

There are several possible goals in mental health intervention with widows, depending on the point in the widowhood process at which intervention takes place. One goal is helping the widow grieve for the lost spouse. A second goal is helping her adapt, focusing on immediate demands for self-care. A third goal is both adaptive and enriching, helping the widow adapt to the realities of singleness and creating a new life. The role of the mental health practitioner will vary, depending in part on the goal or area of intervention and in part on the needs expressed by the widow. At times the role will be that of therapist or counselor, working on aspects of emotional reactions and "unfinished business" in grief. At times the role will be more that of a "listener," allowing the client to ventilate anger or guilt. In the later stages, the role may be more one of guide or teacher, working with the client to develop problem-solving or social skills necessary to adapt to being single.

Bereavement and Initial Adaptation to the Loss   The mental health practitioner may represent a source of emotional support as well as a check on reality for the recently bereaved. For example, the widow who says, "I can't live without him," is likely to be feeling lost or hopeless and unsure how to go on by herself. Allowing ventilation of the hopelessness can be combined with a gentle reminder that the widow can, in fact, live by herself. Similarly, as an "outsider" the mental health practitioner may be one person with whom the widow can resolve feelings of anger and guilt about the death of the spouse. Resolution of these feelings may take time. The focus of such interventions can be on the client's gaining insight and understanding of her or his own needs and wishes as well as coming to grips with the finality of the death of the spouse.

Adaptation to Immediate and New Demands for Self-Care   Three immediate problems expressed by widows upon the death of the spouse are help with funeral arrangements, getting financial matters straightened out, and emotional problems (Lopata, 1979). The decisions about matters such as a funeral and subsequent arrangements should be evaluated in light of existing supports. Is there someone who can help? If there are family members, will they help? The mental health practitioner should work to ensure that resources are available to the widow and may need to meet with family to help communication with the widow.

Beyond immediate concerns, there are likely to be new demands for self-care. For some women this will include paying bills, maintaining a check book, relocating, or obtaining additional financial support, and for some men, preparing meals, shopping, or cleaning. Some widows or widowers may be embarrassed to ask for the help they need to maintain themselves. The mental health practitioner, after assessing needs for self-care, may end up teaching needed skills, referring the client to specific skill groups, or even starting such groups if none exist in the community.

Adaptation to the Social Realities of Singleness: Creating a New Life Perhaps most important, the mental health practitioner can assist the widowed client to create a new life. Ideally, this should be done at three levels: enhancing the client's self-identity and self-worth, creating opportunities for social interaction, and developing the client's coping skills for handling others in the social environment.

How the widowed view themselves and how much they value their abilities are reflections of self-worth. The mental health practitioner, in the dual role of support and reality check, can help the client learn how to challenge statements of low self-worth (using cognitive challenges discussed in Chapter 10). The practitioner can help the widowed develop the necessary self-confidence to venture into the social environment.

The mental health practitioner can aid opportunities for social interaction both by having knowledge of community resources or programs and by facilitating their development. Many widowed people are likely to view their problems as not requiring the assistance of a mental health practitioner. Also, many feel that others give them "bad advice" (Lopata, 1979). One of the most successful programs is peer support or widow-to-widow services, which can be found in many communities. The services sometimes are offered on an individual basis, other times as group meetings. Besides referring clients to such groups, the mental health practitioner can become a resource for such groups by providing training and knowledge about grief and abnormal grief reactions and by acting as a consultant or referral source for widowed clients with particular difficulties.

The mental health practitioner can also act as a "coach" in helping a client make social contacts. Several behavioral techniques, such as charting contacts and outcomes, can help widowed clients appreciate progress in this areas.

The widow or widower is often faced with expectations (voiced or unvoiced) from others that may work against creating a new life. Family and friends may expect the widow to act like "other widows" and not make any substantial changes in living or to socialize only at senior centers. The widow or widower who gets a new job, decides to move, gets a boyfriend or girlfriend, or decides to remarry may hear things such as, "Are you sure you want to go through with this?" or "What would Dad (Mom) say about this?" If significant others are resisting the changes, the widow or widower may need both support and skills to maintain self-worth, limit guilt, and confront others with feelings and reactions to what is being said or implied.

One approach to this issue is to teach the client how to be assertive both in asking for what she or he needs and in sharing feelings. A second approach is to help the client maintain a sense of identity and self-worth that is not dependent on others who may be negatively influencing her or his "new life." Both of these approaches should help the widow or widower cope with negative reactions from others.

The lack of status and other hardships faced by the widowed should be of concern to all who work with the elderly. The mental health practitioner may be in a position of helping the widowed through contact made during death and bereavement for a spouse. Working with widowed clients directly or by referral to self-help and widow-to-widow groups is a logical extension of mental health services.

SUMMARY AND CONCLUSIONS

Four social factors influencing aging are relationships with family, being a member of a minority group, retirement, and widowhood. Each has a different impact on individual older persons, yet each factor carries with it norms or expected circumstances that can be useful in assessing the behavior of the individual client. In addition, aspects of each factor affect and can be affected by mental health intervention. Family relationships are the major source of support for most elderly. Minority elderly have specific cultural patterns that may affect the success of mental health interventions, including culturally determined ways of giving help, low trust of outsiders, and language barriers. The impact of the third area, retirement, may be improved by better planning and preventive services, although most people adapt to retirement without serious difficulties. Widowhood brings with it a series of difficulties. It has several predictable phases that can be positively influenced by interventions to help in bereavement, in adapting to immediate demands for self-care, and in adapting to the social realities of being single.

4

Death, Dying, and Bereavement

INTRODUCTION

An old man is dying. He is sick with cancer and pain. At times he wishes it would end. At other times he cries to himself, wishing he could live long enough without pain to go home from this place, this nursing home.

A woman comes to visit. She sits silently, in tears that cannot be shed now. They have lived for forty years as husband and wife, sharing the same bed, the birth and growth of children, the birth of grandchildren, and the changes of seasons in their lives together. Yet no words find their way to her lips. She only stays a short while and then gets ready to go back to the emptiness of their home, wondering when it will end and how she will live afterward.

A staff member of the facility, it could be you or me, comes into the room as the woman starts to leave. There is a momentary sense that all is not right, that the pain is felt by all three persons in the room. They all know the man is dying, all are unsure how to put words to their feelings. Historically, what has happened at a point like this is that the three will go their separate ways. However, developments over the last two decades suggest there are better alternatives for the dying person, survivors, and caregivers to cope with death.

Death is the end of life. But it is more than that. Death is personal: We all have changing views, perceptions, fears, and senses of death and have lived through deaths of family members, friends, or people we have known. Death is impersonal: It is the statistics on the number of deaths in a given age group or the percentage of persons who die in institutions. Death is cultural: It is the rituals and beliefs about its purpose as expressed in varied religions and customs. Death is societal: There are laws, regulations, and social customs about its definition, impact on survivors, and how the deceased are treated and remembered.

Death is an expected part of old age. However, unlike many other aspects of aging, no matter what our own age and condition, death is also part of our lives. Our personal experiences, feelings, attitudes and idle thoughts about death enter into our work with the aged. Also, our reactions and thoughts about death are likely to undergo change as we live our professional and personal existences. To understand death may be impossible; certainly one chapter will not do the trick. All that we can reasonably do is begin to explore aspects of death.

This chapter begins with some definitions and perspectives about death. Psychological processes involved in the death process and bereavement are reviewed, as are certain social trends and concerns in the death process, including the concept of death with dignity, euthanasia, funeral practices, and the hospice movement. Finally, implications for mental health practice and considerations of the role, function, and approach of the mental health practitioner along the trajectory of death are presented.

DEFINITIONS AND PERSPECTIVES
ABOUT DEATH AND DYING

Death is often considered an event in our culture. Such and such a person died on such and such a date in such and such a place. Within this conceptual framework our resulting focus is on the moment of death, how arrangements are handled, and how smoothly the translation to the death state occurs (Kastenbaum, 1981). Yet, in considering the realities of dying, including its impact on others, anticipation and planning for one's own death, reactions to the impending death of others, and reactions after the death of others, it makes much more sense to think of death as a process that may last for minutes, days, weeks, or years.

Even with this notion that death is a process in mind, it still is difficult or even impossible to "define" death. Death has often been defined in negative terms, such as absence of life or mentation. Other definitions of death focus on what "it" is similar to in our experience, including sleep, coma, or a state in which there is little activity (Kastenbaum, 1981). Views of afterlife (what happens after the moment of death) vary by culture and religion, ranging from beliefs in a heaven and hell to a reincarnation in the form of another body.

There are also those persons who have had what can be called "near-death" experiences, situations in which they have been considered dead by one form of definition or another, but have been revived and report having experienced unusual sensations or feelings. The types of experience reported often include a sense of serenity, leaving one's body, going toward something, and a subsequent turning point of transition (going back to life) (Moody, 1975). However, these experiences cannot at this time be taken as hard evidence for existence of an afterlife or existence of God (cf. Kastenbaum, 1981). There are too many competing explanations for these phenomena, too many persons have been near death without "near-death" experiences, and we have no direct access to information from those who have not "returned."

What we are left with, then, is some ideas about what death might be like, but no exact definition that meets any need we may have to understand the phenomenon more fully. The full experience of death is out of our reach as living beings; we cannot experience it directly (Kastenbaum & Aisenberg, 1972). Perhaps it is this inherent sense of the unknown that has made death and its ramifications intriguing, feared, and difficult to discuss. The following information gives some of the facts about how death is defined and exists, but it cannot by itself answer the questions of the definition and meaning of the phenomenon.

Types of Death

As the technology to extend life has expanded, there has been a great concern about how to define the moment of death. Is it when the person stops breathing? Is it when the heart cannot function without drastic supports? Is it when the brain no longer is capable of response? These three questions underline the generally accepted types of death that have been posited (Schulz, 1978):

Clinical death: cessation of respiration and heartbeat
Brain death: cessation of brain functioning due to lack of oxygen
Biological or cellular death: the actual cessation of organ functioning

Of the three, brain death is becoming the most commonly used for medical purposes.

The Demography of Death

Death Rates   Death rates for the elderly are, not surprisingly, much higher than those of younger age groups. About 6 percent of all older people die each year (Atchley, 1980), with higher rates among the oldest elderly (202 per 1000) (Lerner, 1970). Also, the death rate for males is higher than for females in old age (213 per 1000 versus 194 per 1000 in the old-old—over age 85), leading to increasing numbers of single women in the higher age brackets.

Causes of Death   The most common causes of death in the elderly are somewhat different from those in the rest of the population. The major causes of death in the aged are (in order of incidence) heart disease, cancer, strokes, influenza and pneumonia, arteriosclerosis, accidents, bronchitis (and related emphysema and asthma), cirrhosis of the liver, and kidney infections (Yurick et al., 1980). Heart disease is the major cause of death in over 40 percent of all cases and, with cancer and strokes, accounts for 75 percent of all elderly persons' death. (While Alzheimer's disease may be one of the major causes of death in the elderly, available research on mortality has not included it as of this writing).

There are sex differences in causes of death (men are more likely to have heart disease or cancer). Also, there are some racial differences. While major causes are the same, nonwhites seem more susceptible to kidney infections and diabetes.

Place of Death   Seventy percent of all deaths take place in institutional settings (Fulton, 1976). What this means is that death and dying, for the most part, are no longer functions of the home. The health care system has to be responsive to the needs of the dying elderly if for no other reason than the fact that most are dying in hospitals or nursing homes.

Attitudinal Aspects of Death

Attitudes Toward Death and Dying   Death is an unknown entity. As such it is potentially fear-producing, although it is not clear to what degree the general population fears death. Research has shown that older people do not fear death more than younger people (Marshall, 1971; Kalish, 1976; Conte et al., 1982). This may be due to being prepared by seeing others die or feeling that death is "expected" in old age.

When fears exist, they are generally of the following types (cf. Schulz, 1978):

Fear of physical pain	Fear of not being
Fear of humiliation, loss of control	Fear of punishment in afterlife
Interruption of goals	Impact on survivors
Fear of death of others	

Many of the fears of dying are unspoken or are not in the awareness of the older person, family, or professional. As such, they may lead to avoidance of discussing impending death, sharing feelings, working for closure on interpersonal issues, or even stating what the individual needs from others around him or her.

Professionals' Attitudes Toward the Dying Older Person   The general reaction of the health professions toward the aged dying client has been one of neglect. Older clients receive less effort and care than younger clients (Sudnow, 1967; Simpson, 1976).

Kastenbaum and Aisenberg (1972) found that five types of response were used when a client made a direct statement about dying:

(False) reassurance: telling the client he or she does not have to feel that way
Denial: telling the client she or he is not terminally ill
Changing the topic: talking about something else

Fatalism: dismissing the concern with a statement about the inevitability of death

Discussion: asking for more information

Many professionals unfortunately use the first four response types. This, of course, avoids any discussion of the client's concerns, despite the fact that a substantial number of dying persons want to talk about their condition (Kübler-Ross, 1969).

Perhaps nowhere are the ways in which attitudes toward death made more obvious than in Weisman's (1972) work on pinpointing myths or false assumptions workers make about the dying client:

1.   No one really wants to die, only psychotic or suicidal people are willing to do so.

2.   Fearing death is natural; the closer you are, the more intense the fear.

3.   There is no reconciliation with death, so there is no sense discussing it with the dying. Avoid confronting it.

4.   The dying do not want to be told the truth. If told, they may become suicidal, depressed, and die more quickly.

5.   Doctors should treat patients until all benefits of treatment are gone. Then, with consultation to family, the doctor should withdraw, leaving the patient to die in peace.

6.   It is reckless and cruel to make patients and family suffer. Since the patient will die, no intervention can help. The survivors must realize that efforts are useless and that they will "get over" the loss.

7.   Scientific training and clinical experience give the doctor the right background to handle all phases of dying. The emotional aspects are overrated; there is no need to use psychiatrists, social workers, or clergy (the latter can be called in as death nears). There is no obligation by the doctor after death.

While these fallacies are not always explicity stated, at times professional helpers act as if they were true and inappropriately avoid the dying older person.

Practitioners need to be able to discern when fears may be influencing client, family, or their behavior with the dying person. Examining one's attitudes, beliefs, and fears should be an integral part of training to work with the dying as well as part of the process of intervention with the dying client and family. Suggested methods of examining attitudes and fears include discussion with other persons, such as instructors and people who work with the dying, and participating in exercises designed to uncover one's attitudes and beliefs about death.

THE PROCESSES OF DEATH

The Meaning of Death for the Elderly

As was mentioned earlier, fear of death is no greater for the elderly than for younger people; however, there are two meanings of death that have relevance for the elderly: death as a limit and organizer of time, and death as a loss (Kalish,

1976). Knowledge of impending death (or even limited life expectancy) can bring about a "reorganization of time and priorities" (Kart, 1981, p. 324). That is, there may be little anticipation of future events, a heightened need to leave a legacy of some sort, a desire to straighten out affairs, or a desire to put things in order psychologically.

Death also means loss. Older people have had to grieve the loss of friends, parents, and spouses. Some have outlived children, brothers, and sisters. The dying older person may well be grieving for others, self, or anticipated losses due to her or his own death.

Kübler-Ross's Stages of Death

How do people prepare for death? Is there a "correct" way? Are there patterns of preparation as one confronts his or her own demise? These questions were originally examined by Dr. Elizabeth Kübbler-Ross in her classic book, *On Death and Dying* (1969).

Kübler-Ross's work was based on personal observations of dying clients. She believed that the emotional reactions to one's own death could be characterized by a sequence of five stages: denial, anger, bargaining, depression, and acceptance. The stages are not hard and fast; that is, a client may go back and forth, stay at one, or skip between them.

A person's first reaction to finding out he or she is dying is emotional shock and disbelief that becomes *denial.* Verbalizations about there being a mistake (e.g., "It's not me") are common. Kübler-Ross stated that this initial stage has a purpose (to allow the individual time to marshall other psychological resources) and should be allowed to run its course.

Denial gives way to *anger.* The dying person at this point expresses resentment of the living, hospital treatment, caregivers (particularly doctors and nurses), friends, God, or interruption of plans. The expressed anger is projected; that is, it is placed on others and external events, but it is really a reaction to the internal struggle the dying client faces.

Bargaining, the next stage, is a psychological attempt to postpone death. The client will make "deals" with God, asking for an extension of time or removal of pain in return for good behavior such as prayer. If the extension or pain removal succeeds, another bargain is attempted. Kübler-Ross discussed the case of a woman who bargained to be able to live to attend her son's wedding without pain. On her return to the hospital from the wedding, she immediately began to bargain for enough time to attend her other son's wedding.

As time goes on, the dying person begins to experience a sense of loss due to losses in functioning, increased symptoms, or surgery. At this point, the dying person experiences *depression.* The depression may be focused on past losses (reactive) or on the future loss of loved ones (preparatory) (Kart, 1981). Preparatory depression is a key move towards coming to grips with one's death and can be viewed as a necessary step towards the final stage, *acceptance.* The client has finally come to a full realization and understanding of his or her death. While there is a lack of anger or depression, there is also no joy, but rather a "degree of quiet expectation" (Kübler-Ross, 1969, p. 113).

Despite the attention given to the Kübler-Ross model and the major contribution she made to demystifying the dying process, the stages represent only one way of thinking about a complex phenomenon. They can be misused either as an avoidance by the practitioner who categorizes every word and behavior into a stage to the exclusion of listening and caring for the client, or by the practitioner who attempts to move the client through the stages as if achieving acceptance were a goal to be achieved as soon as possible.

Questions have been raised as to the accuracy of Kübler-Ross's model (e.g., Schulz, 1978). Most older dying clients exhibit signs of depression prior to death, but this may be due to decreased physical ability to cope with the environment or to drug-related reactions. Some older clients do withdraw and await death. Yet other clients, while fully aware of their condition, live each day fully, with new activities as well as relationships (Weisman & Kastenbaum, 1968). Thus, while a stage theory of dying is useful in helping the practitioner think about the client's experience, the "best" way of dying for one client will be different for another (Weisman, 1974).

Another consideration is that the ideas of acceptance and denial have become "all or none" categories that are so broad as to lose meaning in the clinical setting. Many aspects of the dying person's behavior may be inappropriately classified as denial, such as silence. An unwillingness to talk may be as much a reaction to the "listener" as to the illness and pending death. Or perhaps the client is using other mechanisms to avoid confronting death, such as selective attention (focusing on only one or two aspects of the current situation) or compartmentalizing (accepting some aspects and implications of terminal illness while acting in ways that suggest that other aspects are being avoided) (Kastenbaum, 1981).

Perhaps a more realistic view is that there are varying degrees of acceptance and denial of an illness, its consequences, and impending death going on inside an individual—or family and professionals—at any moment in time. These inner states may shift, be in awareness, be out of awareness, be discussed, or be consciously kept as part of the individual's inner experience. As is the case in any living situation of the elderly, the individual's previous experience and ways of coping with loss will influence both inner experience and what is communicated to others. The question of the "best" way to die then takes on added complexity. The client is the final judge and jury for the "best" way to go through the death process.

Bereavement, Grief, and Mourning

Bereavement is the state of having suffered the loss of an intimate, usually a family member. *Grief* refers to psychological and physical reactions directly related to the loss. *Mourning* refers to how the bereaved expresses grief within his or her cultural and religious milieux. Each organized religion has its own specific sets of customs for mourning. However, many people in the United States do not participate in organized religion. Thus, the emotional support of religion is not universally accepted in the process of mourning.

These processes do not necessarily start at the time of death. It is not uncommon for persons to go through a series of phases in preparation for the death of another, such as depression, increased concern for the dying person, rehearsing the death of the other, and attempting to adjust to the consequences of the other's death (Fulton, 1970). This "anticipatory grieving" does not lessen the impact of death of the other. It may, however, decrease the initial response to the actual death.

Also, when there is sudden death, as in suicide or an accident, and no opportunity to rehearse or prepare for the death, there may be a fear in survivors that the same kind of experience could happen again to them:

> "It is not uncommon to find a widow afraid to go out in the evening because her husband was shot at night; or a widower who enters an automobile with trepidation because his wife was killed in an auto accident. . . ." (Schulz, 1978, pp. 141-142).

Symptoms of Grief   Grief is experienced both physically and mentally. Physical symptoms include general somatic distress, tightness of the throat, a sense of choking, sighing, "empty" feelings in the stomach, and weakness. Mental or emotional symptoms include a sense of psychic pain, insomnia, difficulties concentrating, and difficulties remembering (Lindemann, 1944). The symptoms are likely to be experienced in "waves," coming and going for short periods of time. Not all people experience these reactions; their frequency and intensity also vary. Other reactions may occur, including anger, guilt, or seeming indifference.

Stages of Grief   Three stages of grieving and mourning have been posited (Glick, Weiss, & Parkes, 1974). First is an *initial response*—shock, disbelief, feelings of emptiness, numbness, and confusion. Men are likely to experience this as a sense of "dismemberment" while women may feel "abandoned." Much like the initial response of the dying person, this serves temporarily to protect the individual from overwhelming pain; it is followed by feelings of deep sorrow for as long as several weeks, accompanied by crying and weeping (more common for women than men).

At the same time, the survivor may well have a fear that she or he is "not going to make it," that a breakdown is imminent. Responses to this reaction include physical symptoms (loss of appetite, sleep disturbances) and a range of behavioral responses, including taking tranquilizers and throwing oneself into activity to keep busy. An excellent personal perspective is provided in *Widow*, by Lynn Caine (1974).

The second stage is the *intermediate phase*, which starts around three weeks after the death and ends approximately after a year. This phase has three identifiable components: an obsessional review—dwelling on one aspect or situation related to the death (e.g., "If only I had been there to give first aid"); trying to understand the meaning of death (e.g., "Why was it him?"); and a sensing that the dead person is present, at times to the point of having hallucinations that the deceased is actually present or "expecting" the deceased to be there and respond to his or her name.

The third phase is *recovery*. The survivor will often decide that it is time to get on with living, get back into social situations, and develop new skills. Despite the stigma of widowhood, many widows show growth and greater personal strength, having gone through the experience of grieving (Glick et al., 1974).

Some grief reactions can be considered unusual or morbid. Often they are similar to the ones described above, but last longer or are stronger. Severe self-blame, having symptoms similar to those of the deceased, and onset of mental health problems such as alcoholism and depression are examples of morbid grief responses (Parkes, 1972).

One of the concerns often felt by friends and family after a death is that the surviving spouse will die shortly thereafter. Surviving spouses have a greater chance of dying than the nonbereaved, the rate being twice as high (Schulz, 1978). The reasons for this are uncertain. They include higher susceptibility to life-threatening illness because of social stress, loss of "will to live," or not taking adequate care of oneself.

CURRENT CONCERNS IN CARING
FOR THE DYING

Current concerns in care of the dying include death with dignity, euthanasia, funeral practices and the growth of the hospice movement.

Death with Dignity

The idea of a dignified death has spurred debate and legislation about when and how individuals can die. The concept is surprisingly simple—that death should be encountered by structuring the surrounding environment in such a way as to maintain the highest dignity of the individual. Yet, staff in health care facilities rarely have or take the time "for the moments of civility that could impart dignity to the patient" (Schneidman, 1976, p. 470). It also seems that the emphasis on technology, the "antiseptic" atmosphere of institutions, and clinical aspects of health care work can create an inhuman and therefore undignified atmosphere. How can the necessities of care and institutions be brought into line with individual needs and the right to a dignified end of life?

Several sensible goals can be sought to allow the client maximum dignity while dying (Weisman, 1972b):

Reduce pain and suffering
Minimize social and emotional impoverishments
Have the client operate as effectively as possible at the highest level of functioning
Have the client work on existing personal and interpersonal conflicts

Help the client to achieve fulfillment of any wishes given his or her personal and psychological condition

Allow the client to give up control to others if he or she wishes

Allow the client to request or refuse to deal with others (family, staff, friends)

Considering death with dignity at the level of the individual leads to an inevitable conclusion: The client needs to make as many choices over his or her immediate environment, care, and dealings with other people as possible. In addition, a balance must be struck between facility needs, care needs, family member needs, and what the client wishes. Even if the client's wishes are given paramount importance (such as wanting certain people in the room as death approaches), the way in which this gets communicated to others in the environment (including aides, nurses, and cleaning service personnel) has to be done so the wishes are understood and the institution can effectively go about its business. While advocacy for the client's right to die with dignity is certainly needed, the mental health practitioner with a terminally ill client can do the most good by working with others in a supportive manner.

Euthanasia

"Death with dignity" as a concept has also been one of the underpinnings in current debate about euthanasia, or mercy killing. Butler (1975) distinguishes between "passive" euthanasia—allowing a client to die without exercising dramatic measures that will only prolong life in either a vegetable state or a state of constant pain, and "active euthanasia"—actually taking the life of a client because the case is hopeless. Most debate today is over passive euthanasia, active euthanasia being unacceptable in most religious, legal, and professional codes of behavior.

There are five questions to answer regarding euthanasia: What are our cultural values about euthanasia?; If euthanasia is an acceptable option, on what basis would the decision be made?; Who should decide to enact the decision?; When should it be decided?; And, what are the legal implications of acts of this nature?

Our *culutral values* about euthanasia are somewhat unclear. The three major religions in the United States, Protestant, Catholic, and Jewish, have varying values within their sects, although the idea that extraordinary or artificial measures can be either removed or not employed is more acceptable than any other aspect of euthanasia.

Deciding on what basis the decision should be made is not a simple matter. Philosophical issues (do we preserve life at all costs?), medical issues (at what point is a case 100 percent hopeless?), and individual issues (how much does the individual have a right to suffer extensive pain?) need to be included in the decision. The reason or basis for considering euthanasia include: no likelihood or recovery; continued existence in a coma or vegetative state; continued existence in extensive pain and suffering; a personal sense of desiring a "dignified" death, and a personal decision that one would rather die than be a severe financial or emotional burden on others.

Because there are no categorical solutions to the question of euthanasia, another concern becomes *who should decide*? One of the current trends in this area is for right-to-die legislation which allows persons to sign a "living will," a document that clearly states under what conditions they would want extraordinary measures eliminated or not employed in their behalf. At the point where euthanasia is a possibility, several people such as physicians and/or clergy members would jointly decide that the conditions for ceasing extraordinary measures were met. In this way, the individual is involved in the decision before he or she is severely ill and perhaps unable to make any decisions.

The living will also answers the question of *when should the decision be made*? It can provide a series of steps in the decision process; otherwise, the decision has to be established as an institutional policy (which has difficult legal complications) or the decision has to emerge at the time of great stress, while the client is in the process of dying.

A final issue is *legal implications*. Although several states have passed "right-to-die" legislation, because of vagueness in defining key terms such as "extraordinary measures," "no chance of recovery," or "undignified death," there is considerable leeway in interpretation and enactment of right-to-die legislation. The professional or family member who acts on principle to support a passive euthanasia does run some legal risk.

The Hospice Movement

One of the more dramatic institutional responses to the undignified way of dying offered in hospitals and nursing homes was the development of St. Christopher's Hospice in England in 1967, founded by Cecily Saunders (1971-72). Following a tradition of caring for the dying poor, St. Christopher's is dedicated to providing a dignified death for all who come there and support for their families. The work there, as at similar institutions, focuses on controlling pain, maintaining dignity, and providing a caring environment, rather than attempting curative measures. Pain control is managed several ways, including "Brompton's mixture," a mixture of drugs that has received much publicity but in fact has rarely been used by Saunders.

Clients in hospices are encouraged to take their medication at regular intervals and in small enough doses to make them comfortable while maintaining cognitive functioning. This allows clients to avoid addiction, take lower doses of medication, and be less likely to be comatose due to overmedication. Other aspects of pain control include giving the client control over other decisions and working on feelings about personal and family reactions to the impending death.

Clients are given the opportunity to make choices about their dying. At the hospice in Branford, Connecticut, for example, clients can choose the number of roommates they wish, or choose a private room. Perhaps surprisingly, few choose private rooms. Other choices include who visits, when (there are few restrictions on visiting hours), and what personal belongings can be put in a room.

A caring atmosphere is created by availability of staff (the staff ratio is somewhat higher than in other health facilities). Also, staff are encouraged to have physical contact with patients. Families are included as an essential part of the care plan, and bereavement services are offered to survivors. Families can also participate in preparation of the body for burial.

Branford Hospice (the first in the United States) started as a home care program, which is also a major program at St. Christopher's, where the median time in the hospice setting is ten days (Saunders, 1971). Other organizations and consortia in the United States are offering forms of hospice care in communities as well as in institutions, with agencies such as the Visiting Nurses' Association taking a major role (Osterweis & Szmuszkovicz-Champagne, 1979). Each program is autonomous, although standards for training and care are being developed. The hospice team includes clergy, social workers, doctors, nurses, aides, recreation workers, and volunteers.

Hospice volunteers help the dying person and family in a variety of ways, including preparing meals and visiting so that family members can take a few hours off. Volunteers ideally complement the care given by professionals who are tending to the health and emotional care of the dying person.

It is not yet certain that hospice programs are as successful as its proponents claim. Without the ongoing sense of commitment and dedication given by leaders like Cicely Saunders, we could be creating another type of nursing home (Schulz, 1978). Other criticisms include creating fragmented medical care, the high cost of staffing, and taking concern away from reforming hospitals and nursing homes. Finally, there is the unanswered question of how much change should take place in transplanting a British institution to the United States, where the health care system and norms of care are quite different (Osterweis & Szmuszkovicz-Champagne, 1979).

Criticisms aside, hospice represents the first institutional response to the needs of the dying. If it can be shown either to be less costly than hospital and other forms of care, or to provide better options for the dying person and family than currently exist, hospice programs both in institutional settings and the community will become more customary in the United States. The passage of the 1982 hospice reimbursement legislation by Congress may also have an impact on program survival.

Funerals

At first, one might think that funerals or funeral customs have no place in a text on mental health practice. However, since a funeral service can be an important part of bereavement, it is relevant for professional helpers to have some knowledge about funerals.

Funeral practices have been challenged since the 1960s. Jessica Mitford, in her exposé, *The American Way of Death* (1963), discussed how some members of the funeral industry use guilt and deceptive practices to steer the bereaved into costly procedures, such as embalming, sealed caskets, or expensive caskets, none of which are required by law or slow down bodily deterioration.

The processes in the preparation, funeral service, and burial can be used to facilitate mourning. Nichols and Nichols (1975) offer several alternatives that can be made available to the bereaved, provided they fit their religious and cultural backgrounds. The options include physically helping remove the body from the place of death, helping dress the body, deciding who should be a bearer of the casket (as opposed to mortuary provided bearers—an extra cost), and personalizing the service. Personalizing the service may mean having special music played, picking a friend to give a eulogy, or requesting a specific prayer.

Other aspects of the burial that can have meaning to the survivors include being able to see the casket at the gravesite and actually putting dirt on the casket. The goal of the service and burial, even if it is a memorial service without the corpse, is to provide maximum comfort and aid the mourners in going through the grieving process. The funeral industry has historically overemphasized the former to the detriment of helping the mourners grieve.

An alternative to the independently arranged funeral is the nonprofit memorial society. Members are guaranteed a funeral for a low cost, around $300, compared to the national average of $2,000 in 1978 (Butler & Lewis, 1982). The association's address is the Continental Association of Funeral and Memorial Societies, 1828 L Street N.W., Washington, D.C. 20036. (In Canada: Memorial Society Association of Canada, P.O. Box 4367, Vancouver, B.C.). Societies are controlled by their membership, which does its business with one funeral home in a community. Along with being inexpensive, the societies offer their members a dignified burial.

IMPLICATIONS
FOR MENTAL HEALTH PRACTICE

Mental health practice with the terminally ill elderly differs from many other types of therapy in several important ways. First, we are dealing with a phenomenon we do not and perhaps cannot fully comprehend. It is a somewhat feared and mysterious condition. Second, the goal of the work is not curative; we are not out to stop the process of death. Rather, the goal is adaptive—to make what may be a difficult journey as comfortable and meaningful as possible for the client. Third, much of what has been written about counseling the dying client stresses that it is the client who does the leading and the helper who follows to help the client obtain what he or she needs. Fourth, the relationship is time-limited (Schneidman, 1976). Finally, the client has, appropriately so, much more conscious "control" over the course of treatment than in other interventions.

General Approach to Work with the Dying

The major approach to work with the terminally ill has to be one of concern, care, and compassion. The mental health practitioner has to be able to listen, to attend to what the client is saying and conveying through nonverbal communication, and to be aware of implied messages or feelings that may need exploration through appropriate reflection or direct questioning. The mental health practitioner can also work to help the client make his or her death dignified and meaningful by ensuring that the client has as much control over his or her existence as possible—making sure the client's wishes are heeded and that necessary arrangements (food, visitors, funeral arrangements, etc.) are accomplished with minimum delay and no unnecessary stress for the client and family. Thus, the mental health practitioner has a dual role, as listener and as advocate.

The manner in which counseling takes place is not necessarily one of morbid concern or continual sadness. Humor can be as appropriate for the client and mental health practitioner as it is in any other part of living (Koff, 1978).

Initial Preparation and Concerns

The initial preparation of the mental health practitioner takes two forms. First and foremost is being ready to listen to whatever the client, family, or relevant others have to say. This implies a high degree of self-awareness about one's own attitudes and fears about death as well as sensitivity to how concerns and feelings are communicated by others. Methods to improve one's self-awareness and subsequently one's ability to listen include examining personal beliefs about death through discussions with knowledgeable others and going through structured exercises to further awareness of one's own death-concepts, concerns, fears, and anxieties (cf. Kastenbaum, 1981; Luce, 1979; and Koff, 1978, for specific exercises and related materials).

The second aspect of preparation requires the practitioner to have knowledge about the diagnosis, prognosis, and care plan. The practitioner should also know who the other resources are, such as the others caring for the client, friends, clergy, and social supports. Some knowledge of how the family is coping with the situation and how the family had coped with major trauma in the past is useful. Finally, one should have some understanding of the cultural, ethnic, and religious background of the client. The ways in which American Indians, Jews, specific Protestant denominations, Catholics, and Moslems approach and view death differ and may influence how the worker relates to the client. By reading about the relevant issues or consulting with other caregivers with appropriate background (including clergy), the mental health practitioner can gain needed information.

Knowledge of Terminal Diagnosis   One common initial concern is found in question such as: Who should know the client is dying?; How should they be told?; And, who should do the telling? In any health setting, the responsibility for giving a diagnosis falls on the physician. Many physicians are uncomfortable talking about death and will not tell the client. The responsibility may be delegated to a nurse, clergy member, social worker, or other professional.

To tell or not to tell the diagnosis at a particular moment in time depends on three considerations. The first is our own attitudes toward death and dying. To what degree have we, the helpers, come to grips with the reality of our own finiteness? Can we present the news of a terminal diagnosis in such a way as to neither avoid nor deny the likelihood of death without denying hope? Are we responding to the client's concerns or our own fears and anxieties?

The second consideration is a knowledge of the client's personality. One should have some idea of how the client might handle the knowledge of his or her diagnosis. Some clients will want only limited information; some will want more, some will voice their suspicions openly, and some obliquely (Hinton, 1967). Possible ways to approach the topic include asking the client what she or he knows about the illness, allowing the client to speak freely about his or her concerns, or presenting specific aspects of the condition, such as discussing positive and negative parts of the treatment. A final guide in this area is to remember that how the information is given is as important as the information itself. It is crucial to convey that the practitioner is not giving up on the client.

A third consideration of who should know, when they should know, and who should do the telling has to do with family and/or significant others. Again, it is the physician's responsibility to inform the family of the prognosis. Often, it is the spouse who is told first. While it may be important for the physician to do the telling, thus conveying the message that everything that can be done has been, this responsibility can also be delegated.

Handling Reactions by the Client and Family

Denial and Other Forms of Avoidance   The mental health practitioner's role is twofold in working with denial or avoidance of aspects of death. Because avoidance or denial may serve as a temporary respite from realities, in one sense the client has the right to hold on to his or her defenses. When the client is ready to "move on" to a new encounter with uncomfortable feelings or realizations, the practitioner needs to be able to move with him or her. There is a delicate balance between being supportive and being a source of reality. While certain therapists would argue that all irrational beliefs of the client should be challenged as they would be in any situation, the key issue may be one of acceptance—that is, being able to accept that the client is doing the "best he or she can" under the circumstances, regardless of the form denial or avoidance is taking.

The client may need help with the family's or others' denial of the client's impending death (Epstein, 1975). The mental health practitioner can function as a role-playing coach, helping the client practice how to communicate with family and others.

With the family, mental health practice has a slightly different focus in the early stages. One function is to allow the family to take "time for themselves." Another is to facilitate communication among themselves and with the client. The third is to help the family through reactions and anticipation of the death. The family is likely to feel guilt and underlying anger at the client, and these feelings may well benefit from an empathic outsider's attention.

Anger   The mental health practitioner is likely to encounter anger in work with the terminally ill. Anger can be considered a request for time and attention. The angry terminally ill client may need someone to come and talk. Also, it may be useful for the worker to initiate discussion so that an inadvertant reinforcement of anger is avoided.

A second important aspect is to be sure the client is given as much symbolic and real control over his or her life as possible. Some anger may be due to a real but unnecessary loss of independence and individual identity in an institutional setting. Control can include what clothes are worn, when meals and procedures are given, and when to start and stop sessions with the mental health practitioner (Kübler-Ross, 1969). As a rule of thumb, clients should, at the beginning of sessions, be asked if this is a "good time" to talk.

Also, the practitioner should be available if needed before or after working hours. In terms of hospital routine, evenings are usually quieter and allow a greater sense of privacy, which can be quite useful for counseling (Bradley & Edinberg, 1982).

Bargaining   If the client goes through a bargaining stage, the practitioner's general concerns are how to be caring and realistic without breaking down the client's defensive posture. While the futility of the bargaining may be obvious to the mental health practitioner, one can still emphasize with the wish (more time, less pain, opportunity to work through an issue with another family member, etc.). Certain cognitive interventions (see Chapter 10) may be useful at this point.

It is also possible that the family may go through a bargaining stage. While many bargaining statements may be made to God, it does not necessarily mean that the family is requesting consultation by clergy. They may even find clergy intrusive (Epstein, 1975). If clergy are involved at this point, they should be notified of the practitioner's perceptions of underlying dynamics. Clergy are becoming quite sophisticated about psychological processes of death and dying. Like other professionals, some will need very little "extra" education to understand the mental health practitioner's role and work.

Depression   Kübler-Ross (1969) distinguished between depression about an "old" loss (e.g., the loss of a breast through a mastectomy) and depression about current or expected losses with one's death. In the first case, depression due to a loss already incurred, Kübler-Ross suggests helping the client maintain self-worth by emphasizing positive characteristics of the client rather than letting the client dwell on the loss.

In the second case, depression over expected loss with death, reassurance is not as appropriate. Allowing the client to express his or her feelings is more useful. Sitting silently is also appropriate.

At this point the mental health practitioner can also be of help in the real world by responding to client concerns about a will or special arrangements for survivors. He or she may also facilitate expression of needs for intimacy and closeness between spouses and/or family members.

Acceptance   In the final stage before death, much will depend on the client and his or her wishes. Some visits may be quiet and reflective. The mental health practitioner should also pay close attention to changes in the client's behavior that suggest all is not well.

Working with Survivors

The mental health practitioner should consider postdeath work with the survivors as part of death and dying work. Six considerations for practitioners in their work with survivors are:

Attend to the bereaved before the death.
Work with survivors should begin within three days after the death.
Most survivors welcome the opportunity to talk to a "listener."
One of the tasks of the practitioner is to explore negative feelings about the dead person.
The professional respresents a sense of reality and can be used as a sounding board.
Close attention should be paid to physical health and sudden behavioral changes.

Families' reactions to impending death are likely to differ from those of the client. Family members may be guilty, angry, or depressed at the time the client has come to grips with his or her impending death. Some may have difficulty accepting the client's acceptance of impending death.

As the time of death approaches, the mental health practitioner can help the survivors work with the dying client on specifics for funeral arrangements, burial site, people to be informed, preparation of a will, and memorials. By including the client, these arrangements can be made more meaningful for all family members (Koff, 1978).

One structural aspect of mental health practice with survivors deserves comment. Many health care institutions terminate official contact with the family upon the death of the client. Thus it may be difficult for a mental health practitioner in a hospital or nursing home setting to maintain contact on a formal basis due to the psychological sense that the institution is "through" with the survivors. This is unfortunate, as there is value in continuity of care along the dying trajectory. Practitioners should advocate for bereavement services as a standard part of treatment of the terminally ill.

Knowledge of the cultural and ethnic bereavement traditions of the client are important. There is often a period of visitation by friends and relatives. The professional may be able to assess how the survivors are coping during this initial period.

The mental health practitioner can be of help to the survivor in three areas: providing emotional support in the early stages of bereavement, providing support and validation in the first year of bereavement, and reintroducing survivors, especially widows or widowers, to the social system. These were reviewed in Chapter 3 and will not be repeated here.

Another Perspective: Behavioral Approaches with the Terminally Ill

Although most of what has been written about mental health practice in terminal illness can be considered humanistic, a small but growing number of authors (e.g., Sobel, 1981) have begun to develop and refine behavioral methods used in other areas of mental health work with the elderly for work with the terminally ill. (See Chapter 10 for a description of behavioral approaches used with the aged.) Even these authors, however, stress the importance of compassion, care, and concern in working with the terminally ill. At the same time, they argue that compassion, while important, is not always enough to provide maximum aid to the client and/or family. Rather, the mental health practitioner can help the client work through "irrational" feelings or thoughts using "rational-emotive" or disputational techniques (e.g., Ellis, 1981), use active methods to help a client change his or her own cognitive processes that lead to depression (Sobel, 1981), or develop better management of pain and coping with grief (Averill & Wisocki, 1981; Turk & Rennert, 1981). Cognitive approaches (see Chapter 10) may also be effective if the client is "bargaining."

The key to the success and appropriate use of behavioral approaches will lie in the mental health practitioner's sensitivity and capacity to know when such techniques are warranted and when they are being used as a subtle way of avoiding confrontation of feelings or reactions to death by either the client (including family) or the mental health practitioner.

SUMMARY AND CONCLUSIONS

Death is often considered an event but is more appropriately considered a process. Death is difficult to define, as we cannot directly experience it. Of all the possible meanings of death, brain death—cessation of brain functioning—is most commonly used for medical purposes. Older persons have higher death rates than younger persons, usually dying in institutions, but do not seem to fear death any more than the young. Part of the difficulties older persons have had in coping with death have come from the ways in which caregivers have avoided both discussing it and listening to the concerns of the dying patient.

Death may represent loss and serve as an organizer of time for the elderly. In addition, individuals may go through identifiable stages in preparing for death: denial, anger, bargaining, depression, and acceptance. It is not clear how universal these stages are. Also, the terms *denial* and *acceptance* may be too broad to be useful in categorizing the dying person's behavior. Bereavement, grief, and mourning are three important parts of the death process. There are identifiable symptoms and stages in the grieving process.

Current issues in the care of the dying patient include death with dignity, euthanasia, funeral practices, and the hospice movement. Intervention with the dying requires awareness of one's own attitudes, beliefs, and reactions to death and sensitivity to how others may convey their concerns. Both the individual and the survivors may need attention. Approaches to working with the dying emphasize compassion, openness to clients' expressing feelings, and giving clients control over their surroundings. It may be possible to use behavioral and cognitive techniques as part of intervention strategies.

The nature and study of death is complicated. Our personal views, needs, and concerns about dying are likely to continue to change throughout our own lives as well as through our experience in working with the dying.

5

Functional Disorders

INTRODUCTION

Mrs. K., who is seventy-six, has a long history of depression. She has been in and out of treatment for twenty-five years. She has received shock therapy and has been institutionalized several times. She is currently receving medication to control her bouts of elation followed by periods of being blue, sad, and apathetic.

Mr. Y. is an eighty-two-year-old retired manager of a small business. He has recently become highly suspicious of his wife, accusing her of having sexual relationships with other men. Mr. Y. does not trust her out of his sight and becomes anxious when she leaves to go shopping. Mrs. Y. and their two adult children are quite upset about the situation.

Ms. P. is a seventy-year-old resident in a nursing home. She spent many years institutionalized for schizophrenia. She takes medicine to control both agitation and a tendency to talk about bizarre fantasies. Although she manages in the institution, staff are quite leery about caring for her, as she is "different" and, they believe, "dangerous."

These situations, while real and occurring in a certain percent of all elderly, are not normative or expected with age. However, they are representative of a certain segment of the older population, those who can be said to have a mental disorder.

Psychopathology and Aging

It has been suggested that at least 15 percent of the elderly need mental health services (Redick & Taube, 1980). If one considers the numbers of older adults living with organic disorders, depression, alcoholism, chronic illness, in poor living conditions, and in economic hardship, this percentage is surely too low.

There is some evidence that the incidence of mental heatlh problems rises in the elderly. The two most "old-age-related" symptom sets are depression and organic brain syndrome. However, it is difficult to discern if the symptoms of depression or organic brain syndrome reflect a "true" disorder of old age, a reaction to life events and circumstances, or expression of a disorder that has been present for some time. This distinction confounds the problems of accurately diagnosing mental disorders and, along with historical disinterest in the elderly, has hindered accurate epidemiological studies of mental health problems of the aged. This in turn is reflected in the lack of definitive information on many mental health problems of the aged.

Classifying Mental Disorders

The most generally accepted classification of mental disorders is found in the *Diagnostic and Statistical Manual of Mental Disorders*, third edition *(DSM-III)* published by the American Psychiatric Association (1980). Historically, the *DSM* manuals (previously published in 1952 and 1968) reflected psychodynamic and medical thinking; that is, theoretically, disorders are derived from unconscious conflicts and/or intrapsychic disturbances unless a specific disease entity is the cause. *DSM-III*, while it has not moved far from this perspective, has made three important changes: First, the question of the "nature" of neurosis and its classification has been addressed by limiting the definition of neurosis to describing painful functioning in individuals. Second, rather than just having one diagnosis be the description of the client's condition, five areas of functioning are considered. (These five axes are discussed in the following section.) Third, the whole area of organic reactions has been reorganized.

However, there are still several drawbacks in the classification system. Several distinct "types" of disorders may be placed under one diagnosis, such as paranoia (e.g., Zarit, 1980). Also, *DSM-III*, despite its changes from earlier editions, is still based on a disease model of mental illness that implies an unproven course of development and treatment of conditions and an implicit authority of medical treatment and the medical profession over other professionals (Schact and Nathan, 1977). Finally, special concerns or issues of the aged have not been included in *DSM-III*.

DSM-III—Five Axes for Diagnosis

DSM-III has five axes or dimensions on which a client should be evaluated:

Axis I	Clinical Syndromes
	Conditions not attributable to a mental disorder that are a focus of attention or treatment (V. Codes)
	Additional codes
Axis II	Personality disorders
	Specific developmental disorders

Axis III   Physical disorders and conditions
Axis IV   Severity of psychosocial stressors
Axis V   Highest level of adaptive functioning past year
(American Psychiatric Association, 1980, p. 23)

The first three axes are the official diagnostic categories plus a listing of physical conditions that require treatment. The fourth and fifth axes are considered supplemental.

Axis I. Clinical Syndromes, Conditions that are a Focus of Treatment, Additional Codes. The types of disorder found in Axis I include retardation; major disturbances of personality and behavior (psychoses); problems of painful symptoms where "reality testing" is unimpaired (neurotic symptoms); organic disorders (characterized by difficulties in orientation and cognition); substance abuse (e.g., alcoholism); problems in adjustment; specific "focus of treatment" problems such as family problems, antisocial behavior, noncompliance with medical treatment, marital problems; and psychosexual problems such as pedophilia (engaging in sexual activity with young children) or voyeurism.

Axis II. Personality Disorders and Specific Developmental Disorders. A personality disorder can be considered a disorder that bridges the gap between "normal" and "abnormal" behavior (Page, 1971). These disorders are mild defects or exaggerations in personality as exhibited in affect, cognition, perceptions of self or others, responses to situations, or even "orientation to life" (Page, 1971, p. 303). While the resulting behavior may be quite maladaptive, it is not necessarily discomforting to the individual and may exist for a long period of time (Simon, 1980).

Axis III. Physical Disorders and Conditions. Axis III allows formal notation of conditions that can contribute to the expressed mental health problem or its treatment (e.g., hypertension or neurological problems in the case of organic brain syndrome, chronic health problems as they may be related to depression).

Axis IV. Severity of Psychosocial Stressors. Axis IV requires rating the severity of stressors (environmental or situational events related to onset of mental health problems) on a seven-point scale, with 1 representing "no apparent psychosocial stressor" and 7 representing a "catastrophic level." The stressor should have occurred within one year of the mental health problem noted in Axes I and II. The types of stressors include marital, occupational, living circumstances, financial, legal, physical illnesses, developmental, and interpersonal problems. While this dimension has particular relevance for the elderly, the rating guidelines are minimal and criteria are not spelled out, leaving the clinician to base the rating on an opinion about "the stress an 'average' person in similar circumstances and with similar sociocultural values would experience from the particular stressor(s)" (American Psychiatric Association, 1980, p. 26).

Axis V. Highest Level of Adaptive Functioning Past Year.   Axis V allows the clinician to rate the highest level at which a client has been functioning in the last year on a five-pont scale, with 1 indicating "superior" and 5 indicating "poor." Adaptive functioning includes social relations, occupational functioning, and use of leisure time. However, there are few criteria on which to base judgments, and many mental health professionals have neither the knowledge nor experience about aging to ensure a relatively unbiased and relevant rating on Axes IV and V of *DSM-III*.

Functional Versus Organic Disorders

One of the major distinctions in psychopathology of the aging is between functional and organic disorders. A functional disorder is one in which behavioral problems or suffering are not due to an underlying physical disease process. Organic disorders are those disturbances in behavior or affect caused by an underlying physical illness. This chapter focuses on a description of functional disorders and their treatment in the elderly.

SCHIZOPHRENIC DISORDERS

DSM-III does not characterize disorders as "psychotic" or "neurotic." However, psychotic functioning—that is, personality disintegration, trouble testing reality, delusions (belief systems not based on reality) and hallucinations (perceptual distortions)—is a key characteristic in schizophrenia and paranoid functioning, the first two areas to be discussed.

Schizophrenia is characterized by psychotic features and impairment of many psychological processes, including "content and form of thought, perception, affect, sense of self, volition relationship to the outside world, and psychomotor behavior" (American Psychiatric Association, 1980, p. 182). It is not known at present if the nature of schizophrenia is primarily genetic or learned, although there is strong evidence for a genetic component. Nor is it clear if schizophrenia involves several similar disturbances or if it is one "type" of disorder (Post, 1980).

The types of symptoms encountered in persons with a schizophrenic disorder include: having bizarre and fragmented delusions, loose associations, or occasional simple persecutory thoughts ("people" spying on them); hearing "voices," reading minds, or sensing that one's body is changing. Hallucinations may include hearing sounds or having "strange" feelings or sensations.

Cognition is affected by a schizophrenic disorder. For example, thoughts may shift from one topic to another (loosening of associations) without any acknowledgment of the change of topic.

Changes in affect may be characterized by "blunting" (reduced intensity), "flattening" (no signs of emotional expression), or "inappropriate affect" (e.g., laughing when talking of the death of a spouse).

A final set of symptoms involves confusion as to one's identity (sense of self), difficulties in working towards goals (volition), and a withdrawal from the external world into one's own fantasy world. There may also be physical or psychomotor symptoms, such as maintaining a posture for an extended period of time (catatonic stupor) or "purposeless and stereotyped excited movements not influenced by external stimuli" (American Psychiatric Association, 1980, p. 184).

The diagnosis of schizophrenia requires existence of major symptoms (delusions, hallucinations, illogical thought sequences), deterioration from previous functioning, and continuous signs for at least six months.

Schizophrenia and the Aged

Onset of schizophrenia most often occurs before age forty-five. When schizophrenia occurs for the first time in old age (called paraphrenia in Great Britain), there is some question as to whether it is schizophrenic, paranoid, or organic in nature. Late-life schizophrenics generally show differences in symptomology, with their delusions focused more on sex and personal possessions than on the mystical or religious delusions typical of younger schizophrenics. When delusions occur, they are likely to focus on revenge by others in the social environment, such as neighbors (Post, 1980).

Older schizophrenics can be said to be of three types (Post, 1980): those who have had only one episode and were hospitalized for a short period of time; those who show a decrease in symptoms over time (referred to as burnout); and those whose symptoms remain constant throughout the life span. There is some evidence of a certain degree of stability in older schizophrenics; that is, regardless of "type," symptoms do not get worse with time and, if anything, may improve somewhat. However, most older schizophrenics will need some sort of structured care for survival. The national policy of deinstitutionalization over the last two decades has meant that older schizophrenics have been placed in settings other than mental hospitals, including nursing homes, where staff often have neither the training nor interest to respond to schizophrenics' needs, which may well be different from those of most residents.

Intervention Guidelines

Medical Management   So-called *major tranquilizers* are used to control psychotic symptoms in all age groups, including the elderly. The most commonly used antipsychotic drugs are phenothiazine derivities, including chlorpromazine (Thorazine), haloperidol (Haldol), and thioridazine (Mellarill). Depending on the "type" of patient and other medical problems, various major tranquilizers may be equally effective. However, the dosage for the elderly is significantly lower than that for younger persons.

The side effects of major tranquilizers are potentially serious. They include dangerous interactions with alcohol and other central nervous system depressants, drowsiness, confusion, delirium, urinary retention (including bladder paralysis), impotence, vision problems, hypothermia, and nausea (Davis, Segal, & Lesser, 1982). Each drug varies in the type of side effects it is likely to create. Haldol, for example, can create Parkinson's symptoms and should not be used by a person who has Parkinson's disease. A person using Haldol should not be allowed to drive a car.

A final point about maintenance on major tranquilizers has been raised by Davis and his associates (1982). A single psychotic episode does not necessarily mean that long-term medication is indicated. A few weeks of treatment may be all that is needed. Furthermore, the idea of schizophrenic burnout suggests that medication may effectively be decreased in older schizophrenics as symptoms may naturally go towards remission (Bridge, Cannon, & Wyatt, 1978). The medical regimen of individuals should be continually assessed and reviewed.

Mental Health Interventions   The care of older schizophrenics will present great difficulties in the foreseeable future. They will probably not receive the same attention and care as older people with problems that seem to respond better to intervention. It can also be argued that working with these clients take resources away from others who stand a better chance of improving, although medication and appropriate support systems may help many older schizophrenics return to noninstitutional settings. At the same time, staff need to be encouraged to respect the dignity and respond to the individual, not the "schizophrenic patient."

The goals of intervention with older schizophrenics are more likely to be adaptive (training the schizophrenic in skills needed to adapt to the social environment) than curative. The focus is likely to be on behavior and socialization (both increasing useful patterns and decreasing disruptive ones). Suggested approaches include behavioral interventions (see Chapter 10) and the use of small groups to work on skills (Chapter 12).

PARANOID DISORDERS (INCLUDING SCHIZOPHRENIA OF THE PARANOID TYPE)

Paranoid disorders are characterized by persecutory delusions or jealousy; that is, the individual has an unrealistic belief that "others" are out to spy on, conspire, or destroy him or her. Subtypes of paranoid disorders are not clearly distinguished from each other. Furthermore, one of the previously mentioned schizophrenic disorders is "paranoid type"—characterized by "persecutory delusions, grandiose delusions, delusional jealousy and hallucinations with persecutory or grandiose content" (American Psychiatric Association, 1980, p. 191). Ordinarily, the distinction between paranoid schizophrenic and paranoid disorders is made on the basis that in a schizophrenic disorder there is thought and mood disturbance as well as persecutory delusions. In paranoid reactions, the persecutory delusion is often "encapsulated," or contained one single idea, such as that one's spouse is unfaithful. Occasionally, paranoid beliefs are shared by two people *(folie à deux)*, often family members. In the case where one person is submissive, having that person separated from the other will often eliminate the paranoid beliefs.

Belief in delusions can lead to anger, resentment, or even violent acts. Signs of paranoid disorders are often discovered because the individual is continually calling the police, starting legal proceedings against others, or writing letters of complaint about fictitious or distorted events. The paranoid person is suspicious and rarely seeks help. Frequently, others bring the individual for treatment.

The diagnosis of paranoid disorders requires existence of the delusional jealousy or delusions for at least a week along with emotion and behavior fitting the delusions. Also, there should be the absence of schizophrenic symptoms, hallucinations, depressive disorders, and organic mental disorders (American Psychiatric Association, 1980).

Paranoid Disorders and the Aged

Paranoid disorders are relatively uncommon in the aged. Estimates of their occurrence in the aged popuation have ranged between 1 and 3 percent (Post, 1980). Paranoid disorders account for approximately 10 percent of all psychiatric inpatient admissions of the elderly.

The major sensory loss associated with paranoid states in old age is loss of hearing. The loss may be either total or "social," making conversation difficult. The loss may date back to at least middle age (Cooper, Garside, & Kay, 1976). Visual loss, while less predominant, also has been found (Cooper & Porter, 1976).

Post (1980), points out that paranoid phenomena are common in depressive and schizo-affective disorders, that in delirium an illusion may cause a brief paranoid reaction leading to aggressive behavior, and that a more prolonged reaction with little impairment of awareness and olfactory or visual hallucinations can be related to "subacute brain syndromes." Careful assessment is needed to determine the actual cause of paranoid symptoms.

Post also posits three types of paranoid reactions in the elderly (1980, pp. 596-598): One group is *simple paranoid psychosis*, characterized by the existence of a few delusional beliefs, experiences, and hallucinations. This group may never come to the attention of medical or mental health professionals; they are rarely disruptive, and others, including family and spouses, may "cover up" their delusions. Delusions focus on molestation by others, usually in the immediate social environment, who are thought to make threats or disparging remarks about the patient. At times, the content of the delusions will simply be "noises" made by special machines. Also, the older man who unreasonably suspects his wife of being unfaithful falls into this category.

In this group, delusions come on gradually, and the patient feels that the persecution is unjustified. Generally, one's personality is not disrupted by these delusions, but crisis situations may take place. Often, removing the individual from the persecutory situation (including moving in with family if they are not part of the delusion) will lead to a decrease in symptoms, although the individual will still believe that others were persecuting him or her in the other situation.

The second group is those with *schizophrenialike illnesses*. This group shows a greater disturbance of mental functioning, with patients becoming increasingly distressed by their illusions, hallucinations, and loose associations. The symptoms are more "florid and bizarre," with gas lines and electric wiring being part of the delusions as opposed to people simply coming in and stealing. The patient will become more distressed over time and may call for help from the police, family, or politicians. Again, removal from the immediate social situation will lead to a decrease in symptoms (and calls for help) although the delusional system will remain.

The third group is *paranoid schizophrenia states*, characterized by either narrowly defined delusional beliefs or wide-ranging psychotic ideas. There may be depressed affect, indistinct speech, and a high degree of distress over the perceptions of persecution. There is greater likelihood of third-person singular auditory hallucinations, overheard conversations about oneself, in part being maligned, in part being defended, and overt sexual content as well as thought-reading and other evidence of breakdown in reality testing. This group does not benefit from removal from the social situation; that is, agitation will remain. However, in none of the groups is the disorder considered progressive.

Intervention Guidelines

Medical Management   Research on the prognosis or expected change with mental health intervention in the case of paranoid disorders in the elderly is conflicting (e.g., Tanna, 1974; Post, 1980). The general view is that almost all will respond to some degree to a combination of medical and therapeutic intervention. Phenothiazines have been used successfully as a medical intervention (Post, 1980), although there are potentially dangerous side effects such as fever, nausea, and jaundice (Davis et al., 1982). Finally, medication may not be taken appropriately by a suspicious client (Pfeiffer, 1977).

Mental Health Interventions   The goal of mental health interventions with paranoid clients is curative; that is, the desired outcome is decrease of delusionary thoughts and subsequent disruptive behavior. The focus is on both cognitive aspects (thoughts) and behavioral reactions to these thoughts. In some cases a more adaptive stance— that is, a decrease in the negative consequences of the delusional system—may be all that can be achieved.

The following guidelines are suggested as an approach:

1.   *Accept the client without either accepting or attacking the delusional belief.* Many paranoid clients have a desire for the closeness they do not have by virtue of their behavior. Yet they are quite sophisticated at picking up false agreement by others. Thus, "acceptance" of the delusional belief may be seen as "phony," but directly attacking the belief will be seen as distancing or a cause for suspicion. An alternative is to empathize with the anger, loneliness, or frustration the client faces as a consequence of the beliefs. It should also be noted that some "delusions" may have a grain of truth and need to be checked out, including concerns about family members controlling the older person's resources.

2.   *Be honest.* Because paranoid clients pick up on slight miscommunication as evidence that their suspicions are "correct," it becomes important to explain medical procedures, to give names and functions of staff, and to be carefully and precisely honest (Butler & Lewis, 1982).

3.   *Have the client focus on the consequences of behavior rather than truth or untruth of the delusion.* Beck (1976) uses an example of how a therapist pointed out to a husband that his continued accusations of infidelity might cause his wife to leave him, which led to an improvement in the husband-wife relationship. The therapist made no judgment about the "truth" of the accusations but pointed out the negative consequences of their continuation.

4.   *Decrease "secondary gain" or reinforcement received by having the delusions.* Some assessment needs to be made of what the client is "getting" (including attention). Intervention can then focus on making these gains available in a less discomforting manner.

5.   *Provide support to families.* It is hard to imagine the anguish a spouse goes through after 40 years of marriage in having to put up with accusations and suspiciousness over his or her every move. Spouses, sons, and daughters need reassurance that nothing in their behavior is creating the delusion, that there is hope for improvement, and that the family can behave in ways to help the client. Special attention needs to be paid to helping the family avoid inadvertantly reinforcing the delusion through attention, arguments, or strong emotional reactions (Brink, 1980). Addressing questions of "honesty" and "acceptance" may also be the beginning steps in family treatment.

6.   *Tend to sensory deficits.* Hearing and vision exams (done with the client's full knowledge), obtaining aids such as glasses and hearing aids, and good medical/ physical care should be an important part of treatment.

Paranoid older persons can often maintain themselves in community settings with appropriate supports. If their symptoms are discreet—that is, if delusions only occur at certain times and are related to fears of isolation of loneliness—such persons may create few problems for others.

AFFECTIVE DISORDERS

An affective disorder is one in which there is significant disturbance in a person's mood or "feeling" state. Affective disorders are associated with feelings of depression or elation (mania).

It is difficult to distinguish between reactions to stressful events such as death, physical impairment, or other losses (reactive depression) and long-term mood disturbances (endogenous depression) associated with affective disorders. Also, it is possible that an event will trigger a "dormant" depressive disorder, the only sign of the disorder being continually occurring episodes of depression after the event. A further difficulty in diagnosing depression is the problem of determining the cause. Depression may be caused by physiological changes (leading to increased or decreased neurotransmitters), reaction to life events, and reactions to alcohol or drugs given for other illness. Depression could also be caused by an interaction of physical and emotional responses or occur as a by-product of an organic impairment.

Symptoms   Five types of symptoms are associated with affective disorders: feelings of sadness or boredom (dysphoria); reduced behavior or little participation in activities; guilt, anxiety, or doubt about one's abilities; physical (somatic) reactions, such as loss of appetite, headaches, and sleep problems; and cognitive components, including feelings of low self-esteem, worthlessness, and self-blame (Lewinsohn, Biglan, & Zeiss, 1976; Stenback, 1980).

Affective disorders have been classified in *DSM-III* as being *major affective disorders* (major bipolar and major depression) or *"other specific disorders"* (cyclothymic and dysthmic). Cyclothymic and dysthmic disorders are considered less severe and/or of shorter duration than the major affective disorders.

Bipolar Disorders

Bipolar disorders are more commonly known as manic-depressive disorders. Their essential characteristic is a manic stage, in which mood is elevated, expansive, or even extremely irritated. Symptoms include overactiveness (hyperactivity), rapid transition of thought, significantly less need for sleep, self-aggrandizement, and ease in being distracted. Mania may also be expressed symptomatically by participating in many activities, some of which can be dangerous (e.g., reckless driving, speculative investments). Mania may last as long as two weeks. If there are hallucinations or delusions, they are usually consistent with the elevated mood—for example, voices saying the person has special powers or a special attribute. The manic stage is then almost invariably followed by a state of depression. Criteria for diagnosis include existence of the elevated state for at least one week, with at least three of the previously mentioned symptoms occurring. Also, there should be no signs of schizophrenia, paranoid disorders, or organic mental disorders.

Major Depression

The most obvious signs of major depression are a depressed (dysphoric) mood and a general disinterest in pleasure and activities. Other symptoms are loss of weight or appetite, sleeping problems, psychomotor agitation or retardation, loss of interest or pleasure in usual activities (including sex), loss of energy, feelings of worthlessness, difficulties in thinking, and thoughts of death or suicide (American Psychiatric Association, 1980) as well as thinking difficulties. People with major depression will describe their mood as down, blue, depressed, sad, or in the dumps. In the elderly, there may be complaints of memory loss or disorientation, which are also signs of organic brain syndrome.

In addition to depressive characteristics, there may be psychotic aspects. These aspects may be mood-congruent (hallucinations or delusions about death, guilt, disease, and so forth) or mood incongruent (often delusions of persecution or other topics not related to the depression).

Diagnostic criteria for major depression include (a) dysphoric mood and/or loss of interest in activities and (b) occurrence of at least four other symptoms consistently in a two-week period. There should be no evidence of schizophrenic, paranoid, or organic disorders.

Other Specific Affective Disorders

The two types of *other specific affective disorders* are *cyclothymic disorder* and *dysthmic disorder.*

Cyclothymic Disorder   Cyclothymic disorders are characterized as having a duration of over two years, but not being as severe as manic or major depressive disorders. There is also a cyclical nature to the disorder, with periods of depression and elation. These periods can be interspersed with months of "normal" affect.

Dysthymic Disorder (Depressive Personality Disorder)   This disorder is primarily depressive; that is, the major characteristics are similar to those for a major depression. There are no psychotic symptoms and no elevated mood swings. There is no specific or clear onset, and the condition appears to continue over time. There may be other related symptoms such as concern with suicide, irritation, dissatisfaction with life, and a sense of emptiness.

Depression and the Elderly

Depressive symptoms are the most common complaints of the elderly. Several studies suggest that one-quarter of the older population has some form of depressive symptom (cf. Stenback, 1980). There are some indications that physical or somatic symptoms (including hypochondriacal complaints) are more likely to occur than guilt or sadness (Zung, 1967; Epstein, 1976). However, any of the symptoms of depression can occur with the elderly, including reports of recent memory loss.

At the same time, older persons are unlikely to be formally diagnosed as depressed in mental health settings. Possible explanations for this apparent discrepency are that the form depression takes (somatic complaints) does not easily lead to mental health treatment or referral, that depressive symptoms are overlooked by mental health professionals as a "normal" sign of aging, and that older persons who feel depressed may themselves believe that this is to be expected with old age and is therefore not worth trying to change. Finally, it is also commonly assumed that older persons in nursing homes have higher rates of depression than those in the community, although some research questions this assumption (Zemore & Eames, 1979).

Late-Life Depression   Along with the *DSM-III* categories there has been some consideration of depressions of "late-life" onset. In many aspects, they are similar to those of middle age or earlier onset, the most noticeable differences being a preponderance of somatic symptoms. Stenback (1980, p. 625) suggests that the most frequently occurring forms are characterized by "dysphoria, loss of interest in outside matters, and somatic illness, or fatigue." He goes on to argue that this "type" of depression should be considered as a severe and chronic form of what can be considered mild depression. Finally, he points out that depression in old age is influenced by biological, social, cultural, and psychological factors. That is, changes in physiological capacities, loss of goals and roles, lowered self-esteem from a culturally held negative view of the aged, and having to cope with losses can interact to lead to an increase of depressive symptoms in the aged.

Intervention Guidelines

Medical Management of Bipolar Disorder   The most common drug used to control bipolar depression is lithium carbonate (lithium) (Dunner, 1982). In the elderly, side effects include nausea, vomiting, confusion, delirium, hypothyroidism, salt depletion, and renal disease. The relationship between salt and lithium is important. For example, if a patient is told to decrease sodium intake while on lithium, the reabsorption rate of lithium increases, leading to a higher likelihood of lithium toxicity (Dunner, 1982).

Medical Management of Depression

Three types of drugs are used as anti-depressants; tricycle and tetracyclics, monoamine oxidaise (MAO) inhibitors, and stimulants.

TABLE 5-1   Tricyclic and Tetracyclic Antidepressants

	USUAL DOSE RANGE (mg/day)		
STRUCTURAL CLASS	TRADE NAME	YOUNG ADULT	ELDERLY
Tricyclic			
Tertiary Amine			
Amitriptyline	Elavil	100-300	25-150
Imipramine	Tofranil	100-300	25-150
Doxepin	Sinequan	100-300	25-150
Trimipramine	Surmontil	100-300	25-150
Secondary Amine			
Nortriptyline	Pamelor	50-100	10-60
Desipramine	Norpramin	100-300	25-150
Protriptyline	Vivactil	20-60	5-30
Dibenzoxazepine			
Amoxapine	Asendin	150-300	25-150
Triazolopyridine			
Trazodone	Desyrel	150-400	50-300
Tetracyclic			
Maprotiline	Ludiomil	100-300	25-150

Source: R.C. Veith. Depression in the elderly: Pharmacologic considerations. *Journal of the American Geriatrics Society*, 1981, *30*, 581-586, with permission of W. B. Saunders, publishers.

Tricyclics and tetracyclics are suggested for long-lasting depression with sleep and motor disturbances. As is shown in Table 5-1, there are several types, the most common being amitriptyline (Elavil) and imipramine (Tofranil). The side effects of each vary, but many are sedative (except for desipramine and protriptyline), inducing varying degrees of stupor and anticholinergic reactions, which potentially lead to mouth dryness, constipation, blurred vision, delirium, and visual hallucinations. There are also cardiovascular effects (one being an increased heart rate), possible interference with the effects of antihypertensive medication, and postural hypotension, which can lead to falls. Their recommended dosage is one-third to one-fourth of that for a younger adult (Veith, 1981).

MAO inhibitors are mood elevators that include phenelzine and tranylcypromine. They are used to control anxiety, phobias, and increases in appetite and sleep. However, they may lead to serious reactions including hypertension when used in conjunction with certain foods such as cheese, yogurt, beer, wine, or caffeinated beverages (Veith, 1981). Their use with the elderly is debated and should only be considered when there is a good likelihood that dietary restrictions will be followed.

Stimulants include substances such as methylphenidate and dextroamphetamines. With the elderly, they have only short-term results and cause side effects such as cardiovascular problems, paranoid behavior, and, paradoxically, depression upon withdrawal of the stimulant (Veith, 1981).

Drugs versus Therapeutic Intervention   The question of drugs versus therapy has long been debated. One question is philosophical: Can depression truly be "cured" by drugs or is it simply "altered" in some way, with the client being sedated or "not caring"? A second issue is the danger of side effects, mentioned above.

Still a third issue has to do both with efficacy and use of the treatment modality. While there is no question that some older persons would prefer a pill to psychotherapy, proponents on both sides of the question have argued that their approach is more effective. For example, one study (Jarvik et al., 1982), showed 45 percent full remission of symptoms in drug treatment (imipramine and doxepin) versus 12 percent full remission in therapy groups (including a cognitive group). However, in another study (Gallagher & Thompson, 1983), psychotherapeutic interventions led to remission in over half of the elderly clients treated.

One conclusion worth noting is that group therapy (cf. Steuer, 1982) leads to some improvement for the majority of participants whereas drug treatment has a bimodal effect: some patients make significant gains, others are unaffected. This in turn suggests the possibility that certain types of client would benefit more from one form of treatment than the other. However, we do not at this time know how to make that type of determination.

Electroconvulsive Shock Therapy (ECT)   Electroshock therapy is currently under a siege of criticism. While there is no question that ECT has been misused, its relative safety, efficacy, and speed of results may make it a treatment of choice, especially if a client is suicidal, anorexic, or not eating (Jenike, 1983; Gaitz, 1983).

Electroshock treatment is a series of six to ten grand mal seizures electrically induced in the client's brain. The seizure is the therapeutic agent. Side effects come from the electric shock, many of which can be mitigated by medication to help relax the client's body. Shocks are given three times a week, although the frequency varies dependng on symptoms or onset of side effects (Yesavage & Berens, 1980). Side effects include short-term confusion, memory loss, and behavior change. However, there are none of the sedative or anticholinergic qualities of antidepressant medication. Also, patients have few complaints, there is no irreversible brain damage, and ECT has generally had better results than MAO inhibitors and tricyclic drugs (Scovern & Kilmann, 1980; Jenike, 1983; Weiner, 1982). ECT is not recommended if there has been a recent heart attack or cerebrovascular accident (Weiner, 1982.

The controversy about ECT may stem from misinformation (current procedures are unlike those done twenty years ago), fear about the procedure, concern about the short-term side effects (e.g., confusion), concern about overuse, and the same philosophical questions raised about drug therapies. While safeguards need to be maintained or improved to ensure against misuse, the evidence warrents the inclusion of ECT as an indicated treatment, especially when the client is a threat to his or her own life.

Mental Health Interventions   The goal of mental health interventions for depression in the aged is curative; that is, interventions are designed to eliminate depressive behavior and feelings. Their focus varies, depending in part on the theoretical orientation underlying the type of intervention. Cognitive approaches (one of the more validated approaches with the aged) focus on changing thoughts that lead to depressed feelings or changing patterns of behavior that reinforce feelings of low self-esteem. Approaches that emphasize a positive self-concept (e.g., client-centered therapy) focus more on the attitudes and values that lead to a lowered self-image and resultant depressed affect.

The following guidelines constitute a recommended approach in intervention with the aged. It is likely that a practitioner will use only one or two of the specific techniques mentioned.

1.   Conduct a careful assessment of the individual. Key factors are stressors or events that may have triggered or even caused the depression: physical health—impact of either disease or medication on mood; availability and need for social supports; cognitive components—how the client perceives and thinks about events that in turn leads him or her to feel depressed; and how much the depression is rewarded (intentionally or inadvertently) by others.

2.   Appreciate that several types of approaches may be used. The concept of minimal intervention suggests initially tending to some of the more "simple" interventions, such as exercise; letting the client "talk it out" with a friend or supportive relative; or encouraging participation in enjoyable social or work activities (Lewinsohn et al., 1978).

3.   Appreciate the anger and underlying emotional components felt by many older clients. To ignore the sense of helplessness, guilt, or abandonment in the depressed client is to overlook significant aspects of depression. There is a need to let the client express anger or feelings and to uncover underlying dynamics and deal with them directly (Butler & Lewis, 1982). A stance of active listening or a client-centered approach (see Chapter 11) is suggested for handling anger.

4.   Pay attention to "cognitive" aspects of the depression. This is, by carefully sorting out what the client tells himself or herself to become depressed, the mental health practitioner can help the client "correct" the thoughts that lead to feeling depressed. The approaches of Beck (1967, 1976) and Ellis (1962) as well as other cognitive methods discussed in Chapter 10 are useful and recommended.

5.   Consider helping the older client build or develop social skills. It has been shown that depressed individuals have or use fewer social skills (e.g., responding to others, being sensitive to others' feelings) than nondepressed individuals (Lewinsohn, Biglan, and Zeiss, 1976). The mental health practitioner can help clients who have these deficits by encouragement, teaching, role playing, and having the client practice skills in various settings. Assertion training may also be a useful adjunctive method.

6.   Pay attention to the client's interactions and relationships with significant others. For example, an older woman may become depressed over the "fact" that her husband does not "court her" as he once did. It may well turn out not only that the husband is having concerns about his own sexuality but also that the wife's way of respondng to his ambivalence is to become less communicative and withdrawn, which increases the problems.

ANXIETY DISORDERS

Anxiety disorders are characterized by a primary symptom of fear (anxiety). To be classified as an anxiety disorder, the fear or avoidance must significantly curtail social functioning, relationships with intimates, or work.

Physical symptoms of anxiety include dryness in the mouth, sweating, dizziness, upset stomach, diarrhea, rapid shallow breathing (hyperventilation), chest pain, choking, frequent urination, or a sensation of a lump in the throat (Simon, 1980).

Anxiety States   Anxiety that occurs without a specific "trigger" stimulus is considered an anxiety state or anxiety neurosis. Its other symptoms include hot and cold flashes, trembling, as well as fears of dying, losing control, or becoming crazy.

Phobic Disorders   Phobic disorders (or phobic neuroses) are characterized by an irrational fear of objects or circumstances. The degree of fear is much greater than the danger actually posed by the object or activity; the fear interferes with functioning. Phobias may be experienced in social situations (e.g., *agoraphobia*, fear of being in public places with little chance of escaping) or be focused on objects such as snakes, insects, or dogs.

Obsessive-Compulsive Disorders   Obsessive-compulsive disorders have two aspects. The first is obsessions, the continual appearance of thoughts, impulses, or feelings that seem to "just happen." Obsessions frequently focus on issues such as abandonment or losing control over one's life.

The second aspect is compulsion; some specific behavior that the client ritualistically performs to create or prevent a future situation. Carrying out the compulsive behavior relieves anxiety, even though the client knows it serves no real purpose (e.g., excessive cleaning to "ward off" disease).

Anxiety Disorders and the Aged

It has been suggested that anxiety reactions or disorders in the aged arise from the individual's attempts to "deal with psychological problems and stresses that arouse anxiety" (Simon, 1980, p. 655). Although severe anxiety reactions are relatively rare in the aged (Jarvik & Russell, 1979), numerous laboratory tests with healthy aged have found that they have higher levels of anxiety than younger subjects (cf. Botwinick, 1978). This suggests that mild anxiety reactions are the most prevalent form of anxiety reaction in the aged. As is the case for depressive reactions, it is possible that physiological, social, cultural, and psychological factors lead to heightened anxiety in certain older persons as they try to "live up" to performance expectations established at a younger age.

Intervention Guidelines

Medical Management   Minor tranquilizers are used to manage anxiety. The most common are benzodiazepine derivitives: chlordiazepoxide (Librium) and diazepam (Valium is also often used as a muscle relaxant and for arthritis). Minor tranquilizers are widely used with the elderly. However, they have a high potential for central nervous system sedation, leading to drowsiness, falls, and dangers in driving. Other side effects include depression, fatigue, and loss of sexual drive (Greenblatt & Divoll, 1982). Also, many physicians prescribing these drugs do not realize that they have a higher potency and rate of absorption in the elderly than in the young. If minor tranquilizers are used, low dosages are recommended.

Finally, barbiturate sedatives, such as phenobarbital and meprobamate (e.g., Equanil, Miltown) are used in managing anxiety. However, they can lead to dependency and are no more effective than the benzodiazepine derivitives (Butler & Lewis, 1982).

Mental Health Intervention   Psychodynamic procedures and general relationship therapies, while frequently used with the aged, have not been effective in decreasing obsessive-compulsiveness, anxiety reactions, or phobias (Götestam, 1980). Medication in conjunction with certain behavioral and cognitive approaches has been much more effective. The goal of treatment is curative (decreasing anxiety). Treatment may focus on cognitive, behavioral, or physical components of anxiety.

Guidelines for treatment include:

1.   Use specific techniques such as relaxation and desensitization (see Chapter 10). Also effective are homework assignments, in which the client practices new techniques, discovers "new information" about his or her behavior, and either charts or records results. Some older clients will do well with this approach; others may refuse or have difficulty remembering directions.

2.   Build a physical component into treatment. Techniques include breathing (see Chapter 10), relaxation, and physical exercise programs (including walking).

3.   Help the client change internal processes (thoughts, words, pictures, feelings) to avoid thoughts that may lead to the anxiety reactions (e.g., Meichenbaum, 1977; Bandler & Grinder, 1975; Grinder & Bandler, 1976).

4.   Pay attention to the "benefits" (secondary gain) of the anxious behavior. All anxiety disorders serve, in part, to decrease anxiety. That is, by having physical reactions, fear of an object, or even compulsive behavior, tension is somewhat dispelled. Other persons may pay more attention to the anxious person (secondary gain). Clients may be unwilling at some level to "give up" what is a somewhat helpful type of behavior, even though they know it is irrational, because they "feel better" with it.

5.   Be alert for side effects of medications that may cause anxiety reactions in the elderly such as chlorpromazine, thioridazine, and tricyclic antidepressants. Also, be alert to the possibility of overmedication or overdependence in an older person taking tranquilizers for anxiety reactions.

SOMATOFORM DISORDERS

In somatoform disorders symptoms suggesting a physical disease are present, but there is in fact no underlying physical or physiological cause. Rather, the disorder indicates that psychological conflicts are present. There are five categories of somatoform disorders. They are:

Somatization disorders, in which the client may present himself or herself as "sickly," with conversion, pseudoneurological, gastrointestinal, or psychosexual symptoms, as well as menstrual difficulties

Conversion disorders (hysterical neurosis), characterized by specific disease or disability symptoms considered not under voluntary control, such as paralysis, seizures, and blindness

Psychogenic pain disorder, in which the primary symptom is recurring pain

Hypochondriasis (hypochondriacal neurosis), in which the client interprets his or her physical state or reactions as a sign of disease and becomes preoccupied with fear of the illness, finding an "accurate" diagnosis, and, in a sense, living through the disease

Atypical somatoform disorder, a residual category in which symptoms or concerns focus on physical or physiological issues but have no organic basis.

Somatoform Disorders and the Aged

Hypochondriasis is the somatoform disorder most often associated with the elderly (Pfeiffer & Busse, 1973). One complaint associated with this condition is memory loss (Brink, 1981). Any health professional who works with older clients is likely to encounter older persons whose lives seem bound up in trying to get their "illness" diagnosed to no avail. The medical costs incurred in testing, ruling out exotic illnesses, and physician time may be considerable as hypochondriacal clients can be most persistent in "pursuing" health.

However, before a diagnosis of hypochondriasis is accepted, careful consideration has to be given to the possibility that a physical illness is, in fact, present. Unfortunately, the negative attitudes and lack of concern by some medical personnel can make this question difficult to resolve.

Intervention Guidelines

Because hypochondriacs are unlikely to accept a nonmedical basis for their disease, any successful approach is more likely to be adaptive rather than curative.

Specific guidelines include:

1. Attend to consequences of behavior rather than debating the "reality" of the illness.
2. Attempt to understand what the client is avoiding or symbolizing in the "illness" (e.g., making oneself inadquate, self-punishment, controlling others, punishment of others, controlling the environment, or reducing intimacy). Some clients may improve by gaining insight into their problems, although hypochondriacs are unlikely to accept a nonmedical explanation of their illness.
3. Even without interpretation, work with the client to set goals in areas of perceived needs (e.g., feeling good, gaining intimacy) and jointly develop ways the client can meet these "unrelated" goals.

DISSOCIATIVE DISORDERS

Dissociative disorders are characterized by a change in consciousness, identity, or motor behavior. Symptoms include forgetting events, assuming a new identity, or wandering without knowing where one is. Specific dissociative disorders include:

Amnesia, forgetting events when the memory loss is not due to organic mental disorder,

Fugue, suddenly traveling away from home and assuming a new identity without remembering the previous identity

Multiple personality, having two or more distinct personalities, each with its own memories and relationships; each is dominant at times, and the original personality has no awareness of the other personalities

Depersonalization disorder, in episodes of "alteration in the perception of experience of self so that the usual sense of one's own reality is temporarily lost or changed" (American Psychiatric Association, 1980, p. 259)

Atypical dissociative disorder, a residual category for individuals having general symptoms of a dissociative disorder.

Dissociative Disorders and the Aged

Little has been written on the incidence or treatment of dissociative disorders in the aged. The symptoms associated with these disorders are, however, similar to those of organic brain syndrome (memory loss, amnesia, wandering). Care needs to be taken to be reasonably sure that one disorder is not being mistaken for the other.

PSYCHOSEXUAL DISORDERS

Psychosexual disorders are those disorders related to sexual functioning that are considered psychological in nature. There are four groups of psychosexual disorders. In *gender identity disorders*, one's sense of sex role is inconsistent or confused. In *paraphilias*, sexual arousal is linked to objects not usually associated with sexual activity. *Psychosexual dysfunction* is significant inhibition of sexual response or desire. *Other psychosexual disorders* include ego-dystonic homosexuality (unwanted homosexual responses) and psychosexual disorders not elsewhere classified.

Psychosexual Disorders and the Aged

Most of the sexual problems faced by the elderly are not psychosexual disorders but problems of sexual dysfunction, discussed in Chapter 2. However, several points should be made in the discussion of psychosexual disorders as they pertain to the elderly.

First, a psychosexual disorder may be "found" when none is present, due to bias or ignorance on the part of professionals. For example, a disoriented older person needing to urinate may end up being viewed as an exhibitionist. Also, physical contact between elderly (usually men) and children may be considered molestation. Empathy and careful assessment of the older person are strongly urged to compensate for what may be an overreaction by concerned parties when a sexual disorder is suspected. Second, when innappropriate sexual behavior (e.g., public masturbation or exposure of genetalia) occurs, adaptive strategies (e.g., teaching clients where and when such behavior is acceptable or not irritating to others) are suggested (Hussian, 1981).

A final point concerns homosexuality and aging. *DSM-III* has eliminated homosexuality as a disorder in and of itself, except where homosexual impulses are a source of distress to the person having them. What little research has been done indicates that homosexuals are no better or worse than heterosexuals in adapting to age. Many of the issues faced by homosexuals can be best handled by the same principles that would govern treatment of nonhomosexuals.

PERSONALITY DISORDERS

Personality disorders have been given their own diagnostic axis (Axis II) in *DSM-III* because they may be overlooked when they appear in conjunction with a more "obvious" disorder such as those found on Axis I. Generally, these "exaggerated" personality traits are more distressful to others than the person who exhibits them.

Many types of disorder are included in this category, including *paranoid, schizoid, histrionic* (overly dramatic, requiring excitement, drawing attention to self), *narcissistic* (characterized by an exaggerated sense of achievements, exhibitionism—needing constant attention, lack of empathy, exploitiveness), *antisocial* (characterized by acts such as theft, lying, aggressiveness), *borderline* (instability in several areas of functioning), *avoidant, dependent, compulsive,* and *passive-aggressive.* Each has its own sets of characteristics, likely behavior, and type of relationships that can be expected with other people.

Personality Disorders and the Aged

The most common forms of personality disorders in the aged are "depressive, paranoid, obsessive-compulsive, dependent, schizoid, and histrionic personalities" (Simon, 1980, p. 660). These may have existed in the individual for many years, but as the individual tries to cope with physical, social, cultural, and psychological changes of aging, may become exaggerated.

The mental health practitioner should recognize that certain tendencies in later life such as desire to leave a legacy or a strong sense of independence may be incorrectly interpreted as a personality disorder. Later life-cycle issues are not considered in *DSM-III*'s classification system for personality disorders.

Little has been written about treating personality disorders in the elderly. Indeed, the question should be raised as to whether or not a "disorder" that causes little concern to the client should even be treated.

ALCOHOLISM

Alcoholism has been considered a social problem, a crime, a disease, or a mental disorder, depending on the authority examining the phenomenon. According to *DSM-III*, alcohol abuse is a disorder characterized by social and occupational impairment or the "pathological" use of alcohol. That is, social reationships and job performance are impaired by the amount and/or pattern of drinking. Also, there is a regular (daily) need for alcohol, the client is unable to decrease consumption (despite efforts to stop), and there are occasional drinking binges, amnesia, drinking excessive amounts of liquor, and continued drinking in the presence of a physical illness in which drinking will lead to serious complications.

Alcoholism is one of the top three health problems in the United States. While distinctions have been made between *problem drinkers* (persons with some manifestations of alcohol abuse), *acute alcoholism* (a state of alcoholic stupor due to intoxification), *dipsomania* (drinking binges), and *chronic alcoholism*, all represent varying degrees of danger to the person who has the problem.

Alcoholism in the elderly is particularly difficult to uncover for several reasons. Many health professionals are hesitant to diagnose alcoholism in older persons. Older alcoholics may also avoid contact with agencies or professionals who might notice signs of alcoholism. Finally, the signs of alcoholism are similar to those of other physical and emotional problems commonly encountered in the elderly.

A major consideration in the diagnosis of an alcohol abuse disorder is the absence or presence of organic brain disorder. Three clinical subtypes of alcoholic disorder can theoretically be distinguished: alcoholism with no chronic brain damage, alcoholism with brain damage caused by alcohol abuse, and alcoholism existing along with senile dementia of the Alzheimer's type (Simon, 1980). It is possible for alcohol abuse to exist without organic brain damage, to cause brain damage, or to exist along with an unrelated organic brain disorder.

Symptoms of Alcoholism and Alcohol Abuse

The guidelines given in *DSM-III* for the diagnosis of alcohol abuse disorder are general but accurate. Several other sets of symptoms have been proposed both to pinpoint the alcoholic and to serve as soft signs—that is, signs that alcohol problems may be present and further inquiry or assessment is needed. Often, a mental health practitioner who has limited information about or contact with a client and may pick up the alcoholism through one of the soft signs.

Criteria for and indications of alcohol abuse include:

Physical symptoms—shaking, blackouts
Psychological dependency on alcohol
Health problems, including falls
Problems with spouse and/or relatives
Financial problems
Problems at work (performance, attendance)
An "angry" emotional style
Drinking a fifth of spirits or its equivalent a day (for a 180-pound individual)
Withdrawal—convulsions, delirium tremens (DTs)
Blood alcohol level above 150 mg/100 ml without appearance of intoxification
(Calahan, Cisin & Crossley, 1969; Butler & Lewis, 1982, p. 133)

Softer signs of alcohol problems include sleeping problems, falls with no seeming cause, missed appointments, being late for appointments, impotence, rapidly appearing confusion, car accidents, and the use of alcohol to lessen anger, depression, fear, or tiredness (Butler & Lewis, 1982). The mental health practitioner may find only hints of these and may encounter a sense of discomfort on the part of the client when asking the client about personal matters that suggest an alcohol problem. While oversuspicion on the part of the mental health practitioner is not encouraged, a tough minded approach in detecting alcoholism is suggested. It is to the client's long-term advantage because of the increased psychological, physical, and social suffering felt by the alcoholic if the condition goes unchecked or untreated.

Effects of Alcohol

Alcohol is a central nervous system depressant, not a stimulant as many people believe. The false belief comes from the effects of a temporary arresting of higher cortical functioning, which may lead to some "loosening of inhibitions." However, net effect is to depress nervous system and muscular activity.

Alcohol has a more pronounced effect on the elderly than on younger people. This is due to age-related physcial changes that result in alcohol's being metabolized more slowly. Potential physical problems arising from alcohol abuse include organic brain damage, cirrohis of the liver, and heart problems. When alcoholism is suspected, a nutritional assessment may be needed to look for vitamin deficiencies and poor nutritional habits (caloric intake, balanced diet), and the assessment should continue during treatment of the alcohol problem.

Prevalence of Alcoholism in the Aged

Because of the reluctance of older alcoholics to seek (or receive) treatment as well as methodological problems in formal population surveys of drinking, it is difficult to create an accurate picture of alcoholism and alcohol abuse in the elderly. Few elderly, for example, will claim they are "heavy drinkers" in surveys. It is also possible that older alcoholics "burn out" and use less alcohol with age. It does seem, however, that older adults have a lower rate of alcoholism than younger people and that from 10 to 15 percent of the elderly have an alcohol-related problem (Mishara & Kastenbaum, 1980, Schuckit, 1977).

Within the elderly, certain subgroups have a high rate of alcoholism. Older widowers, for example, have the highest alcoholism rate of all age groups. Widows also have a high rate. High rates (up to 60 percent) of alcoholism can be found in veteran's hospitals and nursing homes (Schukit, 1977; Seixas, 1979). At times, family and even staff in such facilities have been known to bootleg liquor in to the alcoholic resident. Finally, one survey of community mental health patients showed a 17 percent alcoholism rate for older patients (Zimberg, 1974). With the current national trend of rising use of alcohol in all age groups and better health of the middle-aged and elderly population, we can expect the number of alcoholics and relative incidence of alcoholism to rise in the elderly in the next decades.

Intervention Guidelines

Older alcoholics do no worse in treatment than younger persons with the same problem. In fact, late-onset alcoholics have a good prognosis (Zimberg, 1974).

Several types of approaches have been recommended for treating the elderly alcoholic. Each includes adequate assessment and attention to diet.

Medical Management   Medical intervention in alcoholism uses Antabuse, a drug that inhibits alcohol intake, and mild tranquilizers to help withdrawal from alcohol dependency (although if the client takes alcohol with the tranquilizers, a dangerous interaction results), coupled with important social support from peers, specifically Alcoholics Anonymous (AA). Alcoholics Anonymous is a national organization of recovering alcoholics who hold regular group meetings and provide personal counseling for others who are recovering from alcoholism. There are also groups for relatives of alcoholics, but there are few AA groups for the elderly.

In a second type of medical treatment, late-onset alcoholism is considered a form of depressive reaction. It is treated with antidepressant medication and by creating a supportive relationship with the older client. It does not require AA or Antabuse and has been reported as being successful (Zimberg, 1974).

Mental Health Interventions   Mental health interventions with older alcoholics are only beginning to be developed. Their goal is curative in that they focus on eliminating alcohol intake. Approaches that focus only on changing the underlying personality are not effective. Zarit (1980), for example, has successfully used behavioral techniques (substituting similar tasting beverages for alcohol, making contracts, carefully assessing the need met by the alcohol ingestion, and substituting other activities) to treat alcoholism in the aged.

In all medical and therapeutic approaches, along with taking specific measures to eliminate alcohol intake, the mental health practitioner needs to develop a strong relationship with the client. Older alcoholics, like those of other ages, will try the practitioner's patience. Some will progress and then go on a binge or otherwise slow up the course of treatment. This inability to follow through may be part of a behavior pattern that is linked to alcoholism.

A final and equally important guideline is to attend to both the stress placed on the family and the ways in which family members inadvertently reinforce the elderly alcoholic's behavior. For many families members, there is a stigma associated with alcoholism. Some will ignore problem behavior, others will deny there is a problem. Family members may reinforce the alcoholic's drinking by placating or accepting excuses for his or her behavior, withdrawing affection, or even bootlegging alcohol into institutional settings.

SUICIDE

Although not considered a specific disorder in *DSM-III*, both the issues and prevalence of suicide among the elderly warrant particular attention.

Prevalence of Suicide in the Elderly

Older persons have a suicide rate about three times that of the general population. Approximately 25 percent of all suicides are by the elderly (Resnik & Cantor, 1970). Males have a higher rate than females, and white males over seventy-five years old have the highest rate of any age group in the population. Surprisingly, black widows, despite their many difficulties, have a relatively low rate.

The rate of suicide among the elderly has decreased in the last several decades (Stenback, 1980), although the rate for elderly women has increased slightly. Also, suicide is responsible for a smaller percentage of deaths among the elderly than among younger persons because the rate of death is so high in the aged.

Older people have a significantly higher rate of completed suicides (one out of two succeed) than younger people (Pfeiffer, 1977; Gardner, Bahn & Mack, 1964). The reasons for this seem to be twofold; older suicides take place when there are fewer social supports, and older suicides are less likely to stage a suicide to hurt another person or gain attention (Zarit, 1980).

It should be noted that the available statistics reflect dramatic, direct attempts to take one's life. They do not necessarily reflect "slow suicide" such as the older person in the nursing home who refuses to eat, the heart patient who stops taking medicine, or the diabetic who goes off his or her diet or insulin regimen (e.g., Nelson & Farberow, 1980).

Theories of Suicide in the Aged

Durkheim (1951) posited four types of suicide: *egoistic, anomic, altruistic,* and *fatalistic.* It has been suggested that much of the suicide in the aged is egoistic; that is, the type of older person likely to commit suicide has a "shallow" personality, with few social ties, little sense of social responsibility, but with a stable personality (Steinback, 1980).

Factors that have been related to suicide in the aged include isolation, being single, being bereaved, living alone, a previous suicide attempt, and feeling helpless. Many older suicides talk about it before the attempt (60 to 80 percent by some estimates). Suicide can also be considered taking control of one's life, although the elderly are less likely than younger people to commit suicide as an impulse (Stenback, 1980; Zarit, 1980).

Other health and mental health problems seem to have a strong impact on suicide in the aged. Pfeiffer (1977) reports that most elderly who commit suicide are depressed (30 to 50 percent), with alcoholism, organic brain syndrome, and untreated illness as contributing factors.

Although it can be argued that suicide in the elderly may be an individual choice in extremely difficult circumstances, many suicides can be prevented. Attempts to help are often well received and the feelings of despair recede. Also, mental health practitioners have an implicit ethical commitment by current legal standards to prevent a client from taking his or her own life (Zarit, 1980).

Guidelines for work with suicidal elderly include the following:

1. Be alert to signs of potential suicide or related factors such as depressive reactions, bereavement, heavy use of alcohol, loss of social supports, and previous attempts at suicide. Also, take all statements and vague hints (e.g., "I just don't feel life is worth living" or "Why bother to try?") seriously. Hints should be explored gently but with concern.

2. Explore suicidal ideas and thoughts carefully. The more depressed the client is, the more complete ideas are, and the more carefully drawn out and feasible the suicidal plan is, the more likely the client is to make a serious suicide attempt.

3. Work to decrease feelings of being abandoned or helpless on the part of the client through cognitive, behavioral, and relationship approaches (see Chapters 10 and 11). As a related issue, the client's major presenting problems (grief, loss of job, onset of illness, adaptation to living in an institution) need attention.

The suicidal older adult needs the concerned involvement of others. Family may need help to be supportive after a suicide attempt as they struggle to feel comfortable talking about it or listening to the client discuss it. Significant others also need to become sensitized to warning signs of future suicide attempts. Socialization and meaningful activities for the elderly are also important in the prevention of suicide (cf. Stenback, 1980; Zarit, 1980; Resnik & Cantor, 1970).

The mental health practitioner needs a general attitude of calmness and concern in discussing suicidal thoughts with a client. The instillation of hope, that something can be done, is an integral building block in establishing trust and working to improve behavioral options and quality of life for the suicidal older adult.

SUMMARY AND CONCLUSIONS

This chapter reviewed major functional disorders, those disturbances of affect and cognition that have no known organic cause. Their incidence and symptomology in the aged can differ from that of younger persons. The disorder most commonly associated with age is depression, although much of the depression in the aged can be considered mild or reactive. Symptomology in the aged differs from that in younger persons in degree (less dramatic symptoms in paranoid and schizophrenic states, some exaggeration of personality traits in personality disorders), and in difficulty of determining the likelihood of there being other conditions, including organic and physical problems.

Many functional conditions in the aged can be successfully treated with either curative or adaptive goals. In the aged, particular attention should be paid to the client's secondary gains and to the impact the mental health problem has on the support system. Too often, the lack of appropriate diagnosis and inavailability of appropriate treatment are the reasons functional mental health problems of the aged do not improve.

6

Organic Brain Disorders

INTRODUCTION

Mr. R. is a seventy-one-year-old retired artist living with his wife in their home of many years. Since he began taking medication for high blood pressure, his wife has noticed that his attention is wandering, he forgets what was just said, and he wakes up in the night, at times thinking it is daytime and wondering where he is. He finds it difficult to concentrate and wonders if he is "going senile."

Mrs. A. is a seventy-eight-year-old widow whose family takes care of her. Since the family is quite well off, they spend three months a year in Madrid at the family villa, where they have been going for many years. One day, however, Mrs. A. is found wandering a mile away from the villa, unconcerned but unable to find her way back, even though she has been there for over two months on this visit. Closer questioning of family members reveals that she has been unable to be on her own over the last year and that she has slowly been losing mental abilities for over two years.

Although depression is the most common mental health problem of the elderly, organic brain syndrome (OBS) is the most feared and least understood. Many people incorrectly assume that any forgetting leads to institutionalization, followed by death shortly thereafter. As was discussed in Chapter 2, some memory loss may be expected with aging, but it is not necessarily a sign of "senility."

However, loss of orientation to person, place, and time, the major signs of organic impairment, are not caused by aging. A multitude of conditions, some of which can be helped and even reversed, lead to this behavior. Only 15 percent of the elderly show signs of OBS. In addition, the onset of organic brain syndrome also does not necessarily create a need for institutionalization. Although some of the underlying conditions of organic brain syndrome do shorten life expectancy, death is not necessarily pending the first time an older person forgets someone's name.

"Organic brain syndrome" is also not a diagnosis. The term refers to a series of symptoms (including lack of orientation to person, place, and time) that imply that brain tissue is not functioning properly. The range of causes of OBS is great. When a client is identified as having OBS, the immediate next question is, "due to what?"

A final point of introduction: Organic brain syndrome can be difficult to distinguish from depression. This problem is confounded by the likelihood that between one-quarter and one-third of all clients with dementia have depression (Epstein & Simon, 1967, Reifler & Eisdorfer, 1980).

DSM-III CATEGORIES
OF ORGANIC BRAIN SYNDROME

DSM-III distinguishes between six types of organic brain syndrome or *organic mental disorder* (when the underlying disease is reasonably identified). In making these distinctions the authors state that "it is often impossible to decide whether the symptoms are the direct result of damage to the brain or are a reaction to (the) cognitive deficits and other psychological changes . . . ." (p. 102)

The six types of organic brain syndrome are:

1. *Delirium and dementia*, characterized by global cognitive impairment
2. *Amnestic syndrome and organic hallucinosis*, characterized by impairment of specific areas of cognition
3. *Organic delusional syndrome and organic affective syndrome*, characterized by behavior similar to schizophrenia or affective disorders
4. *Organic personality syndrome*, characterized primarily by changes in personailty
5. *Intoxification and withdrawal*
6. *Atypical or mixed organic brain syndrome*, a residual category

Symptoms of Organic Brain Syndromes

The general signs of organic brain syndrome are: *changes in judgment*, the ability to make decisions, evaluate options, comprehend; *changes in affect*, either a flat affect or excessive emotionally; *memory impairment*, either in storage, retention, or recall; *loss of cognition*, calculation and learning ability; and *lack of orien-*

tation to time (day, date, month), *place* (current location), and *person* (identity of self and others).

Orientation is often the key to a diagnosis of organic brain syndrome. Time is the first function to be impaired, followed by place, then person. This is not too surprising when one realizes that time (day, date, month) requires active cognition; that is, the day and data change every twenty-four hours. Also, location (where one is—town, address, state) may also include recent learning (for a new address) or memory for numbers, whereas orientation to person (one's own name) is unchanged, linked to many aspects of one's existence, and may be continually reinforced by other persons.

DELIRIUM

Delirium refers to a series of symptoms characterized by a rapid decrease in mental functioning and ability to cope with the environment. There are problems in attention, motor activity, and thought processes as well as disturbances in the sleep cycle. Delirium often starts rapidly and is brief in duration.

There are many causes of delirium. Because each has its own course and prognosis, the "course" of delirium can be said to fluctuate—that is, it may get better or worse; it may go "up and down."

Delirium has been called by other names such as acute brain syndrome, acute confusional state, "pseudodementia," and "reversible brain syndrome" (Libow, 1977; Butler & Lewis, 1982).

Prevalence in the Elderly

Few epidemiological studies have been made to determine the incidence of delirium in the elderly. Misdiagnosis, disinterest, or existence of other dramatic conditions make such studies difficult. It is reasonable, however, to assume that slightly less than half of all older people exhibiting signs of organic brain syndrome have delirium (as opposed to senile dementia) or that between 5 and 10 percent of the elderly exhibit these symptoms.

Delirium can be found by itself or in conjunction with senile dementia, as in the case of an Alzheimer's patient who falls, sustains a head injury, and becomes more confused. Delirium and dementia may occur simultaneously in as many as one in three cases (Epstein & Simon, 1967).

One can also question the diagnosis of delirium in that it may be the only diagnosis given when in fact it is a manifestation of underlying physical problems (Copeland et al., 1975). The postoperative older patient, for example, who is exhibiting loss of orientation to person, place, and time should be categorized as having both delirium and a post-operative reaction. The overmedicated older person should be identified as both delirious and overmedicated.

Delirium in the aged can be caused by many conditions, ranging from psychosocial stressors to specific metabolic disorders. Causes can be classified into twelve categories: medications, metabolic imbalances, depression or actute emotional stress, nutrition, tumors, liver-related conditions, cardiovascular conditions, vascular conditions, fevers, pulmonary conditions, postsurgical reactions, and posttrauma reactions (Libow, 1977). In addition, alcoholism and low pressure hydrocephalus have also been identified as causes.

Medication   It is fitting that medication is listed as the first category. Overmedication, medication interactions, and improper use of medication by older clients are perhaps the most common sources of delirium in the elderly. It should be axiomatic that when faced with a "sudden onset" organic brain syndrome, the mental health practitioner should consider reaction to medication as a likely cause.

Delirium can be brought on by "excessive" dosages of over-the-counter drugs, "normal" dosages of prescription drugs that are in fact too high for the elderly, and/or interactions with prescribed medications. Psychotropic, sedative, and hypnotic drugs (these three being the most frequent in terms of drug-caused delirium) as well as reactions to digitalis, propramolol, or hypertensive medication can also contribute to onset of delirium (Jarvik, 1980; Libow, 1977).

Metabolis Imbalance   Metabolic imbalance refers to a systematic overabundance or underabundance of critical substances in the body. Thus, too high or too low a level of sugar in the bloodstream (hyperglycemia or polyglycemia), high levels of calcium, abnormal thyroid functioning, and problems in urination due to infection or blockages can lead to confusion. Lack of adequate fluid intake can also lead to delirium due to related electolyte problems.

Depression   Depression is difficult to distinguish from organic brain syndrome because presenting symptoms may be similar or the two conditions may coexist. It is important to obtain adequate information on recent losses and personality style for assessment purposes. Also, "testing the limits" in assessment (see "Assessing Mental Health Status," Chapter 7)—that is, asking and encouraging the client to respond—may elicit oriented answers from a depressed client but not from a client with OBS.

Nutrition   About one in ten older adults have deficiencies in at least three of four critical vitamins (ascorbic acid, riboflavin, thiamine, and Vitamin A), which can lead to confusion. Adequate amounts of other vitamins such as B_{12} may be lacking. Illness and economic factors may also lead to nutritional difficulties.

Tumors   Brain tumors can cause behavioral abnormalities, including confusion. These tumors, called intercranial tumors, produce changes in mental

TABLE 6-1   Causes of Acute, Possibly Reversible, Mental Changes in the Elderly

1. Medications
   a. Errors in self-administration.
   b. Chlorpropamide (Diabinese) causes inappropriate ADH secretion leading to water intoxication.
   c. L-Dopa, indomethacin, steroids can induce psychoses.
   d. All drugs with a primary CNS-desired action, e.g., phenothiazines, barbiturates, tricyclic antidepressants, diphenylhydantoin.
2. Metabolic imbalance
   a. Hypercalcemia secondary to
      (1) Carcinoma of lung, breast, and other tissues.
      (2) Primary hyperparathyroidism.
      (3) Multiple myeloma.
      (4) Paget's disease coupled with immobilization.
      (5) Thiazide administration.
   b. Hypocalcemia secondary to
      (1) Malabsorption states.
      (2) Renal failure.
      (3) Hypoparathyroidism: post-thyroidectomy or idiopathic.
   c. Hyperglycemia
      (1) Easily recognized: ketoacidosis.
      (2) Less easily recognized.
         (a) Lactic acidosis; look for the "anion gap."
         (b) Nonacidotic hyperosmolarity syndrome blood sugar above 600 mg/100 ml; serum bicarbonate normal; no urinary ketones.
   d. Hypoglycemia secondary to insulin or sulfonylureas; not with phenformin (DBI) when used alone.
   e. Hypothyroidism: "subacute" onset; low PBI, serum thyroxine (T_4), T_3 resin uptake, and 24-hour I^{131} uptake by thyroid gland; high SGOT, LDH, and CPK; high TSH if primary hypothyroidism.
   f. Hyperthyroidism: may be present in the elderly as depression and/or apathy; termed "apathetic hyperthyroidism"; may also present as dementia.
   g. Hypernatremia: a hyperosmolarity syndrome secondary to
      (1) Inadequate fluid intake in very ill or disoriented patients.
      (2) Cerebral concussion.
      (3) Iatrogenic factors: administration of hypertonic saline by intravenous or intraperitoneal route or tube feeding of high-protein mixtures.
      (4) Excessive sweating without increased water intake.
   h. Hyponatremia: a hypo-osmolarity syndrome secondary to increased antidiuretic hormone secretion; bronchogenic carcinoma; cerebrovascular accident; skull fracture; postoperative period; etc.
   i. Azotemia
      (1) Worsening of a chronic mild nephritis by a urinary-tract infection.
      (2) Medication-induced dehydration or hypokalemic nephropathy.
      (3) "Obstructive" uropathy.
         (a) Benign prostatic hypertrophy.
         (b) Neurogenic
            (i)   Diabetes mellitus.
            (ii) Anticholinergics.
            (iii) Antihypertensives: reserpine, ganglionic blockers, hydralazine.
            (iv) Adrenergics: ephedrine, dextroamphetamine.
            (v)   Antihistamines.
            (vi) Isoniazid.

TABLE 6-1 (continued)

    (4) Potent diuretics causing acute bladder overload.
       (a) Furosemide (Lasix).
       (b) Ethacrynic acid (Edecrin).
    (5) Urate precipitation in treatment of lymphoma or leukemia.
    (6) Calcium precipitation in hypercalcemia syndromes.
3. Depression or acute emotional stress: usually related to "losses."
4. Nutrition: More than 10% of elderly have simultaneous deficiencies of at least three of four important vitamins: thiamine, riboflavin, ascorbic acid, and vitamin A. Deficiencies may play a role in CNS dysfunction and may be due to inadequate intake, or secondary to chronic illness. Pernicious anemia, too, may have CNS manifestations.
5. Tumors
   a. Intracranial:
    (1) Gliomas 50-60% of all CNS tumors, mostly malignant.
    (2) Metastatic, 20-50%; lung, breast, others.
   b. Remote effects of distant cancers: lymphoma, lung.
6. Hepatic conditions
   a. Cirrhosis; onset between ages 40 and 70 years.
   b. Hepatitis; not uncommon in the elderly.
7. Cardiac conditions
   a. Decreased cardiac output secondary to arrhythmia, congestive heart failure, or pulmonary emboili.
   b. Acute myocardial infarction; 13% of patients have confusion as the major symptom.
8. Vascular conditions
   a. Transient ischemic attacks and cerebrovascular accidents.
   b. Subdural hematoma; 20% of all intracranial masses in the elderly.
9. Any febrile condition
10. Pulmonary conditions: Chronic lung disease (emphysema) with hypoxia and/or hypercapnia; pulmonary emboli.
11. Postsurgical dementia
12. Post-trauma dementia
   a. Accidents.
   b. Assaults.

Reprinted with permission from: L.S. Libow, Senile dementia and "pseudosenility": Clinical Diagnosis, in C. Eisendorfer and R.O. Friedel (Eds.), *Cognitive and emotional disturbance in the elderly: Clinical issues.* Copyright © 1977 by Year Book Medical Publishers, Inc., Chicago. Adapted from L.S. Libow, Pseudo-Senility, *Journal of the American Geriatrics Society,* 1973, *12,* 112, with permission of W. B. Saunders, publishers.

functioning about one-half of the time (Libow, 1977). However, because the older brain has atrophied (shrunk) somewhat, the effects of a tumor or even damage from a blow or fall on the head (subdural hematoma) may not show up immediately. A CAT scan (computerized axial tomography) will show the presence of a tumor.

Liver Condition Both cirrhosis and hepatitis, two liver-related diseases found in the aged, can lead to delirium.

Cardiovascular Conditions Several of the heart conditions mentioned in Chapter 3 can lead to delirium. These include embolisms or blockages, which in turn lead to diminished blood flow to the brain and rapid onset of confusion.

Vascular Conditions   While strokes and arteriosclerosis are generally considered under the category of multiinfarct dementias, the client is likely to appear delirious. Care must also be taken to distinguish OBS caused by damage from a fall from that caused by a stroke.

Fever (febrile conditions)   Fevers from several causes can lead to delirium in the aged. Fever can indicate the presence of disease or reaction to infection.

Lung Conditions   Lung diseases, especially emphysema and/or embolisms, can lead to delirium.

Postoperative Reactions   Many postoperative patients may be confused immediately after surgery; however, the elderly are particularly prone to develop a delirious reaction after anesthesia. The reasons for this are unknown. A related cause of confusion has been cataract surgery, although in the last few years it has been discovered that if only one eye is operated on at a time, the incidence of confusion is less. Although the causes of postsurgical reaction are unknown, its relationship to anesthesia suggests that it has some sort of physiological basis rather than being solely a psychological reaction. Impairment in this type of reaction can be permanent (Libow, 1977).

Posttraumatic Reactions   Traumatic incidents for the elderly can include being victimized, being assaulted, or having an accident. Even if there is no direct physical injury, some older adults will experience sudden losses in mental functioning. These reactions, however, are likely to disappear.

Alcoholism   Alcoholism is also a cause of delibrium in the aged, both as an acute reaction (intoxification) and as a contributor to diseases such as cirrhosis. (Alcoholism is discussed in Chapter 4.) Also, alcohol withdrawal symptoms may include delirium (Sloane, 1980).

Normal-Pressure Hydrocephalus   In this condition the ventricles of the brain become large but cerebral fluid pressure remains constant or normal. One characteristic of this condition is a change in gait. This rare condition can be surgically controlled (Adams et al., 1965), although there are serious potential side effects (e.g., infection) that make surgical intervention debatable for the elderly.

The mental health practitioner should realize that in any given case of delirium there are likely to be several causative factors. Textbook cases are rare. In addition, factors other than those mentioned here may contribute to confusion, such as a reaction to physical impairment (especially loss of vision or hearing). Finally, an accurate diagnosis may not be easy to obtain, be it from a CAT scan, a neurological exam for a nursing home resident, or a detailed history from the client, family, or social support system.

Symptoms

With a sense of cautiousness in mind about distinguishing delirium from dementia, the following symptomology has been described for delirium (Jarvik, 1980; American Psychiatric Association, 1980). It is also summarized in Table 6-2.

Fluctuating sense of impairment. The client may show signs of orientation and unimpaired cognition at some moments, yet at other times will not know time, date, place, or person or will show cognitive and judgment deficits.

A sense of agitation and restlessness. The delirious client may be difficult for staff and family to manage because of the agitation.

Difficulty in concentrating and alterness. The client's capacity to stay with one task or subject is limited.

Sleep problems, including insomnia, can be present.

Hallucinations (often visual) may be present. *Delusions of persecution* may also be found. In both cases, there may be anxiety or fear about the delusions and hallucinations.

TABLE 6-2 Differentiating Delirium from Dementia

	DELIRIUM	DEMENTIA
ONSET	Acute, often at night	Usually insidious
DURATION	Hours, days or weeks	Months or years
COURSE	Fluctuates during day; worse at night; lucid intervals	Stable over course of day
ALERTNESS	Reduced or increased, tends to fluctuate	Usually normal
ORIENTATION	Always impaired, at least for time; tendency to mistake unfamiliar for familiar person and place	May be intact
MEMORY	Recent impaired	Recent and remote impaired
THINKING	Slow or accelerated; may be dreamlike	Poor abstraction; often impoverished
PERCEPTION	Invariably impaired; visual hallucinations common	May be intact. Hallucinations often absent
EMOTIONS	Fear or depression	Apathy, indifference, emotional lability, euphoria
SLEEP-WAKE CYCLE	Always disturbed; often drowsiness during the day and insomnia at night	Abnormal; insomnia with rapid transition from sleep to waking; often nocturnal confusion

Source: Z.J. Lipowski, Differentiating delirium from dementia 1982, *1* (1), 9. Reprinted with permission by *Clinical Gerontologist*, c 1982 Haworth Press, Inc. Adapted from Z.J. Lipowski, *Delirium: Acute brain failure in man.* Springfield, Ill.: Charles C Thomas, 1980, with permission.

Memory loss, both remote and recent, will be present.

In delirium, there is *intellectual impairment* as well as orientation difficulties. Clients with delirium may give symbolic mistakes to questions such as "Where are you?" by responding, for example, "I'm in a hotel, (jail, cemetary)" (Kahn & Miller, 1978).

There are no neuropathological abnormalities in the brain. Unlike dementia, delirium and "pseudosenilities" are by definition caused by factors other than brain tissue atrophy, although many of the factors are organic or physiological.

A *rapid onset*, that is, development of symptoms within a short time, is a symptom of delirious states, as well as some dementias.

Prognosis

Unfortunately, the commonly held belief that delirium is a "reversible" condition is not entirely true. Jarvik (1980), for example, reports a 40 percent immediate mortality rate for delirium diagnosed patients. However, if the underlying condition that creates the delirium can be treated or cured, then the delirium can be "reversed"; that is, cognitive, intellectual, orientation, and judgmental functioning can return to their previous levels. However, in some conditions only partial intellectual and cognitive functioning is recovered.

Intervention Guidelines

Because delirium has a series of causes, each with its own medical treatments, only general guidelines are offered.

1.   Careful assessment is needed.

2.   Clients need appropriate reassurance if they express fear or concern about their condition or related hallucinations. The mental health practitioner cannot guarantee that "everything will be all right" or that "you shouldn't worry." Rather, the mental health practitioner can indicate to the client that everything is being done and that he or she is paying attention to the client, is listening, and will "be" with the client (see Chapter 11, "Client-Centered Therapy and Approaches").

3.   Families and support systems also need encouragement and information. If, in fact, the condition is reversible, the family or informal support network may need instruction on how to help the client.

4.   The client's physical environment may also need to be changed so as to accommodate either temporary or permanent cognitive changes due to delirium.

5.   As underlying causes are controlled, the client may need to make life-style changes that require support and active intervention by the mental health practitioner (Wolanin & Phillips, 1981). For example, overdependence on drugs or alcohol may be partially due to underlying psychological or family conflicts that need intervention. Often, cooperation with nursing, medicine, speech pathology, occupational therapy, and other disciplines is critical in helping the client maintain himself or herself at an optimal level of functioning.

DEMENTIAS

The term *dementia* has been used to depict conditions that are inevitably progressive, untreatable, and irreversible. However, while dementias are caused by specific pathology or diseases, some conditions can be stabilized, some can be reversed, and others cannot.

Too often, any older person exhibiting memory loss or confusion has been diagnosed as having dementia. This diagnosis is significantly more prevalent in the United States than in Great Britain, where geriatric medicine is a more highly developed specialty and, perhaps, greater care is taken in diagnosis (Copeland et al., 1975).

DSM-III gives three guidelines for diagnosis of dementia:

1. The impairment is a multifaceted loss of intellectual ability.
2. There is no evidence for a diagnosis other than an organic mental disorder.
3. A diligent search has failed to reveal a specific organic etiologic factor.

There are two primary "types" of dementia: those caused by specific brain disease(s) and those caused by lack of adequate blood flow to the brain, called *multiinfarct dementias*. Most senile dementia is caused by pathological brain diseases, not arteriosclerotic conditions, as is commonly believed.

Senile Brain Disease (Including Senile Dementia of the Alzheimer's Type)

Senile brain disease is a progressive and irreversible condition marked by death of brain tissue. Its impact on the individual is gradual and the person's condition may be stable for a period of time, with small changes in daily behavior and cognition. It may become manifest by stepwise decrements, with changes followed by periods of no change. As the disease progresses, there is deterioration in several areas of cognition and personality. Incontinence and lapses in self-care become evident. Instructions are not followed; clients may become lost in familiar surroundings. The personality of the individual seems to fade as does the ability for self-care in advanced stages.

Senile brain disease, while more common than any other type of dementia, represents the greatest "geriatric" mystery of our era in terms of its course, causes, effects, and treatment. It is not clear whether senile brain disease and senile dementia of the Alzheimer's type are the same or different. For our purposes, it is argued that they should be considered the same as they are not separable by any clinical assessment at present (Katzman, 1976).

It is also important to realize that the clinical picture, the "realities" of a single client, are much more complicated than the following description of causes, symptoms, and course of the condition. All of the classifications of dementia should be viewed as "approximate" at this point. Diagnosis of dementia is still a process of excluding other causes, even with EEG and CAT scans, the latter of which is not a reliable method by itself (Ford & Winter, 1981; Jarvik, 1980).

Finally, the frequency of misdiagnosis of dementia has been estimated at between 15 and 50 percent (Sloane, 1980; Garcia, Reding & Blass, 1981). It is also likely that a large percentage of persons in mental hospitals for a long period of time have unrecognized brain disease (Sloane, 1980).

Prevalence

It is estimated that 15 percent of the elderly show signs of organic brain syndrome. Of these, somewhat more than half (or 8 percent of all elderly) have dementia. From one-third to one-half of all people having dementias have senile dementia or dementia of the Alzheimer's type (Jarvik, 1980). Senile dementia may be considered a contributary factor in about 100,000 deaths per year, possibly making it one of the top five causes of death among the aged (Karasu & Katzman, 1976). Onset can take place anywhere after age sixty. Life expectancy is, on the average, five years after onset. As was mentioned earlier, senile dementia can also coexist with delirium and may be present in this fashion in one-third of all cases.

Pathological Signs

Although a specific "cause" and course have not been found, neurologists, pathologists, and other scientists have discovered several types of pathology or abnormalities in the brain that are related to senile dementia and dementia of the Alzheimer's type.

Low Level of Acetylcholine   Acetylcholine, which seems to be related to memory functions, has been found in lower than normal levels in older persons with dementia (Davies, 1978). This, in turn, has led to some attempts to treat dementia with choline and lecithin, although results have been minimally successful (Levy, 1978). However, if the problem is one of neuronal decay taking place when acetylcholine levels are low, adding more to the system will only stabilize loss, not reverse it.

Senile Plaques   A senile plaque is structure thought to be a sign of neuronal degeneration (Adams, 1980). Senile plaques appear as spherical, and may look different as they "age." While there are several types, the most common has an anyloid core, an abnormal protein not ordinarily found in the brain. In addition, it is surrounded by a "halo" and fibrular substances.

Senile plaques exist in small amounts in all older adults' brains, and the amount is positively correlated with loss of orientation (Roth, Tomlinson & Blessed, 1967). They are found in large amounts in the hippocampus in older persons who have died from Alzheimer's disease or senile dementia (Adams, 1980).

Neurofibrillary Tangles Neurofibrillary tangles are formed between dendrites and axons in the cerebral cortex or hippocampus. The tangles may be related to problems in metabolizing protein (Adams, 1980). They represent degeneration at the synapse, interfere with nerve transmission, and lead to neuronal death (Tomlinson & Henderson, 1976).

Granulovacular Lesions Granulovacular lesions, a correlate of neuronal loss, occur because of formation of granules in the hippocampus. The granules are surrounded by vacuoles and are found inside the brain neurons.

Neuronal Loss While the amount of neuronal loss in Alzheimer's disease has been documented (Terry, 1976), there is some debate about how much loss there is (Tomlinson & Henderson, 1976). The amount of neuronal loss may be less important than the type of cell that deteriorates (Jarvik, 1980). That is, senile dementia may be a qualitative rather than quantitive change in brain functioning.

Causes

Several possible causes for senile brain diseases have been suggested.

Genetic or Heredital Factor The evidence for a genetic or heredital factor comes from several studies that have found a higher percentage of dementia in family members of patients with Alzheimer's disease than in the rest of the population (e.g., Larsson, Sjogren, and Jacobson, 1963; cited in Sloane, 1980).

Cholinergic Factors It is hypothesized that the systems that produce acetylcholine may become dysfunctional and cause memory loss.

Viruses Viruses have been implicated in Alzheimer's disease (DeBoni & Crapper, 1978); however, most attempts to transmit Alzheimer's disease in animals have been unsuccessful (Jarvik, 1980).

Autoimmune System Changes It is possible that somewhere in the formation of autoantibodies a breakdown occurs, leading to the development of senile dementia.

Presence of Metals Aluminum and zinc have been identified found in high or abnormal concentrations in the brains of Alzheimer's patients (Terry & Wisniewski, 1975; Crapper, Krishnan, & Dalton, 1973).

There is little question that the cause of dementia is organic; there is no evidence of psychological or social causes. Whether the disease is due to a virus, a genetic or heredital component, a breakdown in physiological systems, or some combination of these, senile dementia is, as far as we know, a physical and, at present, a progressive illness.

Symptoms

The five major areas in which behavioral symptoms of dementia occur are the same as for delirium: that is, impairment of intelligence and cognition, lack of orientation, memory loss, difficulties in judgment, and changes in affect (Sloane, 1980).

Impairment of intelligence and cognition are generally global. The client with dementia will have difficulty with abstract thinking and will be slow to understand directions or questions.

Lack of orientation to time is more common than to place or person; orientation to person may remain unimpaired. There can be impairment of "spatial orientation," where the patient becomes lost in a familiar setting, such as in a neighborhood or on a nursing home floor (Sloane, 1980).

Memory loss is both severe and clinically significant in that there may be few complaints or concerns about its effects. A tendency for the client to be cheerful or put on a pleasing "front" despite the memory loss and other cognitive impairment, called *presbyophrenia*, may serve to save face or keep the client from becoming depressed (Wells, 1977).

Memory loss for recent events is greater than for remote events. Clients have some tendency to confuse past and present. In terms of memory theory, the problems are in secondary memory rather than primary memory; for example, an individual is able to remember a series of digits but not the content of a story (Zarit, Miller, & Kahn, 1978).

Difficulties in judgment include inability to plan, make decisions, or attend to relevant instructions. Judgmental difficulties may be compounded by lack of interest in the activities of day-to-day living. Lapses in self-care become evident in the course of the disease and present management problems, particularly in the home. Serious questions can arise as to the capacity of the individual to make judgments, which may lead to others' having to assume legal responsibility for the client (conservatorship).

Changes in affect are exhibited in a "flat" or subdued emotional level. In advanced stages of dementia, the individual may lose interest in daily events. Initially, however, he or she may display increased anxiousness, perhaps due to increasing difficulties in handling social situations. The client may also seem more occupied with self than with others, hypochondriacal, and depressed. In the case of senile dementia, it is hypothesized that these changes in affect are the result of a slow disintegration of the client's personality due to physiological and, at present, irreversible processes. It is also believed that strong emotional reactions to the symptoms are a positive sign, that the personality is in better "shape" than if the affective response is one of decreasing interest and intensity.

There are several clinical manifestations that may be related to senile brain disease, such as focal neurological signs (neurologically based physical reactions in a specific area of functioning). These signs include changes in gait, seizures, weakness, and abnormal reflexes (Sloane, 1980; Coblentz et al., 1973). Incontinence, both urinary and fecal, are likely to be present, particularly in later stages. Speech difficulties, although often overlooked or thought to be stroke-related, may also be signs of senile brain disease. Speech problems related to senile brain disease include a limiting of vocabulary and sense of repetition and concreteness in language use (Stengel, 1964). The inability to identify common objects (agnosia) in various sense modalities is also a related clinical manifestation.

Changes in *personal care and personality* include lapses in self-care and/or an increase in expression of personality traits. Sloane (1980), for example, refers to "organic orderliness," in which the client carefully puts everything in place or schedule, sometimes as rapidly as possible, because, at some level, he or she is trying to compensate for the cognitive loss. There may also be increased irritation and temper in a person who originally had a "mild temper."

The disintegration of personality and cognition can lead to insight, anxiety, or the onset of delusions as the client tries to "make sense" out of the world with faulty thinking processes. Delusions are likely to be vague, varying in content, and changeable (Sloane, 1980).

Intervention Guidelines

Medical Management   At this point there is no definitive medical treatment of senile dementia. Central nervous stimulants such as methylphenidate or pentylenetetrazol have been used, but they have significant cardiac side effects and are not recommended (Crook, 1979). Other possible deterrents include ergot derivities (e.g., Hydergine); nootropic agents (e.g., piracetum), which seem useful with "mild confusion"; and "cholonergic-enhancing" agents (e.g., physostigmine, deanol) or increased dietary intake of choline (Kent, 1981).

Other interventions are discussed at the end of this chapter.

Multiinfarct Dementia

Multiinfarct dementia has been known by a variety of terms, including cerebrovascular disease, arteriosclerotic organic brain syndrome, and cerebral atherosclerosis. The major distinguishing characteristic of this disorder is a stepwise loss of mental capacity in which some functions are left relatively intact in the early stages while others show impairment. There are likely to be focal neurological signs and other symptoms related to cerebrovascular disease, especially those related to hypertension. These signs include limb weakness, abnormal reflexes, and a gait with small steps.

In multiinfarct dementia, it is assumed that a vascular disease is present (Adams, 1980). Hypertension, carotid abnormalities, and heart enlargement are frequently found. The vascular disturbance is considered the cause of the loss of mental functioning. As was mentioned earlier, multiinfarct dementia can coexist with senile brain disease.

Prevalence

Between 10 and 20 percent of all cases of senile dementia are due to vascular or multiinfarct dementia (Tomlinson & Henderson, 1976). Onset is between ages fifty and seventy, with men more likely to develop the disease than women. Although onset occurs in later years, the condition itself develops gradually and is closely related to life-style behavior and habits that affect cardiovascular diseases.

Causes

Historically, multiinfarct dementia was thought to be caused by several cerebrovascular problems, including arteriosclerosis, atheroscleriosis, small strokes, and blockage of blood vessels due to leakage or lesions (tissue breakdown). Atherosclerosis in cerebral arteries is not a major factor in diminished mental capacity (Jarvik, 1980). Similarly, a single large stroke without prior smaller ones is not a likely cause of multiinfarct dementia.

Causes of multiinfarct dementia include narrowing of major arteries, small multiinfarcts in the brain, and general death of tissue in subcortical areas (Jarvik, 1980). Because multiinfarct dementia is so closely linked to vascular disease, it is not surprising that causes for the two are quite similar. Multiinfarct dementia and strokes are highly correlated with the presence of hypertension.

Symptoms

The onset of multiinfarct demetia is sudden and noticeable in about one-half of the cases, and it may resemble delirium. In other cases, the onset is gradual.

The major difference between multiinfarct dementia and senile dementia is, as was mentioned earlier, its fluctuating quality, up-and-down progress, or step-wise decline. Cognitive deficits can be patchy, some abilities showing decline while others remain at previous levels. Memory, concentration, and comprehension will deteriorate. Eventually a more general loss of motivation or initiative will be seen (Sloane, 1980). There may even be remission or return of functioning for periods of time.

The degree of insight into and acknowledgment of the condition by the client is much greater than in Alzheimer's disease (Sloane, 1980). The degree of insight is related to the so-called preservation of personality; that is, the older person seems unchanged, without major changes in traits or behavioral style. This aspect may also delay diagnosis of the condition, as the older person does not show dramatic or frequent behavioral changes.

In some cases there may be "emotional incontinence," in which the older person becomes emotionally explosive. With multiple strokes, there may be *pseudobulbar palsy*, with episodes of laughing or crying. Epileptic seizures, usually grand mal, occur in about 20 percent of multiinfarct dementia clients (Sloane, 1980).

Related or secondary symptoms are similar to those of cerebrovascular disease: dizziness, headaches, lack of energy, limb spasticity, anxiety, sleep problems, irritability, and discomfort in the chest, especially if hypertension is present.

Along with difficulties in distinguishing multiinfarct dementia from senile brain disease, its symptoms may also indicate kidney problems, subdural hematoma, or tumors. A careful assessment should include ruling out other related diseases.

Course, Prognosis, and Medical Treatment

As was mentioned above, the course of multiinfarct dementia is uneven. There is a high death rate upon initial onset, but if the client survives the initial episode, remission rates are high and life expectancy is as high as fifteen years (Butler & Lewis, 1982).

Three types of medical treatment have been used with multiinfarct dementia: treatment of the hypertensive condition; surgery for bilateral curotid disease (a rare disorder); and antipsychotic drugs, which have provided some symptomatic improvement (Sloane, 1980).

PRESENILE DEMENTIAS

In addition to the two major dementias, there are several relatively rare conditions that usually occur before the sixth decade but lead to similar cognitive impairment and symptoms as the dementias. Thus, these conditions are categorized as "presenile" dementias and are briefly described below. While they may be differentiated for diagnostic purposes, all are chronic and have a similar course. No cures exist. Alzheimer's disease and Pick's disease are the two most common.

Alzheimer's disease

Alzheimer's disease is virtually indistinguishable from senile dementia of the Alzheimer's type except for age of onset, which is between the ages of forty and sixty (Slater & Roth, 1977). The disease was first noted in the early 1900s by Alzheimer. It is frequently found in Down's syndrome patients. Early symptoms are characterized by fairly sudden mental deterioration and irritableness. Later on, greater disability is seen in all aspects of self-care and mobility. Many clinical features are similar to those of senile brain disease. Like other presenile dementias, the occurrence of Alzheimer's disease creates severe emotional hardship for clients and their families. In one sense, it is "out of phase" in the life cycle. Dementia is seen (and perhaps expected) in late life, not in the forties of fifties. The four or five year's duration of these diseases with their disintegration of personality and cognitive functioning can leave emotional scars on surviving spouses and children, especially if they receive little attention or information about the disease and its course.

Pick's Disease

It is generally accepted that Pick's disease is a different entity than Alzheimer's disease, although both appear similar and are difficult to distinguish in clinical settings. Pick's disease is genetically based (Jarvik, 1980). Its pathological symptoms include atrophy in frontal and temporal lobes of the brain, the presence of what are called Pick and Hiran bodies, but no significant amount of neurofibrillary tangles or senile plaques. Clinical manifestations may include apathy and initial impairment of certain mental abilities, such as learning new information.

Creutz-Feldt-Jacob Disease

This condition is chracterized by global mental impairment along with general apathy and confusion. Although there is a genetic component, it has been shown that it is probably caused by a slow-acting virus (Traub, Gajdusek, & Gibbs, 1977). Creutz-Feldt-Jacob disease is one of the few dementias that has been shown to have a specific viral component.

Considerations and Guidelines
for Intervention with Dementia

Alzheimer's disease or senile brain disease and multiinfarct dementias are physically caused and irreversible; moreover, there seems to be little that can be done to reverse the specific damage they do to the brain. However, this does not mean that nothing can be done for persons who are confused or likely to have a form of dementia. There are three goals to consider in intervening with the client who is labeled as having dementia: assuring adequate diagnosis, curative measures, and adaptive measures.

Assuring Adequate Diagnosis

The label of senile brain disease may be covering depression, reaction to life events, or delirium. Most clients come to a mental health practitioner with the label but not with extensive physical workups and histories. The distinct possibility of an incorrect diagnosis suggests that an initial goal is to ensure that a complete history, physical exam, and assessment have been carried out by appropriate medical personnel, depending on availability of services and types of symptoms.

Curative Measures

Treating Conditions   Any underlying condition that may contribute to or determine the course of the confusion and assumed senile brain disease should be actively treated (Zarit, 1980). This would include medical intervention for certain delirious conditions and mental health interventions for conditions such as depression or anxiety.

Resolution of Other Mental Health Problems   There is no reason to exclude persons with the diagnosis of senile brain disease from consideration as clients with other types of problems and concerns, depending on their degree of cognitive and perceptual ability. The client's problems may include dealing with family members (see Chapter 13), putting one's life in order (see life review and reminiscence in Chapter 9), or coping with delusions, anxiety, or depression unrelated to the senile brain disease. Because senile brain disease is so pervasive in its impact on the individual, we may inadvertently focus on it to the exclusion of other conditions that concern the client.

Adaptive Measures

Coping with Loss of Functioning Clients who are aware of their condition can be helped in coping with their anxiety or fear about present and future losses. The suggested type of approach is similar to that for working with the terminally ill, one in which the practitioner spends a great deal of time listening to the client (see Chapters 4 and 11). Clients may well show denial, anger, or fear over their condition and its consequences for both themselves and their families.

There is also a question of how or even whether to intervene with the client who denies impairment and is cheerful and extroverted. This is not an easily answered question. Too often, the client's defenses can be an excuse for the practitioner to ignore underlying concerns. Yet pushing a client to acknowledge severe deficits without providing extensive support might be considered a small benefit at best. A gentle and firm approach is suggested, offering the client opportunities to talk or ventilate, offering some probes, and giving some orientation to reality— but also giving the client the right not to pursue an acknowledgement of deficits until he or she is ready to do so.

Improving Adaptation to the Loss A range of intervention strategies are available to use with for both the client and support system (usually the family). They are designed to maintain the functioning and the options of the older person with senile brain disease. Several of the most important ones are:

1. Make the environment meaningful (Wolanin & Phillips, 1981). Often, particularly in institutional settings, the environment may be "antiseptic," colorless, and with little personal or general meaning to the client. Surroundings take on personal meaning when the client can identify with them, a goal that is usually accomplished by having personal items in a room. Ideally, the personal belongings should have significant meaning to the client. If the items are of intrinsic value, such as jewelry, care will have to be taken to ensure their not being lost or stolen, as many people have access to nursing home rooms.

In a home setting, it is often assumed that the client will have meaningful items in his or her room This may not be true. Valuables, albums, or other items may be "safely" stored at a relative's apartment. Some careful questioning of client and family may be needed to ascertain if personally meaningful items are, in fact, available to the client.

2. Maintain a sense of body and body image (Wolanin & Phillips, 1981). How clients use and feel about their bodies is related to their sense of self-worth and/or self-perception. At the same time, physical functioning over and above that needed for activities of daily living is overlooked as a legitimate and critical aspect of dementia clients' functioning. Wolanin and Phillips urge emphasizing what the

client is capable of doing, encouraging physical activity, and emphasizing physical comfort, including massage. Also, art and movement therapies may be useful (see Chapter 11).

3.   Provide continuity with prior life history. In addition to having meaningful personal items available to the client, a mental health practitioner can encourage discussion or reminiscence about the past as a conversation topic. The sense of continuity with prior life history is also an important source of identity for a client who is becoming a "patient," an "OBS case," or "senile" in the eyes of others as well as himself or herself.

4.   Maintain continuity in routine. Depending on the degree of impairment, a structured daily routine is a tremendous support to dementia clients as well as a source of orientation (Wolanin & Phillips, 1981). Regular times for bowel and bladder evacuation, appropriate social stimulation (being sure there is some without overwhelming the client), and slow introduction of change are important components of daily routine. A set routine also suggests continuity of nursing home staff or home health aides and regularly scheduled visits from the mental health practitioner.

5.   Encourage independence and self-esteem. Persons with senile dementias become increasingly dependent on others for social and personal care. However, independence can be encouraged by working on remaining faculties. This can be done in many ways, including the use of art and movement. An expectation that the client can achieve or maintain self-worth and attempt tasks is critical. Meaningful activities and discussions are recommended. Reinforcement of successful remembering, completion of activities of daily living, or even attempting these activities can be sources of self-esteem in a client for whom many aspects of the day are a reminder of loss and dependency. Needless to say, the reinforcement should be genuine, not patronizing or demeaning.

6.   Help the client cope with illusions. Illusions refer to perceptual distortions of physical input as well as the resulting emotional reaction to the misperception. Illusions should rarely be reinforced; "going along" with the illusion is neither therapeutic nor sound. Instead, reassurance that the mental health practitioner can help is suggested along with the following strategies:

> Identifying the real physical stimulus that triggers the illusion
>
> Eliminating the stimulus from the client's environment if possible
>
> Teaching the client about the "reality" of the stimulus through discussion and reinforcement of reality
>
> Teaching the client about the reality of the stimulus through contact in sensory channels other than the one causing misperception

7.   Help the client maintain a sense of reality. Maintaining reality implies that the client has access to information about self, others, time, place, and "the world." While formal reality orientation (see Chapter 10) may make no difference in some cases, clients have the right to know who they are and where they are. Confusion should be responded to with facts as well as therapeutic intervention.

8.   Support family members and other caregivers. It is important to realize that families may significantly alter their lives to care for an OBS client and that their caring may last for many years. They may need a range of supportive services, including therapy, counseling, education on how to handle or communicate with their relatives, education on how to pick a nursing home or physician, opportunities to vent frustrations, and training in social skills (Levine, Dastoor, & Gendron, 1983). Peer support groups are growing rapidly in the United States and should be encouraged (e.g., Lazarus et al., 1981).

Communicating with the Confused Older Person

Along with the above guidelines, several specific suggestions for communicating with organically impaired older adults have been developed. They are basic and are intended to serve as effective guides for families and paraprofessionals as well as mental health practitioners.

Respond to a client's confusion calmly.

Respond to confusion with facts (if confusion persists, attempt to uncover meanings).

Ask the client to relax, speak slowly and distinctly.

Explain things clearly—give examples, be prepared to repeat instructions.

Use all sensory channels (visual, auditory, kinesthetic, even olfactory, gustatory).

When asking questions, make them simple rather than complex.

Give clear responses to client questions.

Do not agree to anything that is not understood.

Do not pretend to understand rambling or confused speech.

Avoid unnecessary confrontation about rambling or confused speech. It is more effective to ask the client to repeat because the mental health practitioner does not understand what is being said.[1]

The Care of the Dementia Patient

Zarit (1980) presents a useful model for mental health and physical care of dementia. His four-part model of care is:

Community Care Most authorities are urging care of the client with dementia at home for as long as possible (Sloane, 1980). In most care programs a family member or significant other must take primary responsibilty for coordinating care (Wolanin & Phillips, 1981). We need to make service and support available to families to help keep older persons with dementia in their homes as long as possible.

Service Coordination Given the diverse needs of clients and the realities of how services are given (patchwork, varying quality), a critical factor in care is obtaining and monitoring needed services. Coordinating needed services should be part of care planning for any dementia patient.

Minimum Intervention This concept, originally proposed by Kahn (1975), suggests that the existing caring system be given maximum responsibility and support rather than having providers overprovide services that may not be necessary. The concept also discourages client dependence on service providers. However, this concept should not be viewed as an excuse to do nothing; rather, the least "intrusive" interventions should be considered first, followed by more complicated measures if needed.

---

[1] Adapted from "Help Begins at Home"—International Center for the Disabled, with permission.

Treatment of Reversible Conditions   As was discussed earlier, if a condition is reversible or amenable to treatment, it should be treated. This principle requires an accurate assessment of physical and mental health as well as a commitment to treatment of the elderly.

SUMMARY

There are two major forms of organic brain syndrome, delirium and dementia. Delirium is characterized by sudden onset, a fluctuating course, reduced alterness, impaired perception, and disturbances in the sleep-wake cycle. Delirium has many causes, most of which can respond to medical or mental health treatment if found in time. Dementia (senile dementia of the Alzheimer's type or multiinfarct dementia) represents actual brain deterioration and has a different course and nature, lasting months or years, with gradual onset, intact perception, and apathy or indifference in later stages. Both forms of organic brain syndrome show loss of orientation to person, place, and time. They can occur simultaneously. Often, the clinical picture presents an unclear set of symptoms. At this time, diagnosis is difficult, and frequently not enough information is obtained before a label of senile dementia or Alzheimer's disease is given.

The accurate diagnosis and management of organic brain syndromes are among the most difficult tasks facing the health and mental health professions. Even when a diagnosis of an irreversible condition is made, there is good reason to consider intervention to help maintain the client at the highest possible levels of personal functioning, mental health, and dignity.

7

Assessment of the Elderly

INTRODUCTION

Assessment is one of the most overlooked and misunderstood aspects of mental health practice with the aged. This is in part due to greater interest in treatment than in assessment, the lack of suitable assessment instruments for the elderly, and a response to the "overselling" of assessment in the past (Miller, 1980). However, without systematic evaluation of client functioning and progress, we have no accountability for our endeavors as mental health practitioners.

This chapter approaches questions of assessment by examining several issues. The first is the general purpose of assessment. Then, general considerations in assessment are discussed, including differences in the practitioner's approach to assessment and to therapeutic intervention, the use of tests, the availability of age norms to help interpret test scores, and yardsticks by which tests or assessment tools should be evaluated: reliability, validity, and base rates. Commonly assessed aspects of the older person's functioning are presented along with examples of tools and approaches used in their assessment. Finally, some guidelines are presented to help the practitioner in choosing assessment and screening procedures.

The instruments reviewed in this chapter are those that have widespread use and application and do not require significant clinical training to administer. Most can be considered screening tools. Assessment in areas such as cognitive functioning, personal dynamics, and neuropsychology is not reviewed, although there are many instruments used in these areas with the elderly, often by psychologists. The reader seeking information in these areas is referred to reviews by Miller (1980), Lawton et al., (1980) and Sloane (1980).

WHY ASSESS?

Consider the following situation: A woman, age seventy-eight, has been recovering from a hip operation. In the course of her recovery, she has been cheerful, responds to questions, and seems quite alert. The medical staff concludes that she is "oriented" because she is so alert. However, when the social worker in the hospital goes in and asks her specific questions as to the day, date, year, her age, address, and who she is, the woman cannot answer all of them. In fact, she may give the wrong answers to four out of ten questions. On the basis of her responses to a test of mental status the social worker concludes, quite correctly, that the woman is moderately confused, and can begin to uncover the cause of the confusion. In this case, the use of a systematic approach (a test of mental status) helped discover an important sign that all was not well with client.

Assessment represents a systematic approach to uncovering and describing client problems. In any assessment the information obtained is assumed to represent the individual's general condition. Assessment has several purposes. One is to decrease the amount of extraneous information about a client's functioning. Another is to decrease incorrect judgments about the client's status and functioning. A third is to provide common language or frameworks by which findings can be shared.

GENERAL CONCERNS IN ASSESSMENT

The assessment of an older client's problems is an important part of the intervention process. Four issues to consider in assessing client functioning are: how assessment differs in approach from intervention, how tests and instruments can be used and misused, on what basis tests and instruments should themselves be evaluated, and the likelihood of incorrect decisions (false positives and false negatives).

Approach and Practical Considerations

Approach　Assessment is, by nature, somewhat different from therapeutic intervention. The purpose of assessment is to determine the nature and type of problems, the client's strengths and weaknesses for handling problems, how the client thinks, and what the client is feeling. The mental health practitioner who is performing assessment obviously needs to establish rapport and a trusting relationship with the client, both to make assessment go well and to pave the way for future mental health work. However, it is important that the client have the opportunity to answer questions or provide information. Some mental health practitioners will be tempted to encourage socially acceptable or correct responses by hinting, giving clues, or even providing answers: "I'm sure you know your name. It's Millie, right?" While encouraging a response may be appropriate, giving hints is not, especially if a standard test instrument is being used.

Another concern in testing and evaluation procedures is inadvertently reinforcing correct or desirable responses, either verbally (e.g., responding with "good," "OK," "right," "um-hmm") or nonverbally (nodding, smiling). A person administering an evaluation instrument would do better to reinforce the act of responding or the attempt to respond ("Thank you for trying," or "Some of these are harder for you than other").

Practical Considerations   Older people may feel uncomfortable or anxious in assessment sessions, which can lead to poor or decreased performance. Establishing rapport and explaining the purpose of the session thus take on added meaning for accurate assessment. Also, privacy, physical comfort, and compensation for physical impairment need to be considered. Finally, especially with ill or old-old (over eighty-five) elderly, sessions may have to be kept short, since clients may be tired or heavily medicated.

Uses and Misuses of Test Instruments

The use and misuses of psychological testing has aroused considerable controversy over the last two decades. Test scores have been misused in a number of ways: Scores on one type of test (e.g., intelligence) are assumed to be comparable to those on a test of a different area of functioning (e.g., life satisfaction); scores have been used to provide arbitrary and inappropriate criteria for decisions such as institutionalization; scores on specific measures (e.g., personality) have been used to predict functioning in unrelated areas (e.g., "Can the individual maintain himself or herself in the community?"); and scores have been assumed to represent a prediction as to how the individual will function in the future on measures that are meant only to assess current level of functioning. The unanswered question in much asessment is "How do the measures used relate to the question at hand?" (Botwinick, 1978).

Tests should not be used by themselves to make decisions about the care and living circumstances of older persons. Rather, they should be considered as one part of the assessment process. One way to ensure accurate and appropriate use of tests is to have both the person administering the test and the person interpreting results (they can be one and the same) be trained and knowledgeable in the specific measures being used, their strengths, drawbacks, and limits.

Age Norms, Validity, and Reliability:
The Value of Assessment Tools

People who have developed testing instruments of all types have devised a series of yardsticks against which the instruments can be measured: age norms, validity, and reliability.

Age Norms One concern in using a particular test with the elderly is whether or not there are norms—scores from a representative sample of the aging— against which test results can be compared. Most personality tests and assessment devices in current use were neither developed nor normed for the elderly (Botwinick, 1978). The question of norms becomes even more difficult when working with minority elderly for whom English is a second language, or elderly with dramatic life situations, such as institutionalized older adults or older adults with severe health problems. While there has been an effort to develop measures for the aged or determine normative scores for the aged, many instruments without appropriate age norms are being used.

Validity One yardstick for evaluating an assessment tool is its *validity*. Any assessment tool obtains a select group of answers or behaviors. The degrees to which these behaviors relate to broader, important aspects of functioning determines the validity of the instrument. In other words, an instrument is valid if it actually measures what it claims to measure. A test name does not by itself mean that the measure has meaning.

Reliability Reliability refers to consistency in test performance. In other words, to what degree does the same person test the same on a measure over time (test-retest reliability), or the same on a measure with similar items (internal consistency, split-half reliability)? If the instrument requires ratings, how similarly do different judges perform ratings (interrater reliability)? Obviously, if an individual's test scores on an instrument vary on different occasions without any real change on the part of the individual, the instrument is not particularly consistent.

Categorization and Decisions:
False Positives, False Negatives, and Rates

Often, assessment is done to determine whether or not an individual has a specific disorder, needs institutionalization, or even is competent to manage her or his affairs. Three areas of concern in such decisions are:

1. How often does the instrument or procedure categorize people as having the disorder, incapacity, or inability when in fact they do not (false positives)?
2. How often does the instrument or procedure "miss" or not detect problems it is supposed to detect (false negatives)?
3. Does the instrument or procedure do a better job of detection for the target group than no assessment at all (effect of base rates)? For example, assume that we

were to use a test of mental status that is accurate two-thirds of the time for a group of ex-mental patients over eighty years old who are nursing home residents. There is an 80 percent incidence of OBS in such patients. Using the instrument would yield errors 33 percent of the time. However, if we simply assumed that all have OBS, we would have only a 20 percent error. In this situation, the base rate is a better predictor than the instrument.

ASPECTS OF FUNCTIONING TO BE ASSESSED AND EXAMPLES OF SCREENING TOOLS

The types of function that assessment procedures address in the elderly are:

Physical/Medical Functioning   This type of assessment usually focuses on functional abilities, such as Activities of Daily Living (ADL), including ability to bathe, toilet, eat, prepare food, or go shopping.

Mental Functioning   Four areas of mental functioning are addressed in geriatric assessment: mental status (orientation to person, place, and time as well as certain mental skills related to organic brain syndrome); cognitive ability; mental health problems; and social skills, such as ability to relate to others. The discussion below focuses on mental status and mental health problems.

Social Functioning   This area has two focal points: (1) personal satisfaction with life or circumstances, and (2) measures of social support, the relationships and indices that show how the individual is engaged in society. Although assessment of social functioning is important, tools or scales in this area are not usually used in mental health practice and are not addressed in this chapter.

Assessing Physical Status

Ideally, assessment of physical health should include evaluation of body systems, autonomic nervous system functioning, activities of daily living, mobility, and capacity to do chores in the home (Leering, 1979).

The most common way to assess health functioning, other than through a physical exam, is to take a health history, which should consist of both an interview and compilation of a record of the client's past health problems. In addition, several instruments have been developed to assess current physical status of the elderly. They focus more on determining functional capacity than on diagnosing illnesses underlying current symptoms (cf. Granger, Sherwood, & Greer, 1977). Three examples are the Older American Resources and Services Program—OARS (physical health), the Index of Independence in Daily Living Scale, and the Instrumental Activities of Daily Living Scale (IADL).

Physical Health: OARS   The OARS instrument (Duke University, 1978) is a multidimensional tool for assessment in community settings that includes a section on health care. It consists of a series of check lists and rating scales to assess a range of dimensions from days in the hospital to medications. It is widely used, has had respectable research to demonstrate reliability and validity, but the person administering the instrument needs training to ensure proper usage.

Activities of Daily Living: Katz Index of ADL   The Katz Index of Activities of Daily Living (Katz et al., 1963) is one of the more commonly used methods of assessing capacity to perform activities usually encountered on a daily basis: feeding, continence, transfer, toileting, dressing, and bathing (see Table 7-1). Each dimension can also be rated on a scale from 0 (no help needed) to 3 (completely dependent).

Instrumental ADL Scale   The IADL (Lawton & Brody, 1969) assesses maintenance tasks such as use of the telephone, shopping, food preparation, laundry, and managing finances (see Table 7-2). Each area should be scored separately rather than attempting to devise a single score for a given client. A score of 1 indicates at least minimal functioning in each area. Cooking and housekeeping, traditional female roles, are not included for males. Records and interviews can be used to determine level of functioning. The IADL is a reliable and valid instrument.

Assessing Mental Status

Mental status is considered part of overall cognitive functioning. It has particular importance in work with the elderly because of its relationship to organic brain syndrome. Mental status refers to orientation to person, place, and time. Some measures of mental status not only assess these functions but also include items designed to tap into memory, perceptual ability, and ability to abstract.

Over twenty tests have been devised to measure mental status (Gurland, 1980; Kane & Kane, 1981). Many use a direct question and answer format to determine orientation to person, place, and time (e.g., What is your name? What is your date of birth? Where are we now?). Some use specific cognitive tests, such as counting backwards from 100 by sevens or doing simple arithmetic. Psychiatrists will check the client's abilities to interpret proverbs (e.g., "In which way is a lion and a dog alike?"), although the validity and reliability of this method is questionable. Three of the most easily administered, commonly used, and valid screening tools are discussed below.

Mental Status Questionnaire (MSQ)   The administration of the Mental Status Questionnaire (Kahn et al., 1960) consists of asking ten questions, eight of which can be easily woven into an intake interview. The ninth and tenth questions—Who is the president and who was president before him?—may require a bit more explanation or lead-in, such as asking if the client pays attention to politics or if he or she has any memory problems. Scores of 0 to 2 wrong suggest no or minimal signs of OBS, 3 to 8 wrong indicate moderate OBS, 9 or 10 wrong suggest severe OBS (see Table 7-3).

TABLE 7-1 Index of Independence in Activities of Daily Living

The Index of Independence in Activities of Daily Living is based on an evaluation of the functional independence or dependence of patients in bathing, dressing, going to the toilet, transferring, continence, and feeding. Specific definitions of functional independence and dependence appear below the index.

A	Independent in feeding, continence, transferring, going to toilet, dressing, and bathing.
B	Independent in all but one of these functions.
C	Independent in all but bathing and one additional function.
D	Independent in all but bathing, dressing, and one additional function.
E	Independent in all but bathing, dressing, going to toilet, and one additional function.
F	Independent in all but bathing, dressing, going to toilet, transferring, and one additional function.
G	Dependent in all six functions.
Other	Dependent in at least two functions, but not classifiable as C, D, E, or F.

Independence means without supervision, direction, or active personal assistance, except as specifically noted below. This is based on acrual status and not on ability. A patient who refuses to perform a function is considered as not performing the function, even though he is deemed able.

BATHING (Sponge, shower or tub)
Independent: assistance only in bathing a single part (as back or disabled extremity) or bathes self completely
Dependent: assistance in bathing more than one part of body; assistance in getting in or out of tub or does not bathe self

TRANSFER
Independent: moves in and out of bed independently and moves in and out of chair independently (may or may not be using mechanical supports)
Dependent: assistance in moving in or out of bed and/or chair; does not perform one or more transfers

DRESSING
Independent: gets clothes from closets and drawers: puts on clothes, outer garments, braces; manages fasteners; act of trying shoes is excluded
Dependent: does not dress self or remains partly undressed

CONTINENCE
Independent: urination and defecation entirely self-controlled
Dependent: partial or total incontinence in urination or defecation; partial or total control by enemas, catheters, or regulated use of urinals and/or bedpans

GOING TO TOILET
Independent: gets to toilet: get on and off toilet: arranges clothes, cleans organs of excretion: (may manage own bedpan used at night only and may or may not be using mechanical supports)
Dependent: uses bedpan or commode or receives assistance in getting to and using toilet.

FEEDING
Independent: gets food from plate or its equivalent into mouth; (precutting of meat and preparation of food, as buttering bread, are excluded from evaluation).
Dependent: assistance in act of feeding (see above); does not eat at all or parenteral feeding.

Name _____ Date of Evaluation _____

For each area of functioning listed below, check description that applies. (The word *assistance* means supervision, direction of personal assistance.)

TABLE 7-1 (continued)

BATHING—either sponge bath, tub bat, or shower

☐ | ☐ | ☐

Receives no assistance (gets in and out of tub by self if tub is usual means of bathing)	Receives assistance in bathing only one part of body (such as back of a leg)	Receives assistance in bathing more than one part of body (or not bathed)

DRESSING—gets clothes from closets and drawers—including underclothes, outer garments and using fasteners (including braces, if worn)

☐ | ☐ | ☐

Gets clothes and gets completely dressed without assistance	Gets clothes and gets dressed without assistance except for assistance in tying shoes	Receives assistance in getting clothes or in getting dressed, or stays partly or completely undressed

TOILETING—going to the "toilet room" for bowel and urine elimination: cleaning self after elimination and arranging clothes.

☐ | ☐ | ☐

Goes to "toilet room," cleans self, and arranges clothes without assistance (may use object for support such as cane, walker, or wheelchair and may manage night bedpan or commode, emptying same in morning)	Receives assistance in going to "toilet room" or in cleansing self or in arranging clothes after elimination or in use of night bedpan or commode	Doesn't go to room termed "toilet" for the elimination process

TRANSFER—

☐ | ☐ | ☐

Moves in and out of bed as well as in and out of chair without assistance (may be using object for support such as cane or walker)	Moves in or out of bed or chair with assistance	Doesn't get out of bed.

CONTINENCE—

☐ | ☐ | ☐

Controls urination and bowel movement completely by self	Has occasional "accidents"	Supervision helps keep urine or bowel control; catheter is used or is incontinent

FEEDING—

☐ | ☐ | ☐

Feeds self without assistance	Feeds self except for getting assistance in cutting meat or buttering bread	Receives assistance in feeding or is fed partly or completely by using tubes or intravenous fluids

---

Reprinted with permission from S. Katz, A.B. Ford, R.W. Moskowitz, B.A. Jackson, and M.W. Jaffee, "Studies of illness in the aged. The Index of ADL: A standardized measure of biological and psychosocial function," *Journal of the American Medical Association*, 1963, *185*, 94 ff., American Medical Association, publishers.

TABLE 7-2   Scale for Instrumental Activities of Daily Living (IADL)

MALES' SCORE		FEMALES' SCORE
	A. *Ability to use telephone*	
1	1. Operates telephone on own initiative; looks up and dials numbers, etc.	1
1	2. Dials a few well-known numbers	1
1	3. Answers telephone but does not dial	1
0	4. Does not use telephone at all	0
	B. *Shopping*	
1	1. Takes care of all shopping needs independently	1
0	2. Shops independently for small purchases	0
0	3. Needs to be accompanied on any shopping trip	0
0	4. Completely unable to shop	0
	C. *Food preparation*	
	1. Plans, prepares and serves adequate meals independently	1
	2. Prepares adequate meals if supplied with ingredients	0
	3. Heats and serves prepared meals, or prepares meals but does not maintain adequate diet	0
	4. Needs to have meals prepared and served	0
	D. *Housekeeping*	
	1. Maintains house alone or with occasional assistance (e.g., heavy-work domestic help)	1
	2. Performs light daily tasks such as dish-washing and bed-making	1
	3. Performs light daily tasks but cannot maintain acceptable level of cleanliness	1
	4. Needs help with all home maintenance tasks	1
	5. Does not participate in any housekeeping tasks	0
	E. *Laundry*	
	1. Does personal laundry completely	1
	2. Launders small items; rinses socks, stockings, etc.	1
	3. All laundry must be done by others	0
	F. *Mode of transportation*	
1	1. Travels independently on public transportation or drives own car	1
1	2. Arranges own travel via taxi, but does not otherwise use public transportation	1
0	3. Travels on public transportation when assisted or accompanied by another	1
0	4. Travel limited to taxi or automobile, with assistance of another	0
0`	5. Does not travel at all	0
	G. *Responsibility for own medication*	
1	1. Is responsible for taking medication in correct dosages at correct time	1
0	2. Takes responsibility if medication is prepared in advance in separate dosages	0
0	3. Is not capable of dispensing own medication	0

TABLE 7-2   (continued)

MALES' SCORE		FEMALES' SCORE
	H. *Ability to handle finances*	
1	1. Manages financial matters independently (budgets, writes checks, pays rent and bills, goes to bank); collects and keeps track of income	1
1	2. Manages day-to-day purchases, but needs help with banking, major purchases, etc.	1
0	3. Incapable of handling money	0

Reprinted with permission from: M.P. Lawton and E. Brody, Assessment of older people, self-maintaining and instrumental activities of daily living. *The Gerontologist,* 1969, *9,* 179-186, Gerontological Society of America, publishers.

Short Portable MSQ (SPMSQ)   The Short Portable MSQ is also part of the OARS battery (see p. 136) but it can be used as a separate scale (Pfeiffer, 1975). A correction factor has been established for different racial and educational groups. The scoring is similar to the MSQ in that a 1 to 10 point score is given. Administration consists of asking the questions or giving instructions (e.g., Item 10: Subtract 3 from 20 and keep subtracting 3 from each new number you get, all the way down). Fewer than 2 errors suggests no impairment, 3 or 4 errors suggest mild

TABLE 7-3   A Comparison of the MSQ and SPMSQ

MENTAL STATUS EXAM	SHORT PORTABLE MENTAL STATUS EXAM
1. What is the name of this place?	What is the name of this place?
2. Where is it located (address?)	What is your street address? OR: What is your telephone number?
3. What is today's date?	What is the date today? What day of the week is it?
4. What is the month now?	
5. What is the year?	
6. How old are you now?	How old are you?
7. When were you born? (month)	When were you born?
8. When were you born? (year)	
9. Who is the president of the United States?	Who is the president of the United States now?
10. Who was president before him?	Who was president before ?
	What was your mother's maiden name?
	Subtract 3 from 20 and keep subtracting 3 from each new number all the way down.

Adapted from B.J. Gurland, The assessment of the mental health status of older adults. In J.E. Birren and R.B. Sloane, (Eds.), *Handbook of mental health and aging.* Englewood Cliffs, N.J.: Prentice-Hall, with permission.

impairment, 5 to 7 errors suggests moderate impairment, 8 to 10 errors suggests severe impairment. The instrument has been validated (Smyer et al., 1979).

Face-Hand Test Originally developed by Bender, the Face-Hand Test (Kahn et al., 1960) determines how well an individual can discern simultaneous touch on her or his cheek (left or right) and back of the hand (left or right) while seated with hands on knees (see Table 7-4). Ten trials are given . Mistakes in trials 7 through 10 indicate brain damage. The face-hand test is useful in distinguishing psychotic clients from brain-damaged clients; it also requires little understanding of English, little verbalization and is culture-free. It may not, however, give any more information than the MSQ or SPMSQ.

Administration of the Face-Hand Test allows a rehearsal sequence to familiarize the client with the procedure (trials 1 to 4 in Table 7-4). Then two teaching trials are administered, with both cheeks and both hands being touched. The four test trials are then repeated. Any errors after the first sequence (four test trails and two teaching trials) suggest organic impairment. Errors include naming other parts of the body (displacement) or omitting one of the touches.

Assessing Mental Health Status

The assessment of mental health status implies uncovering the degree and nature of symptoms of distress or psychopathology in the individual. The method most commonly used to assess mental health status is the interview, a relatively unstructured interaction between the client and a practitioner. The purposes of diagnostic interviews vary, depending on the nature of the situation, the client's known conditions, and the interviewer's theoretical point of view. Interviews can

---

TABLE 7-4 Face-Hand Test

A. Trials consist of simultaneously touching cheek and dorsum (back) of the hand while client is seated with hands on knees. Client is asked: "Where were you touched?" (on Trials 1-4, if client only says one place, probe: "Where else?")

B. Ten trials are given:
   1. right cheek: left hand
   2. left cheek: right hand
   3. right cheek: right hand
   4. left cheek, left hand
   5. right cheek: left cheek   (Teaching Trials-reinforce correct response or tell client that
   6. right hand: left hand   there are two touches)
   7. right cheek: left hand
   8. left cheek: right hand
   9. right cheek: right hand
   10. left cheek: left hand

C. Trials are given two times, once with client's eyes closed, once with eyes open.

Adapted from R.L. Kahn, A.I. Goldfarb, M. Pollack, & A. Peck. Brief objective measures for the determination of mental status in the aged. *American Journal of Psychiatry*, 1960, *117*, 326-328 with permission of American Psychiatric Association.

be held to explore underlying defense mechanisms and degree of reality testing (a psychodynamic approach), to uncover irrational beliefs that lead to current undesired behavior (a cognitive or behavioral approach), or to get a sense of the client's self-concept (a humanistic approach). Interviews are also useful in obtaining the client's perceptions of his or her difficulties; obtaining needed history of medical, social, economic and psychological concerns; and assessing the client's capacity for verbalization or his or her willingness to enter into a therapeutic relationship. The kind and amount of information uncovered in the interview thus depend on both the client and interviewer.

A range of tools and instruments are also available to assess cognition, personality, and degree of pathology in individuals. Cognitive and personality tests are being developed for use with the elderly; however, the need for advanced clinical training in their administration and interpretation as well as questions about their utility in many settings serving the elderly warrant their exclusion from this discussion (cf. Zarit, 1980). Even with the exclusion of these tests, there remain several instruments that can be easily administered, are reliable and valid, and give potentially useful information on existence and severity of mental health problems. Examples include:

OARS Mental Health Screening Scale   This is part of the OARS Battery used primarily for screening. It consists of fifteen Yes/No questions about mental-health-related concerns but has no guidelines for interpreting scores (see Table 7-5). It is best used as part of the total OARS instrument.

TABLE 7-5   OARS Mental Health Scale

OARS MENTAL HEALTH SCREENING QUESTIONS

1. Do you wake up fresh and rested most mornings?
2. Is your daily life full of things that keep you interested?
3. Have you at times very much wanted to leave home?
4. Does it seem that no one understands you?
5. Have you had periods of days, weeks, or months when you couldn't take care of things because you couldn't "get going"?
6. Is your sleep fitful and disturbed?
7. Are you happy most of the time?
8. Are you being plotted against?
9. Do you certainly feel useless at times?
10. During the last few years, have you been well most of the time?
11. Do you feel weak all over much of the time?
12. Are you troubled by headaches?
13. Have you had difficulty in keeping your balance in walking?
14. Are you troubled by your heart pounding and a shortness of breath?
15. Even when you are with people, do you feel lonely much of the time?

Source: *Multidimensional Functional Assessment: The OARS Methodology* (2nd Ed.) 1978. Edited by Duke Center Staff, Center for the Study of Aging and Human Development, Durham, N.C. 27710, with permission.

Sandoz Clinical Assessment This instrument, The Sandoz Clinical Assessment (Shader, Harmatz, & Salzman, 1974) requires that an observer rates a client on eighteen items using a seven-point scale for each. A rating of 1 means "not present;" a rating of 7 means "severe." While overall average scores of less than 3 are considered normal, raters are likely to vary considerably on their scoring of certain items (e.g., irritability, anxiety, and fatigue). Also, no criteria are given for making judgments.

The Geriatric Depression Scale (GDS) Brink and his associates (1982) have developed a thirty-item yes/no forced choice scale in which an expected "normal" score is ten or less (see Table 7-7). A point is scored by answering "no" to items 1, 5, 7, 9, 15, 19, 21, 27, and 30; or answering "yes" to any other item. Their initial study showed acceptable validity and item-total reliability. This instrument may be useful in clinical settings.

Self-assessment Scale-Geriatric (SAGE) The SAGE is a self-assessment scale in which older persons rate themselves on seven-point scales in several areas: confusion, mood, self-care, orientation, and lability of affect (Yesavage el al., 1981). This scale may provide useful initial screening data but it can be used only with older adults with low to moderate impairment.

TABLE 7-6   Sandoz Clinical Assessment-Geriatric

1. Mood depression
2. Confusion
3. Mental alertness
4. Motivation, initiative
5. Irritability
6. Hostility
7. Bothersomeness
8. Indifference to surroundings
9. Unsociability
10. Uncooperativeness
11. Emotional lability
12. Fatigue
13. Self-care
14. Appetite
15. Dizziness
16. Anxiety
17. Impairment of recent memory
18. Disorientation
    Overall impression of the patient

Source: R.I. Shader, J.S. Harmatz, & C. Salzman. A new scale for clinical assessment in geriatric populations: Sandoz Clinical Assessment-Geriatric (SCAG). *Journal of the American Geriatrics Society,* 1974, *22,* 107-113, with permission of W. B. Saunders, publisher.

TABLE 7-7 The Geriatric Depression Scale (GDS)

1. Are you basically satisfied with your life? . . . . .yes/no
2. Have you dropped many of your activities and interests?   yes/no
3. Do you feel that your life is empty?   yes/no
4. Do you often get bored?   yes/no
5. Are you hopeful about the future? . . . . .yes/no
6. Are you bothered by thoughts you can't get out of your head?   yes/no
7. Are you in good spirits most of the time?   yes/no
8. Are you afraid that something bad is going to happen to you?   yes/no
9. Do you feel happy most of the time?   yes/no
10. Do you often feel helpless? . . . . .yes/no
11. Do you often get restless and fidgety?   yes/no
12. Do you prefer to stay at home, rather than going out and doing things?   yes/no
13. Do you frequently worry about the future?   yes/no
14. Do you feel you have more problems with memory than most?   yes/no
15. Do you think it is wonderful to be alive now?. . . . . .yes/no
16. Do you often feel downhearted and blue?   yes/no
17. Do you feel pretty worthless the way you are now?   yes/no
18. Do you worry a lot about the past?   yes/no
19. Do you find life very exciting?   yes/no
20. Is it hard for you to get started on new projects?. . . . . .yes/no
21. Do you feel full or energy?   yes/no
22. Do you feel that your situation is hopeless?   yes/no
23. Do you think that most people are better off than you are?   yes/no
24. Do you frequently get upset over little things?   yes/no
25. Do you frequently feel like crying?. . . . . .yes/no
26. Do you have trouble concentrating?   yes/no
27. Do you enjoy getting up in the morning?   yes/no
28. Do you prefer to avoid social gatherings?   yes/no
29. Is it easy for you to make decisions?   yes/no
30. Is your mind as clear as it used to be?   yes/no

Multidimensional Assessment

Several instruments have been developed that give some indication of functioning within separate areas (physical, social, mental) as well as a single score or profile of the older individual. While cumbersome, they are gaining in popularity and usage. Examples include:

OARS Instrument The OARS (Duke University, 1978) assesses functional activity level in five areas: social resources, economic resources, mental health, physical health, and activities of daily living. It takes at least an hour for the 105 questions to be asked. The interviewer then rates the client on the five dimensions on a six-point scale (1 being a "high" rating, 6 being "totally impaired"). Pfeiffer, Johnson, and Chiofolo (1980) have reported on a shortened form of the OARS that may also be effective. The instrument has been validated (Fillenbaum & Smyer, 1981). Training is needed to ensure appropriate administration.

CARE Instrument The CARE Instrument (Comprehensive Assessment and Referral Evaluation) is designed to assess functional levels of activity and presence of clinical syndromes. It uses an interview format with a series of yes/no self-report and rating items. It was designed with a psychiatric emphasis. Gurland and his associates (1977) describe the instrument in detail. Although it requires highly trained administrators, it may be useful because of its psychiatric focus, especially in an interdisciplinary setting.

An Alternative: Behavioral Approaches

An alternative related to functional assessment is behavioral assessment. Rather than focusing on intrapsychic concerns, a behavioral approach asks such questions as: "What conditions (reinforcers, self-statements, environmental factors) maintain this behavior?" "What conditions (reinforcers, new associations, or learnings) can lead to a change in behavior?"

The term *applied behavioral analysis* has been used to describe an assessment of patterns of behavior that reveals an "antecedents-behavior-concequences" (ABC) design. By accurately analyzing each part of the pattern, antecedents or consequences can be altered, with a subsequent change in behavior.

Kanfer and Saslow (1965) have developed a comprehensive set of guidelines and parameters for behavioral assessment that not only pinpoint behavioral aspects of problems to be assessed but also the social and cultural context in which they occur.

In this system seven areas are assessed:

1. *Analysis of the problem situation.* This area has three components: (1) a specific and accurate description of the behavior (when, how often, how much); (2) a determination of whether the problem is one of excesses or deficits; and (3) a determination of how severe the problem is.

2. *Analysis of antecedents and consequences of the problem behavior.* This area details what is going on immediately before the problem behavior occurs (including internal thoughts) *and* what happens as a result of the behavior. These events need to be looked at to determine both the "sequence" of the behavior pattern and how the events strengthen or maintain the problem behavior. Benefits arising from problematic behavior may need to be linked with other behaviors before the problem ceases. For example, a paranoid isolate who receives attention from others only when she calls the police may need to develop other social contacts before the calls will cease.

3. *Assessment of other assets and deficits in functioning.* Rather than simply tending to the presenting problem, a more complete assessment of social skills and deficits is suggested. Clients with few other skills may need additional help if they are to improve in the one problem area. For example, a widow who is continually anxious may need to learn how to be assertive in social situations as well as how to relax in order for anxiety to subside.

4. *Analysis of social relationships.* The quality of relationships as well as their impact on the client's behavior should be determined. Direct intervention may be needed to help the client develop support networks and appropriate "expectations" about social relationships.

5. *Motivational analysis.* The client's motivation to change, her or his "goals" in seeking treatment, and even his or her philosophical views in related areas (e.g., "Man is born to suffer," or "We need to accept what cannot be changed") should be considered in devising treatment.

6. *Analysis of the social-cultural-physical environment.* One can ask "What are the expectations of the social or cultural group?" and "How well is the client handling these?" as an important aspect of assessment. A client may not be handling them well because the expectations are unreasonable in the specific situation or the client does not have the resources to handle them.

7. *Developmental Analysis.* A developmental analysis consists of obtaining a history of the client's major life events and how he or she has coped with them, as well as a history of the problem being treated.

This last approach is useful because behavior and problems are specifically spelled out, and the interpersonal, social, and cultural contexts in which they occur are acknowledged. However, much of the specific information has to be developed through interviews, a procedure that requires considerable time and judgment on the part of the evaluator.

DEVELOPING STRATEGIES FOR ASSESSMENT

Assessment can serve several potential objectives and functions for the elderly (cf. Kane & Kane, 1981):

Documenting an individual's problems

Pinpointing conditions that need additional services or support

Documenting small changes in functioning

Screening older adults who need help or further assessment

Providing accurate diagnosis/description of problems

Providing an efficient monitoring of progress

Providing an efficient monitoring of conditions in which there is no intervention

Aiding prediction of outcomes or decisions in case management

Obtaining critical information in an efficient manner

As has been mentioned previously, assessment of the aged is often overlooked or may be done haphazardly. An assessment "strategy" should be developed by answering each of the following questions:

What is the specific purpose of the assessment, and what questions need to be answered?

If the client's situation is assessed, is new information likely to be discovered?

Is the new informtion going to be useful? How?

What methods (interview, assessment tool, psychological testing, medical evaluation) would most efficiently provide answers to relevant questions about the client?

How much will these methods cost in terms of time and money?

What resources are available (including staff, time, and money) that can be used for assessment?

If resources are not sufficient for full assessment, what alternatives can be implemented?

The assessment strategy used in any setting will be influenced by the needs of the client, the resources available in the system, and subsequently, the degree to which a compromise can be reached when the two do not match, which is frequently the case. The choice of a given approach or tool should be determined through a careful consideration of what information is being gained and at what cost.

SUMMARY AND CONCLUSIONS

Assessment of the elderly is an important step in the intervention process. It can be used systematically to uncover client problems and make appropriate decisions about treatment. The mental health practitioner's approach in assessment, while working for rapport, also has to allow the client to answer questions or perform assessment tasks on his or her own.

There is considerable controversy about the use of tests in assessing the elderly. The lack of age norms, validity, and reliability limit the utility of some instruments. Some instruments produce too many incorrect categorizations to make them useful in the clinical setting.

Areas commonly assessed in the elderly include physical health, mental functioning, and social functioning. In each area, there are several types of tools commonly used for screening. Behavioral assessment of problem behavior is a useful alternative to formal testing.

Assessment of the aged is a complex undertaking. A variety of procedures and instruments have been designed to assess aspects of the older person's functioning. The decision about which to use in a given clinical setting depends on the specific information or questions to be answered as well as the resources available to carry out desired procedures.

8

General Considerations in Mental Health Practice with the Elderly

INTRODUCTION

This chapter addresses some general questions and issues encountered in all approaches to intervention with the aged: How is mental health practice with the aged different from its practice with other groups? What are the important considerations in developing helping relationships with the aged? What are some of the common dynamics likely to be encountered with the aged? What ethical concerns are likely to arise? The chapter then ends with a description of a general approach and steps to use in designing interventions and a paradigm to compare varying approaches to mental health intervention with the elderly: goals, focus, targeted groups, and strengths and weaknesses.

HOW IS MENTAL HEALTH PRACTICE WITH THE ELDERLY DIFFERENT?

Differences Between Older and Younger Persons

The earlier chapters of this text suggest several differences between old and young that may affect mental health interventions with the elderly. There are, however, no differences that suggest that mental health practice with the elderly is

140

impossible or that it is dramatically different from similar work with younger people.

One set of differences is the likelihood of physical changes due to impairment or decrement. The mental health practitioner needs to know how well the client hears and sees, how fast the client can process information, and how well the client remembers from session to session (Wolff & Meyer, 1979). A related issue is the close relationship between mental health problems and physical status. Mental health interventions may focus on helping the client adapt to physical and health problems.

Even beyond health problems, older people are likely to have many interrelated economic, social, and personal concerns. Mental health intervention by itself will be much less effective than intervention that is integrated with social, economic, and advocacy efforts (Zarit, 1980).

A third difference concerns the issue of loss. While all people experience losses in their lives, the losses typically faced by the elderly are multiple. The theme of coping and accepting loss is a dominant one in work with the elderly.

Another difference is the likelihood of a client's having negative self-stereotypes because of being old. Negative attitudes can impede or even effectively counter the potential benefits of mental health intervention.

The client's generational values and values related to "being old" may also differ from those of the mental health practitioner. This may be reflected in the client's feelings about what matters are appropriate to discuss as well as their views about what constitutes appropriate behavior with family members. Minority group elderly are often quite reluctant to broach certain topics when talking with a professional who is not from their group.

The Role of the Mental Health Practitioner

There is general agreement that for any age group one of the mental health practitioner's roles is therapeutic or facilitative rather than prescriptive. That is, the mental health practitioner does not simply prescribe or give advice; rather, he or she works with the client to obtain mutually agreed upon goals.

Within this general view, however, there are differences of opinion. Insight-oriented approaches emphasize a facilitative role with interpretations of behavior being offered by mental health practitioners; client-centered approaches emphasize a more strictly facilitative role; and behavioral or cognitive approaches emphasize a teaching or challenging approach to intervention. In no instance, however, is it acceptable for the mental health practitioner simply to "tell the client what to do." Even the most radical approaches to intervention are based on a client's integrating new behavior, learnings, insights, or cognitions and depend on an assumed capability of the client to respond, learn, and integrate whatever is done in the course of therapy.

A related aspect is what mental health practice can realisticallly offer an older client. The mental health practitioner can offer a helping relationship, the ability to identify and understand thoughts and feelings, as well as the ability to explore feelings and help clients derive appropriate and useful ways to cope with problems

(Wolff & Meyer, 1979). The mental health practitioner can thus be a sounding board or source of reality, challenging clients to begin to change irrational beliefs or to develop goals that will improve the quality of their lives.

Still another potential role is that of resource. The mental health practitioner can offer knowledge about services, benefits, agencies, and living situations. Because the mental health practitioner may be the only person the client trusts for information, the practitioner should be knowledgeable about benefits, current services, and housing options for clients.

The mental health practitioner can also function as an instructor. Clients and their families may need information on aging, environmental aids, or even problem-solving strategies to help them solve problems that contribute to emotional distress.

At times, the mental health practitioner is a negotiator. He or she may be called on to help clients and families or clients and systems work out differences or learn to communicate more effectively.

The mental health practitioner often has the role of case manager. At times, he or she may have to track a client's progress through legal, health, or social systems—because no one else is available to take charge of the case.

A final role is that of advocate. Successful advocacy to change legislation, attitudes, or service availability for older clients is needed in many areas of the United States. The mental health practitioner can also set up needed "nontraditional" services, such as support groups, widow-to-widow programs, peer counseling, and outreach.

These potential roles overlap and may even be performed simultaneously. Particularly in community settings, the practitioner may be called on to play several roles in succession, depending on the range of client needs and the availability of other components of the service network. Because of the multiple nature of older persons' problems, the likelihood that adaptive interventions are needed, and the lack of other services, mental health practitioners working with the elderly can rarely confine themselves to playing a single preferred role (often that of therapist). They will often be required to display a high degree of flexibility, geared to the specific needs of the clients.

The Need for Nontraditional Services

In traditional mental health care, a "patient," a person with an identified mental health problem, seeks help from a therapist and is usually treated in a hospital, psychiatric clinic, private office, or even a community mental health center. However, the utilization of noninstitutional services by elderly is low (2 to 6 percent of patients are seen in outpatient settings) compared to the estimates of need in the community (15 percent at a minimum) (Redick & Taube, 1980; Vanden Bos, Stapp, & Kilburg, 1981). One reason for low utilization is that many older people avoid traditional mental health settings and are reluctant to accept formal help (Sargent, 1980).

One suggested solution is to offer "nontraditional" services—ones that are informal, nonthreatening, and establising a personal relationship and rapport—before other mental interventions take place (Sargent, 1980). There are several reasons for this suggested change in initial approach to treatment. First, traditional approaches do not seem to meet the needs of most elderly. Second, the nature of traditional treatment implies that the person receiving help is less than capable, a "patient." Nontraditional approaches, those that first establish a nonhelping relationship, may be necessary to reinforce the notion that older persons are capable of being independent, can solve their own problems, and can carry on after the mental health intervention is finished. Finally, nontraditional approaches encompass several relatively inexpensive treatment approaches that can be successfully integrated with the mental health practitioner's focus, such as peer counseling, adult day care, outreach, and support groups (see Chapter 15 for a description of these approaches).

Direct Versus Indirect Services Most clinicians and mental health practitioners are trained in direct service, with practitioner and client (or family) sitting face-to-face for a period of time. However, indirect services can be beneficial to more people (G. Cohen, 1980). Examples of indirect services include instructing the teaching staff in a nursing home in the principles of behavioral analysis or teaching a support system how to manage older person with OBS. The skills, "payoffs," and values inherent in indirect mental health services are not always in the forefront of clinicians' training. However, the mental health practitioner should consider how to provide indirect as well as direct services to maximize both client functioning and provide impact (Glasscote, Gudeman, & Miles, 1978).

Illness Versus Wellness Approaches Much of the traditional focus of mental health health care is on curing or solving problems, an "illness" approach (G. Cohen, 1980). This focus is valuable and useful. However, given the nature of problems faced by the elderly, consideration should als be given to "wellness" approaches, those that emphasize building on existing strengths, adaptation, and coping mechanisms.

Length of Sessions Mental health practice with the elderly often cannot be confined to fifty-minute sessions. Mental health practice takes place in nursing home rooms, in private homes with outside interruptions, and with clients who do not initially understand the nature of mental health interventions. Also, clients may be medicated, have limited attention spans and limited energy. The mental health practitioner needs to be flexible in terms of how much time is spent in a single session. Initially, daily visits of ten minutes may create better rapport with a nursing home resident than a fifty-minute visit once a week.

DEVELOPING HELPING RELATIONSHIPS
WITH THE ELDERLY

For many older people the relationship formed with a mental health practitioner is not simply one of a series of professional or personal relationships they encounter in their personal environment. As was mentioned earlier, there are many potential roles for the mental health practitioner in working with the aged. When there is a restricted social environment, the mental health practitioner may need to fulfill needs such as intimacy, social contact, or friendship (Wolff & Meyer, 1978). Also, the mental health practitioner, as one of the few professionals who will spend time talking to an older person, may become extremely influential without being aware of it. For these reasons, practitioners need to examine their own motivation, needs, and attitudes toward the clients with whom they work.

Needs, Motivation, and Attitudes of the Mental Health Practitioner

People enter the helping professions for a variety of reasons, ranging from a "discovering why I am the way I am" to "wanting to help others." There are also many reasons for choosing to work with the elderly (cf. Butler & Lewis, 1982). Some motives and needs are:

1. Having had close relationships with older relatives (including being raised by them)
2. Attempting to conquer either one's own fears of aging or one's guilt about relationships with elders
3. Attempting to cope with a personal sense of inferiority by identifying with a group generally considered inferior
4. Admiring or emulating another person who works with the elderly (having a mentor who works in the field)
5. Needing to feel loved or powerful by being important in others' lives
6. Preparing oneself for old age
7. Attempting to redress social injustice or discrimination against the aged
8. Feeling a sense of achievement in helping others

Several of these motives may lead to undesirable outcomes. For example, the mental health practitioner who needs to feel powerful can unintentionally create dependence. The mental health practitioner who needs to be "liked" by everyone will work for client approval rather than client change (Huber & Wolff, 1981). Because the relationships that develop can be so important to the elderly, the mental health practitioner needs to be able to assess her or his varied motives and their impact on the client, relationship, and process of mental health practice.

Attitudes of Mental Health Practitioners Towards the Aged The generally negative view of age and aging is in part reflected in how mental health professionals have responded to the needs of the elderly. Too often there has been an assumption that the problems of the elderly are untreatable (Butler, 1975). The reasons for such an assumption include fear of one's own aging, a belief that older people cannot be helped, ignorance about mental health problems and old age, a negative bias against the aged, and lack of prestige in working with the elderly. From the perspective of mental health practice, however, it is more important to consider how attitudes may influence care once the decision to intervene has been made.

Both overly positive and overly negative stereotypes about the elderly can influence treatment. For example, the practitioner who believes that older persons can handle all problems on their own or that all problems faced by the aged are merely the result of how others treat them (an overly positive view) may pay little attention to changes in behavior that indicate severe emotional or physical problems. Similarly, the practitioner who believes that older persons cannot significantly change their ways (the rigidity myth) is likely to overgeneralize the first sign of "resistance" or ambivalence as rigidity and "give up" on the client.

The degree of belief in any of the myths discussed in Chapter 1 may be slight and its influence may be subtle, appearing only in terms of lowered expectations for change in older clients. Because mental health practitioners can influence decisions such as institutionalization or access to other services, it is important for them to assess the impact of their beliefs about the aged as a regular part of supervision and practice.

Helpful Versus Friendly Relationships

Because the mental health practitioner can fulfill many needs with older adults, there is often a conflict between having a friendly or a helping relationship. In a helping relationship the client and mental health practitioner focus on problem solving, insight into self, and behavioral or cognitive change (Brammer, 1981). Part of the conflict comes from the mental health professional's search for alternatives to the "doctor-patient" relationship. Friendship and mutual respect are important, but the mental health practitioner needs to maintain perspective and retain the right to draw discussion into significant issues for the client. In this regard, *self-disclosure*, which implies that the mental health practitioner share her or his personal life, is appropriate to create trust or credibility, but it should not be used indiscriminantly or become the dominant theme of the relationship.

Providing an Appropriate Setting

Many settings are not conducive to mental health practice. Nursing homes are particularly difficult settings in which to find a quiet and private place to talk. When clients are bed-ridden, staff or roommates may be present during sessions unless an assertive request is made for privacy. In private homes, noisy televisions and radios should be turned off. Other family members may need to be invited in or out of sessions, as appropriate.

Forming Helping Relationships with Minority Aged

As was discussed in Chapter 2, minority elderly suffer from a double jeopardy—being old and from a minority group. Also, each minority group has its own culture and values; these have an impact on how services are best given. Lawrence

(1981), for example, suggests several tips for working with specific populations. They stem from language, history, and family patterns. It is important to realize that these are anthropological guides and cannot be followed mechanically.

Blacks

1. Give formal respect to the client. Use titles and last names, appreciate the value of self-sufficiency, and present services as a right, not as a need.
2. Be alert for signs of overcompliance (the client's saying "yes" when, in fact, there is no understanding or agreement). The client should also set the pace.

Hispanics

1. Tend to concerns about politeness in language (using formal forms of "you," asking how to refer to the client's ethnic group).
2. Allow a social relationship to develop. This includes asking personal questions only with permission, sharing coffee and tea, and participating in talk about the client's family, pictures, and so on.
3. Allow the client to set the pace. Conversations may focus more on a service than an underlying problem.
4. Learn the language—more than just a few words. This is a sensible goal if you are going to have contact with Hispanics over time. It also shows some commitment to the client group and respect for their background.
5. When possible, arrange to have mental health practitioners treat clients of their own sex. This will make sharing easier.
6. Use aspects and strengths of the culture (roles, values) as part of an intervention plan (Szapocznik et al., 1981).

Pacific-Asians

1. Slow the pace of the helping process. It will take time for relationships and formal services to be accepted or developed.
2. Pay attention to cultural differences signaling respect (using titles, carefully tending to issues of politeness as opposed to confrontation, reassuring clients about confidentiality when issues involving shame are discussed, limiting eye contact—a sign of respect, avoiding touch in many situations, not interpreting a polite nod as agreement).
3. When possible, match mental health practitioners with clients of the same sex.

American Indians

1. Appreciate tribal differences. Each will vary in terms of the meaning of touch, eye contact, and value of mental health practitioners of the same or opposite sex.
2. Take time and care in building relationships. The mental health practitioner comes in untrusted and is likely to be tested for his or her commitment.

3. Solving specific problems and being honest are critical.
4. Form relationships with formal and informal leaders in the community.
5. Avoid aggressive behavior and excessive talking. Listening is a valued skill.
6. Other cultural differences include respecting experience and age (an older helper has an advantage), the importance of sharing (accept refreshments if offered), and not looking around people's homes when invited in (a sign of disrespect).

All of these tips focus on how to develop a helping relationship with a person from another culture. They are only general guides and cannot be used as a "cookbook" approach. The helper must also be congruent and genuine, not aloof, disdainful, or self-depreciating. Much of the work with any minority group can be made easier by first establishing contact and a relationship with formal and informal leaders, intermediaries, or "brokers" in the specific community. They can lend their credibility to your efforts if they believe you can be of help.

DYNAMICS ENCOUNTERED IN WORKING WITH THE AGED

In the course of treating any emotional problem of the aged, certain behavior or behavioral patterns (dynamics) may occur. Some of the most frequently encountered are resistance, dependency, transference/countertransference, anger, and difficulties in termination.

Resistance

Many times in the therapy or counseling process, it appears that the client is not working towards agreed upon goals and is, in fact, slowing the process or even negating changes. This tendency to go against help is called *resistance*. Some schools of thought consider resistance a stage in which defenses are working against needed change because the client does not want to give up the rewards of having problems (secondary gains). Resistance can also be considered an implicit statement that the client does not believe there is a problem, does not want to admit there is one, does not find help effective, or does not trust the helper (Blake & Bichekas, 1981).

Suggested methods for handling resistance in the older client include (Blake & Bichekas, 1981):

Focusing on unwanted outcomes of current behavior and thoughts

Identifying the rewards of current behavior (e.g., attention, care) and working on making them available to the client in other ways

Maintaining a supportive, warm, nonjudgmental approach

Guaranteeing privacy and confidentiality

Exploring which aspects of mental health practice are uncomfortable or ineffective

Openly discussing the difficulties the client is having

Not giving help when none is needed.

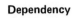

Dependency

Dependency is a common issue in mental health practice with the elderly. Many older people have expectations of being dependent (a "patient") when treated for any problem. That is, they do not take full responsibility for their own care but depend unrealistically on the helper to solve problems for them. The implicit inequality of helping relationships reinforces dependency in initial stages of intervention. Also, mental health practitioners who feel somewhat ambivalent or unsure about working with the elderly may use an advice-giving approach (which reinforces dependency) as a way to avoid a deeper therapeutic relationship.

While a dependency relationship can become the focus of therapy (i.e., the client can be led to gain insight about his or her needs from others), in most other circumstances it is not a healthy state of affairs. It should be directly discussed by both parties when it occurs, the goal being a more realistic understanding of the relationship. Giving people control over their lives is one goal of mental health treatment. In institutional settings this may be the most important goal a mental health practitioner can have. Fostering independence in even simple activities can have long-term beneficial results (e.g., Rodin & Langer, 1977; Langer & Rodin, 1976). A dependency relationship left unresolved is potentially harmful to the client.

Transference and Countertransference

Transference refers to client feelings or perceptions about the mental health practitioner that are, in reality, based on conflicts or issues in the client's life. *Countertransference* refers to the mental health practitioner's reactions and perceptions of the client that are significantly colored by relationships or fears in the mental health practitioner's life. In classical psychoanalytic theory, transference is expected and is, in fact, critical to the success of therapy because successful analysis of the tranference relationship leads to insight and subsequent change. Countertransference, however, needs to be "worked through" outside of the therapeutic relationship so that the therapist can accurately interpret and work with the client's problems. Other schools of thought do not place as much emphasis on the transference relationship (behaviorists or cognitive therapists may consider it of very minor, if any, importance). However, all would agree that mental health practitioner biases or misperceptions of clients work against effective intervention.

In addition, it has been suggested that for analytically oriented workers transference and countertransference relationships with the aged may need to handled differently than with younger age groups (e.g., Verwoerdt, 1976). If the two are positive, without neurotic components, and fit well, the resultant relationship, despite its basis in nonreality, can be beneficial for the client (cf. Goldfarb's Brief Therapy, Chapter 9). Also, the transference relationship is used less as a vehicle for therapy, whereas supportive and realistic approaches are encouraged.

Anger

Mental health practitioners are at times surprised by the amount of anger found in older clients. Anger has many sources in the elderly, including reaction to medication; feelings of helplessness about increasing impairment, institutionalization, or dependence on others; guilt about previous life experiences; or even a reaction to the implied role of being "old" (lack of status, sexuality, individuality, and power). Anger can stem from the client's feeling tht he or she is not understood, appreciated, or treated with dignity, or it can be a transference of anger from earlier situations (Blake & Bichekas, 1981).

The angry client needs support and attentive concern as well as help in either exploring underlying causes or developing ways of decreasing unwanted results of anger, such as withdrawal of significant others or negative reactions of staff. The best time to explore the client's anger is not while the client is expressing it. Also, severe forms of expression such as swearing at staff, hitting, biting, or throwing objects may need specific behavioral interventions (see Chapter 10) to decrease their occurrence.

Difficulties in Termination

Termination refers to the ending of the helping relationship. Termination can be difficult for both the older client and mental health practitioner. Because the relationship may be one of few if any where there is intimacy and trust, termination can represent another irreplaceable loss for the client. Time may need to be spent discussing this and preparing the client for the ending of the relationship. In addition, creating additional meaningful social contact (groups, activities, having another person continue as a visitor) can help the transition and maintain therapeutic gains.

It is also possible for the mental health practitioner to continue the relationship upon termination on a different basis. A helping relationship may have to end, but a friendship may continue with the two parties on a more equal basis and with a different focus of discussions.

ETHICAL CONSIDERATIONS

As mental health interventions have become more widespread, questions about ethics and values of the mental health practitioner have been raised. Professional organizations such as the American Psychological Association, American Personnel and Guidance Association, National Association of Social Workers, and the American Psychiatric Association have developed codes for professional behavior. Certain ethical principles have particular relevance for work with the elderly and are discussed below.

Obligations to the Client   Mental health practitioners have a primary obligation to the client to maintain him or her at the highest possible level of functioning. Conflicts of interest may arise with family, whose goals may vary from those of the mental health practitioner. These conflicts can become difficult to resolve when one's job is on the line or a family with considerable influence in a community tries to influence a case plan.

Limits of Expertise   Mental health practitioners are obligated to acknowledge the limits of their abilities, neither overselling their abilities nor promising more than they can deliver. This principle also mandates referral when the problem is beyond the mental health practitioner's range of knowledge or expertise. At the same time, it should be recognized that mental health practitioners can find themselves "over their heads," but have to stay with the client because of lack of referral sources or the client's refusal to seek other service.

> *Case:* An outreach worker had finally made contact with Mrs. Goldberg, an obese woman in her early seventies. After several weeks, Mrs. Goldberg had let the worker in for two sessions. It became obvious that Mrs. Goldberg had health problems (i.e., hypertension) and was moderately disoriented, consistently forgetting the date and the worker's name. However, whenever the worker suggested that Mrs. Goldberg go to a physician or discuss her problems with family, Mrs. Goldberg became agitated and refused. Despite being in "over her head," the outreach worker continued to visit Mrs. Goldberg for a year, during which time there was slight deterioration in Mrs. Goldberg's condition.

There is little question but that the worker needed to make a referral in this instance. However, the client's refusal to see a physician meant the worker had to continue in a situation that required more skills than she had.

Confidentiality   This principle covers several areas of mental health practice. Confidentiality implies that whatever the client says to the mental health practitioner is said in confidence, that no one, without the explicit permission of the client, will have access to this information and its public use should not identify the client. Confidentiality is a concern in professional writing, public speeches, discussions with colleagues and intimates, and discussions with family members. Obvious exceptions are supervisors and persons with legal access to records.

There are several related concerns about confidentiality. First, there is a question of exactly how much family members have a right to know. Second, in some settings, including nursing homes, there is at times an air of casualness about confidentiality among staff that will overstep ethical boundaries. It is hard to know when to draw the line and, unfortunately, it is frequently easier to forget one exists.

Third, practitioners should be aware that they cannot always guarantee the confidentiality of their records. Many mental health practitioners do not come under protection of the law for privileged communication; that is, their records and they themselves can be subpoenaed to testify in court that a client is incompetent to handle his or her affairs (conservatorship) or needs an institutional placement.

Fees Fee setting is the responsibility of the individual mental health practitioner or agency. However, private practitioners should be willing to see some clients for a nominal or no fee.

Unduly Influencing Clients with One's Own Values All people have personal values or guides for evaluating behavior, goals, and relationships. In Western culture, some likely values include instrumentality (the value of work or activity) and a belief that problems can be solved. As Okun (1982) points out, one's values are influenced by views about family, relationships, and roles (including parent, child, older adults). At the same time, mental health practitioners are requested to be nonjudgmental in their professional behavior. Being nonjudgmental, however, does not mean giving up one's values but rather not letting them subtly and unduly influence the client.

For example, the views of some elderly clients about "obligations" due to them from family members will differ from the views of the mental health practitioner. This is particularly true for older Hispanics and American Indians. The mental health practitioner needs to be able both to clarify the value disagreement and then be able to focus on the mental health aspect of resultant behavior, such as discussing hurt feelings when a family does not take a parent in to live with them.

The impact of values can be great in mental health practice with the elderly because the mental health practitioner has tremendous influence in the relationship as an authority figure and professional. Care and self-awareness are needed to prevent inadvertent influence by personal and cultural values.

Contracts A contract is an agreement between two people. In mental health practice it exists on two levels, an *explicit* level where both parties openly agree; and an *implicit* level, where agreements and commitments are not openly aknowledged. Ethically, there should be an explicit understanding of how often meetings will take place, over how long a period of time, the purpose of the sessions, and limits of confidentiality. Because many elderly are unaware of the nature of therapy, it will also be useful to spend some time instructing them about their role in treatment, which is usually considered an implicit aspect of the contract.

Implicit aspects include a commitment by both mental health practitioners and clients to work for change or growth, the right of the client to terminate, and that personal concerns of the client are the focus of the relationship, as opposed to social concerns.

GENERAL APPROACHES
IN WORKING WITH THE AGED

Empathy Versus Detached Concern

Empathy, genuineness, and "unconditional positive regard" for the client are perhaps the cornerstone of counseling in any age group (e.g., Carkhuff, 1969; Wolff & Meyer, 1979; Brammer, 1981). Even critics of approaches that rely primarily on these aspects would agree that supportive, caring concern by the mental health practitioner is usually an appropriate approach. The critical point of disagreement is whether or not warmth, empathy, therapeutic relationships, and unconditional positive regard are both *necessary* and *sufficient* for mental health interventions to lead to desired changes. Client-centered therapists (see Chapter 11) would argue yes; behaviorally oriented therapists (see Chapter 10) would agrue no.

The question of a general approach to the aged has been considered somewhat differently by Verwoerdt (1976). Verwoerdt does not endorse a solely empathic approach, but rather one of "detached concern," in which the mental health practitioner is realistic, consistent, gentle, yet firm. The ability to have insight into client problems is as critical as being supportive. This is also in line with the approach advocated by Pfeiffer and Busse (1973), that the therapist be more active and directive with the aged than in traditional treatment.

In part, the type of disagreement mirrored above reflects some theoretical differences in schools of therapy. It may also reflect differences in the "type" of person who becomes a client-centered therapist, a more analytically oriented therapist, or a behavioral therapist. A possible but imperfect solution to this issue is that a given approach is more effective when it is consistent with both the theoretical views and the style of the mental health practitioner. Nothing is worse than an "empathic" worker who comes off as phoney or a "detached but concerned" worker who comes off as professorial or uninvolved. Genuineness and concern for the client can be expressed in many ways. At the least they are important building blocks in developing trust; at best they are the key to successful mental heath interventions with the elderly.

A closing concern on the issue of general approach is an exhortation to use touch with older clients as is appropriate and comfortable for both client and mental health practitioner. Handshakes, holding hands, or hugs convey care and concern (Voerwoerdt, 1976). Touch is also reassuring and shows regard for the other person.

Steps in the Intervention Process

Regardless of type of intervention strategy, certain steps take place in the design and implementaton of mental health interventions. Ideally, each step is carefully considered, and the results of each step in turn influence choices made in the steps to follow. In reality, however, some of the steps may be ignored or glossed over due to lack of resources, knowledge, or time. When an intervention is unsuccessful, it may well be due to deleting or not paying enough attention to the steps and not a statement about ability of either the practitioner or the client.

Entry   Entry is an initial stage in which the older person becomes a client or is identified as having a mental health problem. She or he may be self-referred, referred by others, or even coerced into seeking mental health care by family and/ or the staff of an institutional facility. An important concern here is how the older person views himself or herself—as a person seeking aid, as a "patient," or as a "victim" of others' manipulations.

Initial Exploration of Problems   In the beginning, information will be given by the client and others as to the nature of the problem, its course, onset, manifestations, and possible causes. Some information and perceptions will be withheld until the client develops trust in the mental health practitioner. The practitioner's job at this point includes helping to clarify problems, winning the client's trust, and providing the client with some understanding of the nature and limits of the helping relationship.

Extensive Exploration of Problems   In this phase the problems are formally assessed. Underlying dynamics, parameters affecting the problems, and/or the client's symptoms are analyzed to obtain a complete understanding of the situation. Although there are systematic differences in approach to the assessment of mental health problems between major approaches to psychotherapy, the following areas are recommended for the elderly, due to the multifaceted nature of most problems they face. Assessment should include health information and history, including medication; a social history focusing on family relationships and past experiences; an examination of physical and psychological losses and how they have been handled; current family relationships and informal support systems (friends, neighbors); social, housing, and economic status; analysis of the symptoms (e.g., frequency, degree, discomfort, secondary gains); and an analysis of the client's abilities for change, including motivation, cognition, and ability to learn. Appropriate assessment instruments can be used to aid in gathering information in these areas.

Changes in any of these areas may contribute to or determine onset of symptoms or discomfort. There are times when the problem is the family's or the institution's rather than the client's. Uncovering probable causes, contributing factors, and client abilities for change are necessary prerequisites to designing appropriate interventions.

Exploration and Establishment of Treatment Goals   Treatment goals should be explored and established collaboratively with the client and relevant support systems. One standard goal should be integration of mental health care with other forms of support. The goals should be realistic and clearly stated and should not violate any rights of the client. Mental health interventions may have many possible goals; at times interventions may be designed to meet several concerns (see the following section for a paradigm describing potential goals for treatment). Court rulings in Massachusetts in the early 1980s about schizophrenics' rights to refuse medication suggest that all clients have the right to know the goals of treatment and refuse treatment without recrimination from any party.

Working Towards Treatment Goals At this point, the mental health practitioner needs to make choices about the methods to be used to meet treatment goals. One guideline is the concept of minimum intervention, that is, trying the least intrusive and disruptive methods to induce change while maintaining the client's independence and reliance on existing supports before resorting to extensive or dramatic strategies to solve all of the client's problems (Zarit, 1980). The methods used and their impact on the individual should be evaluated on a regular basis.

The practitioner can expect to encounter dynamics of resistance, dependency, transference and countertransference, anger, and difficulty preparing for termination and should be prepared to discuss them with the client and minimize their potential negative influence. The amount of time necessary for goals to be realized will vary considerably and depend on the nature of the problems and goals, the abilities of the client, the form of treatment, the practitioner's skills, and logistical realities.

Termination At this point, the mental health practitioner has finished her or his work with the older client. Ideally, there has been a final assessment of the impact of intervention, the client is ready to move on to other problems and relationships, and the utility of further intervention is minimal.

These steps do not necessarily progress in a smooth and orderly fashion. Even with the best of intentions information may be ambiguous, some diagnostic work may not be able to be done, goals may not be understood, evaluation of interventions may be overlooked, intervention strategies may not be well implemented, and termination may be unclear or premature. However, the steps provide a guideline for planning interventions with the elderly and may provide a key to understanding where interventions fail to improve mental health functioning.

A PARADIGM FOR COMPARING
AND EVALUATING APPROACHES
TO MENTAL HEALTH INTERVENTION
WITH THE ELDERLY

In the previous section, reference was made to choosing an intervention to meet treatment goals. The following six chapters describe a range of theoretical and specific approaches that have been used with the elderly. One source of difficulty in understanding and being able to choose a type of intervention stems from the lack of a framework for describing and evaluating intervention approaches. The following framework has been developed for this purpose. (It is based in part on the work of Huyck & Hoyer, 1982.)

Four areas will be used to summarize intervention approaches are goals, focus of intervention, targeted population, and strengths and weaknesses.

Goals There are four general goals of intervention, several of which may be present in a given approach: *Cure* removes identifiable symptoms or pathology; *adaptation* enables the client to compensate for losses that cannot be replaced; *enrichment* brings the client's level of functioning beyond a minimally acceptable level (this includes goals such as improved social functioning or "self-actualization"); *prevention* decreases likelihood of onset or impact of problems in persons considered "at risk."

Traditionally, psychotherapy has focused on curing mental disorders. Adaptive goals have been seen as somehow less than optimal, and adaptive treatments have been viewed as less sophisticated forms of cure. Many of the problems and concerns in the first part of this text are adaptive, as are many of the suggested interventions for functional and organic disorders in the aged. Working to help individuals maintain their functioning at the highest level, cope with physical and mental losses, handle the death of and mourning for a spouse, or prepare for their own death should be viewed as highly complex interventions and be considered as extremely important in the mental health of the aged. It is probably a disservice to the elderly to continue to consider adaptive interventions as "second rate." We would do much better to consider adaptive and curative interventions as having qualitatively different goals, neither being "better" or "more sophisticated" than the other.

Focus of Intervention An approach may focus on one or more of these areas: *health, cognition* (e.g., memory, intelligence, decision making, thought processes, problem solving), emotions (e.g., anxiety, feelings of depression), *behavior, socialization,* and *attitudes and values* (inner thoughts related to self-image or outlook). These areas overlap and have different relative value in varying theoretical approaches to treating mental health problems.

Targeted Population An approach may be designed for a specific group (e.g., persons with senile dementia) or have different application in community and institutional settings.

Strengths and Weaknesses Approaches vary in their *proven scientific validity,* the *flexibility* with which they can be applied, the *clarity* of their concepts and techniques, and the *degree to which they can be applied to the multifaceted problems of the elderly.*

SUMMARY AND CONCLUSIONS

Mental health practice with the elderly differs from that with younger persons in several ways. Physical impairment, health problems, social functioning, and a theme of coping with loss are likely to be present in elderly clients. Negative self-images of being old and generational differences are also likely to occur.

Although there is a sense that intervention with the elderly is more directive than intervention with younger persons, a range of roles are available to the practitioner: facilitator (therapist), sounding board, resource, instructor, negotiator, case manager, and advocate. These roles may overlap and they may have to be utilized in "nontraditional" services, services that develop an informal and nonthreatening relationship before intervention takes place.

The formation of a helping relationship is an important step in the intervention process. Helping relationships may take on special meaning for older persons with limited opportunities for intimacy. Forming relationships with minority aged may require particular sensitivity on the part of the provider.

Several dynamics are likely to be encountered in any intervention: resistance, dependency, transference/countertransference, anger, and difficulties in termination. In addition, the practitioner has ethical responsibilities in working with the elderly that should be carefully understood by both parties.

A general approach to working with the elderly should include empathy or perhaps detached concern. Steps in the intervention process include: entry, exploration of problems, formal assessment of problems, establishment of goals, working towards goals, and termination.

Many strategies and approaches can be used in intervention with the elderly. One way of evaluating approaches is to examine their goals, focus, targeted population, and strengths and weaknesses.

9

Psychodynamic Approaches

THEORETICAL PERSPECTIVE

Psychoanalysis is the treatment modality most often associated with psychodynamic approaches. This therapeutic approach is based on several premises: that personality systems (id, ego, and superego) interact to determine current behavior; that maladaptive behavior stems from unfinished resolution of prior conflicts (e.g., the Oedipal relationship); that defenses (ineffective patterned responses that partially decrease anxiety arising from unresolved early conflicts) are unconsciously controlled; and that the way to improve functioning is to help the patient uncover his or her unconscious conflicts in order to achieve insight and to strengthen the patient's ego so that he or she has more options in handling reality.

The approach of traditional psychodynamic therapy is unstructured. The therapist lets the client talk about whatever comes to mind, using free association to allow unconscious thoughts to emerge. The therapeutic relationship is very important and should be viewed as a recapitulation of other troublesome relationships in the patient' past (transference relationship). Through accurate and timely interpretation of the patient's reactions to the therapist, the patient's free associations, and the patient's dreams, the therapist guides the patient to achieve conscious understanding of both defensive behavior and underlying conflicts (insight). Then a process of reeducation takes place; that is, the patient learns new and more useful ways of coping with reality and with his or her own needs and drives.

Few analysts seriously consider a full analysis or personality restructuring with elderly clients. In part, this is due to beliefs that older persons cannot effectively achieve insight and work through issues that are many years old, that the aged ego (or part of the personality that interacts with the real world) is too rigid to change, that the process of change is too long, and that defense mechanisms are too ingrained in the aged. It may also be due to fears or unresolved issues the analyst has about her or his own aging, grandparents, or death. However, aspects of traditional psychoanalytic approaches have been used with the elderly.

For purposes of this text, *psychodynamic approaches* presuppose that events in the past influence how an individual views current reality. Also, gaining an understanding and appreciation of "old" conflicts (insight) can lead to substantive changes in feelings, self-concept, and behavior. The symbolic relationship with the therapist (transference relationship) is an important tool in dynamic approaches, as a source of either insight or support to the client.

Insight Versus Supportive Therapy

Insight   Achieving insight is a major step in psychodynamic therapy. The major ways of gaining insight are through discussing current problems and viewing the transference relationship in light of earlier experiences. By understanding that past experiences have lead to the current situation and to how he or she interprets or perceives current reality, the client achieves insight into his or her behavior and emotional reactions. Insight, while not the end of the therapeutic process, is a benchmark of successful treatment in psychodynamic therapy.

There are two questions to be asked of the value of insight to older clients. The first is whether the older client is capable of achieving insight: Does the client have a degree of awareness and the mental ability to achieve an understanding of how he or she has responded in "historic" and defensive ways to current situations? Some older clients may have great capacity for insight. For others, especially those with dementia or whose current life situation is so stressful that they cannot "free" any energy for an examination of their unconscious motives and patterns of behavior, insight may not be appropriate as a treatment goal.

The second question is to what purpose insight might be used by an older person (Verwoerdt, 1976). If a person has lived his or her life in a manner that can be considered "defensive" and has few options to change it, it can be argued that insight would lead to depression rather than significant change in behavior.

Supportive Therapy   Alexander (1944) has suggested that a particular form of treatment not involving insight is appropriate for the elderly. The underlying personality dynamics are not explored with the client nor are they interpreted or altered; rather, the therapist works to provide supports so that the client achieves maximum comfort and adaptation to his or her problems.

For example, in cases of anxiety, a supportive approach focuses on establishing a positive relationship and then working on ways to decrease anxiety such as providing services, social contact, or encouraging a style that gives the client a sense of mastery over his or her environment (Verwoerdt, 1976). The key aspect of supportive therapy is developing a relationship that has positive transference; that is, the client gains strength from what he or she perceives to be a powerful, healing, or warm therapist.

It can be argued that supportive therapy encompasses everything included in humanistic and behavioral approaches. However, it differs philosophically in that personality dynamics are viewed as the critical aspects of mental health problems. The specifices and step-by-step application of supportive therapy have not been well spelled out, leaving much of "what to do" in the hands of the mental health practitioner. Acknowledgement of a non-insight approach does, however, allow dynamically oriented mental health practitioners a bridge to alternative approaches.

PSYCHODYNAMIC INTERVENTIONS WITH THE AGED

Goldfarb's "Brief" Therapy

Goldfarb developed one particular form of psychodynamic treatment specifically for use with the elderly (Goldfarb & Turner, 1953). Goldfarb argues that a brief and simple approach is necessary, especially with older clients who have few resources and a limited life expectency.

His approach was to use short sessions (no more than fifteen minutes) spaced as widely as possible. The goal, not unlike that of "supportive approaches," was to provide emotional support and build high self-esteem. The key to this treatment was that the therapist not only accepted the role of powerful, protective parental figure but actually encouraged the client to project the role on him (transference relationship). Then, rather than working through this relationship to increase insight, Goldfarb suggested using the relationship as a way of giving the client strength through avenues such as "defeating" the therapist (venting anger and still having the therapist show concern).

Goldfarb also pointed out that staff in facilities needed to be included in respecting the therapist's role as a powerful authority. In addition, he emphasized the need to use a "continuous or recurrent reinforcing technique" (p. 918) with brain-damaged patients and pointed out that specific strategies of using this approach may have to be expanded for nonorganically impaired clients.

Goldfarb's method, while not stringently validated or widely used today, has potential value in work with organically impaired elderly. The data in his study were encouraging in terms of clients' improvement (about half of a small number improved) with a minimal investment of therapists' time. The power of the mental health practitioner-client relationship should not be overlooked in working with older adults.

Evaluation The goal of Goldfarb's approach is adaptive, helping the older person cope with disability or decline. It focuses on self-concept in that its goal is to improve the client's sense of power. It is targeted towards a specific group (institutionalized patients who have verbal ability). Its strengths are its efficacy (requiring little time), ease of implementation, ease of use in hospital or nursing home settings, and some sense of proven value. Its disadvantages are a lack of clarity on specifically how to apply its principles, limited flexibility (its goals and focus are on certain "broad" issues, but it may not be effective for more specific problems in other areas), and a lack of scientific data on its validity.

Butler's Life Review Therapy

A somewhat different approach to providing mental health service and support to the aged has been suggested by Butler (1963). His approach is called life review therapy. Other elaborations have been described by Lewis and Butler (1974).

Life review therapy is a systematic review of a client's life, done either individually or in groups. While many older persons will reminisce or review their lives without prompting, both the methods and purposes of life review therapy are somewhat different from this natural tendency.

The process is not necessarily introduced by the mental health practitioner during treatment; rather, it should be developed around whatever type of analysis of previous events the client is doing. The goal is to have the older client use an analysis of her or his personal history to resolve current conflicts, old conflicts, and preoccupations. Also, the client may marshal unrealized strengths to cope with life cycle issues and integration of the totality of his or her life.

Butler and Lewis suggest the following methods to aid the life review: autobiography (either taped or written); visiting locations of significant events in one's life; reunions (both formal and informal); developing a family tree or geneology (see Edinberg, 1978, for a therapeutic approach to creating family history); using albums, letters or scrapbooks; having the client formally summarize his or her life (this can turn into poems, books, or publishable works); and emphasizing an ethnic or racial identity.

Through these methods a client can be encouraged to review significant events in her or his life. Unresolved conflicts may be brought directly into the review or ignored. The mental health practitioner needs to be aware of obvious omissions and distortions, such as talking about only one parent and never mentioning the other or "glorifying" a spouse or child. Some aspects of life will be painful for the client to review, but the hope is that they can be "worked through" or resolved in the process of life review. This also suggests that persons who have had particularly difficult lives may not be good candidates for life review.

The mental health practitioner's role in this review is multifacted: to aid the client in achieving new insight (and resultant peace of mind); to put closure on troublesome events from the past; to view earlier events from a new perspective; and to help rekindle lost interests or abilities. The mental health practitioner thus needs to use both empathic and interpretive skills in life review therapy.

Chubon (1980) has used a "bibliographic" approach to life review. She describes a case where a client read a novel with several similarities to her life and then discussed the novel and her life in counseling sessions. Greene (1982), in another variation, has used life review with a daughter and father present together is sessions. Through the father's review of his life, both he and the daughter were reported to clarify their roles in the family and understand the family's dynamics.

While the purposes of life review are explicit, the techniques are somewhat general and require significant variation for each individual. Because many formats and approaches can be used, life review can also be adapted for use in many settings and circumstances, such as nursing homes, senior centers, or college oral-history projects.

Evaluation   The goals of life review therapy are curative (resolution of old conflicts) and adaptive (marshalling forgotten strengths to handle current circumstances). The focus is on attitudes and values and, subsequently, affect. The target group is clients who have sufficient verbal skills and cognitive ability both to recall previous events and achieve some insight into them. It is also aimed at persons who have had enough positive experiences in life so that the life review will not be a depressing experience.

One of the main strengths of this approach is that it encourages clients to "get their life in order." Few other interventions have this purpose, an important task of aging. Also, the approach is quite flexible, allowing the therapist ample freedom to tailor it to the individual client or client group.

Its disadvantages are a lack of clarity in how to apply its procedures and techniques, an overreliance on "clinical judgment" on how to use it, little scientific validity, and its limited utility in handling specific problems, such as adapting to organic dysfunction. It is unclear how life review might benefit persons with reactive depression or conflicts with others (e.g., family members). In part, the answer to its usefulness lies in the degree to which one believes that understanding historical conflicts leads to improvements in current functioning.

Reminiscence

Butler's life review therapy is based on a well-accepted "fact," that older adults are capable of and interested in remembering previous events and talking about them. This tendency to reminisce is occasionally a source of irritation to others (e.g., "Grandma's telling that same old story again"). However, mental health professionals have begun to appreciate two aspects of reminiscence that have been overlooked: (1) that reminiscence can serve a positive purpose for the client; and (2) that it be used as a vehicle for promoting self-worth and shared experiences, goals that might not be accomplished through other techniques or approaches (Ebersole, 1978a, 1978b; Ellison, 1981; Lesser et al. 1981).

In analytic theory, early memories have a certain power—the power of the forces and conflicts that cause them to be imprinted and remembered or forgotten (repressed). Repressed memories may be the source of drives in middle life. Verbal review of memories can be "cathartic"; that is, the process of remembering and talking has a potential therapeutic value. By discussing old memories and achieving a "new perspective" on them, a client can make substantial internal changes (Ebersole, 1978a; Kaminsky, 1978).

At the same time, some cautions should be noted: Reminiscing has not been clearly tied to specific affective and cognitive processes. We do not know if it is the process of remembering or the actual memories that have value. Nor is it clear that people who are "good" at reminiscing are any more adjusted than those who are not. It is thus important to consider reminiscence a tool rather than an end in itself (Merriam, 1980).

Purpose   In addition to possible cathartic or therapeutic values, reminiscence can be used as an approach to working with the elderly for the following purposes:

Creating a sense of age identity for clients.

Bringing forth strengths, resources, or affect not found in current life circumstances. For example, the author (as well as others) has used reminiscence and "imagination" to recreate the feelings of being at a dance hall for wheelchair-bound elders.

Passing on values, impressions, or reactions to "old" events (sense of legacy).

Socializing and social participation, especially in groups of the same age. Having lived through certain historical events (the Great Depression, World War I) or local events and changes creates an opportunity for sharing.

Stimulation. Many institutional environments are somewhat unstimulating. The use of reminiscence can temporarily stimulate memory and other cognitive abilities (e.g., discussing why certain events took place, or what would have happened if some local event had happened differently).

Enjoyment. Sharing old jokes, vaudeville routines, or humorous events in the past can be therapeutic in drab or sad present circumstances.

Observing others. In groups where reminiscence is used, clients can gain from each other as observers as well as participants. There is potential benefit in listening to others' lives as a way of gaining perspective or insight into one's own.

Providing a framework for understanding or adapting to current problems and new situations.

Raising self-esteem by participating in reminiscence as an equal or a "resource" to others. By having access to information that others do not have and by remembering successes and positive experiences, self-esteem can be enhanced.

Structures and Techniques   While reminiscence can be used as an adjunct technique for several therapeutic approaches, the following discussion focuses on reminiscence as a major format or approach in work with the aged.

Reminiscence may take place spontaneously (e.g., at a social occasion or meal) or formally, often in groups. The duration of a group will have a strong effect on its goals. Short-term groups (fewer than ten sessions) should focus on immediate, specific group or member needs rather than attempting to resolve long-standing problems. Short-term groups should be small (fewer than seven numbers) for maximum input from members (Ebersole, 1978a, 1978b).

Along with general considerations in group work with the elderly (see Chapter 12), there are several issues and techniques in reminiscence that should be considered before beginning reminiscence work. The first question is whether to structure the content and focus of sessions. In part, this will be influenced by clients' understanding of the purpose of the sessions as well as the goals of reminiscence. A group (or individual clients) who expect to simply sit around and talk about "the old days" will respond differently from a group that expects to review past experiences to learn to appreciate themselves better. In addition, it would appear useful to provide structure when the groups are going to meet for a short time or when group members are reticent to share because they are inexperienced in groups (Ebersole, 1978a, 1978b).

Methods of structuring can include choosing a specific topic (or having clients think about a topic before the session), picking an area (historical events, holidays, seasons, etc.), having one client decide on a topic for the session, or even using a developmental framework such as early childhood, childhood, adolescence, adulthood, middle age, and old age. There should be a balance between specificity and generality. If the structure is too specific, some clients may not have any relevant memories at hand (e.g., "Remember June 4, 1936?"). If the structuring is too general, there will be little commonality and basis for sharing.

A second issue is how to handle "negative" reminiscences. Most people have both positive and negative memories. Feelings of guilt, anger, despair, regret, or sadness will be parts of reminiscence sessions. The mental health practitioner has several options when "negative" memories are expressed: to comfort (either physically, visually, or verbally), to encourage further expression of feeling (using silence, minimal reinforcement such as "um hm," or focusing on feelings), or to move the client away from the memory (subtly changing the topic, changing the focus of the client from affect to specifics of the situation, or asking others in the group for related memories). The type of approach (comfort, deepening the feeling, moving away) should depend on the mental health practitioner's assessment of the client's needs. Some clients need to vent or express pent up feelings, some need to be comforted, some need to learn how to distance themselves from overwhelming experiences (Ingersoll & Goodman, 1980). The mental health practitioner also needs to be sensitive to the timing of interventions. When comfort is given can be as important as how it is given. Finally, the mental health practitioner needs to be able to assess whether or not an intervention is done out of his or her own anxiety about the client's situation (countertransference) or is done for the client's benefit.

A third issue is how to introduce topics. There are many aids that can be used to introduce and guide reminiscing. The following list of approaches is not exhaustive. Mental health practitioners will have to adapt it to particular circumstances as well as create their own approaches. Aids in introducing reminiscence include:

1. Music
   Sing-a-long (with our without accompaniment)
   Records
   Entertainer
   Discussing dance halls, big bands, etc.
2. Scents
   Spices
   Having a snack food, discussing food and special occasions
   Flowers
   Perfumes
3. Imaging based on affect
   Asking group members to remember a particular event—when they were happy, sad, scared, etc.
4. Imaging based on social interactions
   Asking clients to remember a holiday get-together, a time when they went out with other people, a time when they were alone, etc.
5. Cohort events
   Asking clients to remember how they lived through the Great Depression, World War I, World War II, etc.
6. Memorabilia
   Pictures from magazines
   Clothing
   Models (old automobiles)
   Household appliances (butter churns, meat grinder)
   Antiques
   Election buttons
   Old newspaper headlines (copied from a library)
7. Personal items
   Photograph albums
   Knick-knacks
8. Movies, slides recordings of old political speeches, news, etc.

An additional issue is the potential dangers in reminiscence. The concern, also present in life review therapy, is that a client may "uncover" unpleasant memories or become "stuck" in the past with a resultant loss of confidence and self-worth and an increase in feelings of depression. In part, this concern may be a projection of the mental health practitioner's fears that he or she cannot help a client or that the client's pain is overwhelming. Yet there is a risk and responsibility in going into the past that cannot be overlooked. The risk is that unpleasant memories will be stirred up without positive change. The responsibility is for the mental health practitioner to take the necessary time to instill hope, a new perspective, confidence, and a helping relationship to minimize the dangers and maximize the positive benefits of reminiscence.

Other Approaches   Ryden (1981) suggests four guidelines in reminiscence work: (1) *initiating reminiscence* by using open-ended questions and involving clients in activities that lead to reminiscence; (2) *reinforcing reminiscence* by praise or nonverbal behavior; (3) *helping the client cope with feelings* uncovered in reminiscence; (4) *helping family* cope with both the act of reminiscence and the feelings that are brought up in the process.

Fry (1983) found greater gains in ego strength and decreases in depressive symptoms by using a highly structured approach to reminiscence rather than unstructured reminiscence. The purpose of the structuring was to help clients come to grips with strong feelings and unresolved concerns that may be avoided in a less structured experience.

Fry's steps are:

1. Relating both positive and negative feelings about the event being discussed
2. Reviewing reactions to persons, events, or objects related to the event
3. Relating thoughts and images that came to mind while reminiscing
4. Relating "hopes, anxieties and fears associated to the event" (p. 22)
5. Relating dreams connected to the event
6. Relating wishes for (or against) interaction with others in the event
7. Relating "unresolved" feelings (e.g., guilt, anger, desire to avoid others)
8. Relating specifically what was done during the event

Although the work of Fry and Ryden overlap the approach used by Ebersole, one advantage of using their more structured approaches is that the client is given tools to "go after" unresolved issues in a systematic manner that may move therapy along more efficiently than if no structure is given.

Evaluation   Because reminiscence is as much a tool or technique as a therapeutic approach, it can be used in curative, adaptive, and enrichment interventions. Its focus is on attitude/values and affect, although one can argue that it can be used to help people use their "memories." In the latter case, it may be difficult to decide the validity of the events "remembered." Ideally, reminiscence promotes a feeling of self-esteem and can be used to elicit pleasant feelings. In group settings, it also can lead to increased socialization and give the client a positive role, that of storyteller. It can be used with older persons of all degrees of social, physical, and mental abilities, although some variations are needed for persons with cognitive difficulties, usually in the form of providing a more highly structured experience.

The strengths of reminiscence are its flexibility, ease of application, potential integration into many types of interventions, applicability with various groups, and capacity to instill curative factors (e.g., hope, positive roles, self-esteem) in settings where there are few opportunities for such attributes to develop. Its weaknesses lie in some uncertainty about its scientific value and a related uncertainty about the specific values and processes involved in "reminiscence."

EVALUATION
OF PSYCHODYNAMIC INTERVENTIONS

Goals

The goals of psychodynamic interventions are either curative or adaptive. Most literature addressing the elderly argues for an adaptive approach, rather than focusing on substantial reorganization of the older person's personality.

Focus

Psychodynamic interventions focus primarily on attitudes and values, that is, uncovering and achieving insight into prior conflicts and unconsciously determined defenses in hope of developing more effective ways of coping with current realities. Insight, while limited in Goldfarb's approach, should be considered an important objective in life review and reminiscence. The power of the transference relationship is also important and should be considered as affecting the therapeutic process regardless of the type of intervention approach used.

Targeted Groups

Depending on the type of intervention used, psychodynamic interventions can be used with many different groups of elderly. Goldfarb's approach is designed for impaired older persons. Life review is more likely to be useful with clients who have capacity for insight and good verbal and cognitive ability. Reminiscence can be adapted for any level of functioning.

Strengths and Weaknesses

The strengths of psychodynamic approaches lie in their potential flexibility and focus on areas not directly addressed by other types of intervention. The past is viewed as a source of potential strength and personal resources that can be marshalled to handle current difficulties.

One weakness of these approaches is that the techniques and strategies are rarely spelled out with any specificity, reminiscence being one exception. It becomes difficult for the individual who does not have extensive psychodynamic training to understand how to use interpretation or analyze defenses and unconscious functioning.

Also, there are some inherent difficulties in evaluating dynamic approaches and interventions with the aged. Because the focus of dynamic interventions is change and insight into internal events (personality structure), any measure of change should ideally address these events rather than symptoms or behavior. Much of the evidence supporting psychodynamic approaches are single case studies rather than scientific analysis of treatment with appropriate controls.

In a review of studies of dynamic approaches, Götestam (1980) points out that few use control groups. Almost all rely on clinical ratings by experts (therapists, nurses). Only two studies (Wolff, 1967; Godbole & Verinis, 1974) can be considered scientific, and of these two, the latter used patients with physical rather than emotional problems and the former was not well designed. A more recent study (Lazarus et al., 1982) found that "brief dynamic" treatment can be effective with older persons.

Concepts and aspects of dynamic interventions do enjoy a certain degree of popularity and use in many settings serving older adults. Reminiscing, formal or informal life review, focusing on internal dynamics, and insight approaches are undoubtedly employed by many mental health practitioners as one part of their treatment. These approaches are theoretically well grounded. Their efficacy, however, is unproven at present.

A final note should be made about Goldfarb's brief therapy approach. The idea that very brief encounters over a period of time that use the curative power of the therapist-client relationship seems supported by clinical evidence (Götestam, 1980), as well as current thinking about placebo effects and other aspects of healing relationships discussed in Chaper 2.

SUMMARY AND CONCLUSIONS

Psychodynamic approaches are based on several assumptions about maladaptive behavior: that it is the result of unconscious conflicts of historical origin; that insight into unconscious motives is important in changing behavior; and that the relationship with the therapist, the transference relationship, is important as a recapitulation of prior conflicts in the individual's life. Through interpretation and review of historical (past) experiences, the client is made aware of unconscious conflicts and can develop new ways of coping with reality.

Psychoanalysis and the resolution of major unresolved conflicts in the past are usually not treatments of choice with the elderly. However, older persons have the capacity to gain varying degress of insight into their problems. Life review and reminiscence are two therapeutic approaches that capitalize on insight and the tendency for older persons to discuss the past. Goldfarb's brief therapy approach was developed to use a positive transference between patient and therapist to provide a source of strength and identity to persons with cognitive and physical loss.

There are a range of applications for psychodynamic approaches. Some evidence suggests that brief therapy approaches may have value, but the goals of treatment (internal changes) are hard to verify, leading to a lack of scientific evidence supporting their efficacy. Life review and reminiscence have particular value in that they focus on areas not usually considered in other systems of therapy and can be incorporated into other approaches.

10

Behavioral and Cognitive Approaches

THEORETICAL PERSPECTIVE

The major theoretical tenets of traditional behavioral approaches are: mental health problems are learned by the same principles that all behavior is learned; the principles by which all behavior is learned are the appropriate ones to change "abnormal" behavior; overt behavior, not the subjective, internal experience of the client, is the focus of treatment; and problems are resolved by learning different and less distressful responses or behavior (Bandura, 1969; Craighead, Kazdin, & Mahoney, 1976; Rimm & Masters, 1974). Behaviorists have also begun to include thoughts and thought patterns (cognition) as a focus of therapy (e.g., Mahoney, 1974). However, rather than focusing on the interpretation of thoughts or uncovering their meanings, a cognitive-behavioral approach attempts to change or eliminate maladaptive thought patterns by working directly on the pattern, by substituting other patterns, or by decreasing the frequency of the maladaptive pattern.

There is also a spirit of pragmatism and parsimony in behavioral and cognitive therapies. That is, certain methods, such as imagery, will be used because they can be shown to work. Methods that do not work are not used. Parsimony implies initially using the least intrusive and simplest methods to solve problems and moving to more elaborate procedures only if these fail.

A final theoretical concern is that of the scientific approach; that is, the methods and techniques of behavioral and cognitive therapies should be rigorously tested and be replicated to prove their value.

BEHAVIORAL APPROACHES WITH THE AGED: TECHNIQUES AND STRATEGIES

In theory, a behavioral approach used with an older client should not be any different from that used with a younger person. The principles by which learning takes place are the same and can theoretically be applied with any clients of any age. Appropriate assessment of a problem should lead to a treatment plan that uses reinforcement of incompatible responses, shaping desired behavior, or learning new skills by applying the concepts described in the following sections. The following principles and examples of strategies are discussed in light of their potential and actual use with the elderly.

Assessment

An accurate assessment of the problem and client are critical for effective behavioral intervention. An excellent general framework for assessment, that of Kanfer and Saslow (1965, 1969), was reviewed in Chapter 7. Along with the issues addressed in that chapter, the following concerns need to be examined before behavioral interventions:

Antecedents of Behavior   The antecedents of behavior are the events and circumstances immediately preceding the problem behavior. Some antecedents are *temporal* (e.g., a certain time of the day). Some are related to *location*: the behavior occurs at a certain place. Others may be *cognitive*—that is, the client may think a certain thought pattern or feel a certain way. Still others may be *social*—that is, others may act in a way that triggers problem behavior. Any or all may be important in maintaining problem behavior.

Consequences of "Problem" Behavior   One key question about any problem behavior is: "If it is such a problem, why is it being maintained?" It is critical to examine the positive rewards resulting from the client's behavior. One approach is to change "outcomes" until the problem behavior ceases. Take, for example, the case of an older client in a nursing home who continually stands, holds a rail in a hall, starts to teeter, and screams, "I'm going to fall, I'm going to fall." He creates excitement in that several staff run over to catch him. However, when one staff member stays with the resident, is the only person to respond to the teetering and crying for help, and does so calmly, the teetering and calling for help disappear (are extinguished). In this case changing the "positive" consequences (now there is no big commotion) extinguished the problem behavior.

Specifying Problem Behavior   More than any other approach, behavioral interventions attempt to specify the problem behavior *before* intervention takes place. How often does the "problem" behavior occur? How intense is it (or does it feel)? What specifically does the person say, do, or feel that is the problem?

Classical Conditioning Techniques

Classical conditioning approaches have been used with a range of behavioral problems of the elderly (e.g., Cautela, 1969). Classical conditioning refers to the learning process by which neutral cues (or stimuli) becomes associated with emotional reactions. Two techniques that are frequently used in reconditioning emotional responses are systematic desensitization and relaxation.

Systematic Desensitization

The techniques used in desensitization are among the most carefully researched behavioral approaches to mental health problems. They are ordinarily employed to help clients handle anxiety-provoking situations (Kanfer & Phillips, 1970; Rimm & Masters, 1974; Wolpe, 1958). The idea behind desensitization is that by introducing an incompatible response (usually relaxation) to anxiety-provoking situations, the degree of anxiety diminishes. By slowly reconditioning the client to relax in increasingly difficult situations, the anxiety-provoking situation can become anxiety-free.

The process of systematic desensitization has three steps (Craighead, Kazdin, & Mahoney, 1976):

1. *Developing an incompatible response to anxiety.* Usually, the incompatible response is one of deep muscle relaxation, although assertion or other responses can be used. Establishing incompatible responses can take several weeks of practice.
2. *Developing a hierarchy of anxiety-producing situations.* Usually, client fears are around a single event (fear of elevators, airplanes, etc.) or a class of events (talking to other people, going out in public). The mental health practitioner and client need carefully to break down classes of events into discrete graded steps (hierarchy). Each step should represent an increasing degree of anxiety, the initial step being one with little or no anxiety for the client. The hierarchy may include time, proximity or thematic aspects. One rule of thumb is that if a client has subsequent trouble moving from one step to another, additional steps or variations may be needed, such as presenting the scene for a shorter period of time or altering it.
3. *Presenting the hierarchy with the new incompatible response so that anxiety is inhibited.* Usually, this is first accomplished in imagination, starting with the client being relaxed (incompatible response to anxiety) and then moving in imagination up each step of the hierarchy, relaxing before each scene is imagined. The client should be relaxed before imagining a specific scene and should not be moved to a subsequent scene until she or he feels completely relaxed imagining the current scene.

Some clients seem able to go through the steps of a hierarchy in their imagination and remain relaxed, yet they still exhibit anxiety in real-life situations. In such cases the mental health practitioner might include real-life steps (actual encounters with the feared object) as part of the hierarchy and have the client go through them, relaxing before each one, and again only continuing up the hierarchy if the client is completely relaxed in the current step. The practitioner may also participate as a model or source of reassurance in both imagining and real-life steps. The pacing of scenes, time spent with each scene, and session spacing may be varied to ensure maximum benefit.

Evaluation   The goals of desensitization are curative within the philosophical position of behaviorism. That is, by decreasing and elminating symptoms, the disorder is "cured." The focus is on physiological behavior and, secondarily, cognition, as the techniques attempt to decrease the experience of anxiety. The targeted population would be those who have anxiety reactions and have the mental capacity to construct a hierarchy. A further consideration is that the client be willing to practice desensitization on his or her own, suggesting a high level of motivation for change. The strengths of the approach are its proven efficacy with all age groups and the specificity of techniques and outcomes. Its weaknesses are that it requires substantial abilities on the part of the client and can be used in a mechanistic manner, ignoring other more pervasive problems.

Relaxation

Relaxation training is an integral component in many systematic desensitization programs. It can also be used to relieve sleep problems and certain physiological and psychosomatic symptoms, including hypertension and pain control.

Relaxation training is done in several ways. One is to teach the client to associate the feelings of being relaxed with cue words, such as "calm" or "meditate" (e.g., Paul & Bernstein, 1976). This is accomplished by having a client relax and repeat the cue word while exhaling. After several such pairings, the cue word can be used to elicit the feelings of relaxation in a real-life situation.

The method most frequently used in behavioral approaches to help clients relax is based on Jacobson's (1938) successive relaxation techniques. In this approach, groups of muscles are systematically tightened for about ten seconds and then relaxed for a slightly longer period of time. Clients should be told to focus their attention on the muscles being tightened while the rest of the body relaxes and not to exert any painful muscle groups. At the end of the relaxing sequence, the client should be instructed to go back and "redo" any tight muscle groups. Clients can also signal by hand how much tension they feel at the end of the session as the mental health practitioner counts from one to ten (ten representing maximum anxiety) (cf. Rimm & Masters, 1974, for a more complete description of the procedure.)

Although it is not necessary to follow a particular pattern, it is beneficial to include these muscle groups:

1. Head (turn to right to tense, back to relax)
2. Face
3. Eyes (open wide, then relax; close, then relax)
4. Mouth (open, then relax; close tightly, relax)
5. Neck (move head to chest, then up; drop head back, then up)
6. Shoulders (forward, then relax; back, then relax)
7. Arms (biceps, then triceps)
8. Forearms
9. Hands
10. Chest
11. Back
12. Stomach
13. Buttocks
14. Pelvic area
15. Upper legs
16. Lower legs
17. Feet

Relaxation training can take as long as an hour; the length of a session will depend on the client's ability to tense and relax muscle groups. Some older clients will have difficulty focusing on one area, in which case initial sessions might be spent on working on a few muscle groups. Also, one implied concept of relaxation training is that clients can learn to discriminate between tension and relaxation, become aware of muscle tension, and learn to consciously relax tense necks, backs, arms, stomachs, or arms. The process of learning to focus on a tight muscle group and relax it has benefit in and of itself.

A final consideration is the use of prompts in relaxation training. The mental health practitioner can talk the client through relaxation, telling the client directly to clench or tighten muscles, feel the tension, then relax and feel the relaxation as the client goes through the process. The mental health practitioner can use both verbal cues and nonverbal aspects of the voice (pitch, speed, volume) to help create the sense of tension or relaxation for the client. Also, the pace and speed of instructions must to be slow enough so that the client can experience both the tensing and relaxing feelings.

The following case is an example of how a mental health practitioner used some of these concepts:

Case: Mrs. Spinoli, and Italian-born woman in her late seventies, spoke broken English and was relatively isolated, having one friend visit and not going anywhere by herself. She had few social contacts and lived in her own house. Mrs. Spinoli wanted to go out by herself; however, she became extremely nervous when she even considered the possibility. The first step in intervention was for the practitioner to introduce the idea of relaxation. "I have learned a method of relaxing that is both good exercise and one other people use to relax. Would you be interested in trying it next time? Think it over." At the next session Mrs. Spinoli did not discuss the question of relaxing until the end, when there was not time to do it. In the third session the practitioner raised the topic and, together with Mrs. Spinoli, went through systematic relaxation, reassuring Mrs. Spinoli that the exercise was safe and that no other demands were to be made of her at that time. During the next several sessions the client and practitioner talked and did ten to fifteen minutes of relaxation.

Eventually, the practitioner introduced both the idea of a hierarchy and desensitization: "Mrs. Spinoli, I know you can relax with me. I would like to see if you can learn to relax while thinking about the things that trouble you about going out. What I want to do with you is put them in order so that the least troublesome is first." A hierarchy was soon developed, which included going out with the practitioner, going to a senior center with the practitioner, sitting in the center with the practitioner, and, finally, talking to others in the center without the practitioner being present. The practitioner was able to combine imagination and real-life steps and get Mrs. Spinoli to a senior center where she was able to make new friends.

Evaluation Relaxation is more of a technique than an approach to treatment. As such, it can be used in curative, adaptive, enrichment, and preventive interventions. Its focus is primarily on individual internal behavior or affect, that is, the decrease of anxiety. Depending on the philosophical view of the practitioner, it can be argued that a relaxed state is a "natural" way of being, that is a step to "self-awareness," or that it is simply the absence of undue anxiety.

Relaxation has been used as part of treatment interventions with a wide range of older persons (e.g., Luce, 1979; Edinberg, 1975). With certain adaptations, parts of the technique can be used with persons of limited cognitive abilities, as well as with those who are "healthy" and functioning quite independently. With impaired elderly, care has to be taken to keep instructions clear and simple and not to require significant memory of detail.

Relaxation's strengths are its flexibility, specificity of techniques, and proven effectiveness in conjunction with other forms of treatment. Its weaknesses are few, perhaps including a theoretical concern that relaxation can be used in institutional settings to reinforce complacency when other types of treatment and stimulation are more appropriate.

Homework

Classical conditioning programs rely heavily on clients' practicing skills on their own (e.g., relaxing ten minutes a day, working on developing a hierarchy, or counting how often troublesome behavior occurs). Homework has several advantages. First, it actively involves the client in a meaningful way. Second, it gives the client a sense of control over what was previously an "unsolvable" problem. Third, it can serve to reinforce or teach useful skills in the client's home environment.

At the same time, homework tasks may be avoided or not carried out successfully. In this case careful assessment of the noncompliance is urged. Questions the practitioner should consider include: Did the client understand the assignment? Were instructions clear? Was the task one that the client is capable of doing successfully? Are intermediate steps needed? Has too much or too little time been allotted to the task? Does the client find the homework task meaningful or does he or she view it as not useful? The mental health practitioner may need to explain, convince, change instructions, change tasks, or renegotiate the client's understanding of his or her role in the process (one of "learner").

A final thought about homework is that some elderly, particularly those with little formal education, have negative feelings about their own schooling. The practitioner needs to be sensitive to any negative self-perceptions that may sabotage the effectiveness of homework.

Operant Approaches

Operant approaches have been successfully implemented with the elderly in a range of areas, including incontinence, verbal interaction, social interaction, sign-language training, walking, and activity (e.g., Libb & Clements, 1969; MacDonald & Butler, 1974; Wisocki & Mosher, 1980; Hoyer et al., 1974; see also Götestam, 1980, and Hussian, 1981, for extensive reviews). The general approach in operant procedures is:

1. Specify behavior to be changed and an acceptable/appropriate alternative
2. Identify antecedents-precursors to problem behavior
3. Identifying reinforcers (conditions taking place *after* behavior occurs that influence its frequency of occurrence) for the individual client such as:
   Food
   Social rewards (praise approval)
   Activities
   Negative reinforcers (unpleasant stimuli that can be removed upon completion of appropriate behavior)
4. Develop a strategy to facilitate learning of adaptive or alternative behavior through shaping (rewarding increasingly accurate approximations of desired behavior) and reinforcing alternative behaviors.

Several issues bear consideration in implementing these procedures with older clients:

1. *Appropriateness of desired behavior.* Especially in institutional settings, older clients are at the mercy of others for basic needs such as food, toileting, and medical care. At the same time, behavior problems may be defined by the degree to which they upset floor routine, staff sensitivities, family members, or others in the community. The practitioner should be alert to the distinct possibility that interventions will be focused on eliminating management problems rather than relieving personal discomfort or suffering. Behavioral approaches should not be used solely to create "good" (i.e., passive and quiet) patients.

2. *The client's understanding of new contingencies.* For both ethical and practical reasons, every effort should be made to inform and explain to the client what is being rewarded and how it is to be done, even if rewards are not self-initiated. An understanding of contingencies improves performance, helps internalize learning, and respects the client's rights.

3. *Involvement of significant others.* Involvement means that everyone is consistently rewarding desired behavior. Family members, staff on all shifts in institutions, friends, nonprofessional staff (including housekeeping), and other residents in long-term care settings may need an explanation of what is being done as well as training to encourage desired behavior and prevent inadvertent reinforcement of undesired behavior.

4. *Use of punishment.* Punishment is *generally* not as effective as positive reinforcement, for several reasons. Punishment can elicit strong emotional reactions. The client may avoid the person who "gives" the punishment. And, by itself, punishment does not help the client learn a new behavior.

However, when a client is self-destructive or endangering others, few practitioners would hesitate to take measures to decrease behavior such as head banging, hitting, scratching, or biting, either by verbal statements ("No!" being one of the more polite) or physical restraint. Forms of unpleasant stimulation have been successfully used with adults to help them stop smoking or overeating and to change unwanted sexual responses (cf. Kanfer & Phillips, 1970; Craighead, Kazdin, & Mahoney, 1976; Yeates, 1970).

If punishment is to be used (including taking away privileges if certain behaviors persist), it has to be considered effective only if the undesired behavior decreases. Ways to accomplish this include: punishing all occurrences of undesired behavior; telling the client the contingencies; and encouraging, shaping, and reinforcing desired responses that are incompatible with the undesired response.

Case: An aide in a nursing home was having difficulty overcoming a resident's refusal to eat. On examining the situation the aide determined that a major positive reinforcer of the problem behavior was the aide's presence and a related punishment was the aide's leaving the client. The aide then told the client, "If you are not eating, I will not come in to talk to you. Also, if we are talking during a meal and you stop eating, I will leave. I will stay with you as long as you are eating. I want you to eat and I want to be able to talk with you." After very few meals, the client self-fed and eventually the aide "faded" her presence for most parts of meals.

A Case in the Literature   There is a growing literature that describes how operant principles can be used to help older people in a variety of ways (cf. Reidel, 1974; Götestam, 1980; and Hussian, 1981). The work of MacDonald and Butler (1974) is a good example of how operant procedures can be used for a specific problem (walking) that has implications for the client's general functioning.

MacDonald and Butler demonstrated that behavioral principles can be applied to reverse certain behavior (loss of walking) that is often considered "irreversible." They argued that often this loss is induced by conditioning from others and an acceptance of the "sick role" by the patient and others. That is, the patient is passive, dependent, and not expected to regain former functioning. MacDonald and

Butler considered the acceptance of the sick role as conditioning. They then took the following steps:

1.   Collection of base line data. The authors walked to meals wheeling two clients in their wheelchairs, talked with them in the elevator, and silently wheeled them to the dining room. There was no self-initiated walking by the clients over seven days.

2.   Treatment. The authors then asked the clients to stand and helped them to walk. If a client complied, the experimenter gave praise for standing and talked with the client about topics the client enjoyed as long as the client continued walking. This took place during an elevator ride and all the way to the dining room where the experimenter would once again compliment the client for walking. With this treatment clients walked to practically every meal over twenty days. When treatment was stopped (a "reversal" condition), clients ended up in wheelchairs. Treatment was resumed again and clients began walking again.

This study gives a clear indication that the treatment package (prompting, praise, social interaction, praise upon completion) was successful. The reversal condition also demonstrated that, with twenty days of training, the new behavior did not persist without reinforcement, suggesting it was neither internalized nor likely to transfer to other situations unless the pattern of reinforcement was continued. We also do not know which parts of the package (prompts, compliments, discussion) were the key to success. Finally, the clients were not informed of the contingency. It is interesting to speculate whether or not the clients would have improved their response by being told that discussion would only take place when they walked. Clearly, how this message was conveyed would be critical in terms of whether the client interpreted it as a put-down, manipulation, or involvement in self-care.

For a similar program to be effective in the long run, two additional steps might have to be taken: (1) involving others (aides, family, staff) in giving praise, instructing the patient, and engaging in conversation in a dignified, caring manner; and (2) setting up other types of rewards so that the client would want to walk and would do so on his or her own. Sometimes a client can be encouraged to practice walking because a dance class is being held or a trip that requires some walking is being planned.

These additional steps appear simple but can be time-consuming. Getting families and staff to change their customary behavior is not necessarily easy. However, an operant approach can work for many problem areas.

Evaluation

The goal of operant approaches is often thought of as curative, that is, decreasing undesired behavior or increasing desired behavior. However, operant approaches can be adaptive, as in token economy programs, where clients, upon completing specified tasks (e.g., talking, socializing, dressing) are given rewards in the form of tokens that they can use to "purchase" desired rewards (food, goods).

The distinction between "cure" and "adaptation" becomes blurred in that there is not necessarily an attempt to "cure" the underlying "cause" of dysfunctional behavior. The theoretical stance of the behavioral approach is that the underlying cause is irrelevant to behavioral change.

Operant approaches focus on behavior, although they can be used to decrease "undesired" thoughts and increase "desired" thoughts as well. One technique used in this area is that of "thought-stopping," having the client learn to shout (internally) "stop" when an undesired (fear-producing or depressing) thought occurs. Operant techniques can be used with clients at any level of functioning, as all observations can be made without reference to any internal processes on the client's part.

Strengths include flexibility of approach, the scientific validity of the techniques, and the success with which operant approaches have been applied in institutional settings. Also, operant programs can include environmental and institutional factors that may significantly influence problematic behavior, such as wandering (Hussian, 1981). The weaknesses are similar to those of other behavioral areas, specifically the potential for misapplication in the service of institutional goals rather than the well-being of the client. Also, the nature of the approach eliminates certain areas of the client's functioning as a primary source of concern (e.g., self-concept or "putting one's life in order"), a decision that should not be made lightly.

Examples of Behavioral Programs

Reality Orientation

Reality orientation, developed by Folsom and his associates (e.g., Folsom, 1968), is a behavioral approach to working with clients with organic brain syndrome. Although the people who developed the procedures for reality orientation were not behaviorists (in fact, many were aides and nonprofessional staff), the specific procedures they developed are pragmatic, focus on behavior, and use principles of reinforcement to help clients maintain a sense of who they are (person), where they are (place), and the time of day, date, and year (time).

Reality orientation focuses on maintaining clients at their current level of functioning and actively orienting them to reality through three approaches: environmental management; teaching/training methods, and staff and family attitudes (Taulbee, 1976; *Guide for Reality Orientation*, 1974; Folsom, 1968).

Environmental Management The physical environment should be arranged so that people with organic brain syndrome have access to relevant information without continually having to ask (and annoy) staff, family, or others in the environment. This, in turn, suggests a variety of aids such as names on doors (names of rooms on doors in a house or apartment); calendars, clocks, and other reminders of time and date; and props such as notecards with instructions and information or a "reality center" in the home where keys, medication, telephone numbers, and such are kept.

Along with physical props and reminders, it is extremely helpful to develop and maintain a consistent daily routine and to create a "calm" environment. Excessive stimulation (too many visitors or too many new activities at once) may be overwhelming. Major daily events such as group meetings, meals, and daily living activities should take place at the same time each day.

Teaching/Training Methods   Along with environmental management, several teaching/training methods are used in communicating with clients to orient and reinforce oriented behavior from the clients (*Guide to Reality Orientation,* 1974; *Help Begins at Home,* undated). The procedures include:

1. Telling or reminding clients who they are, where they are, and what day, date, and time it is.
2. Talking to the client directly and distinctly, using simple sentences.
3. Correcting mistakes in orientation and rambling in a caring but direct manner.
4. Giving simple instructions one step at a time.
5. Asking for one answer at a time.
6. Immediately praising oriented responses (this may require some shaping; that is, initially praising attention to a question, then praising closer approximations to an oriented response). If a client has difficulty remembering his or her name or where he or she is, prompting, giving the answers, and asking the client to repeat them are appropriate.
7. Allowing time for the client to respond.
8. Reinforcing the attempt to respond.
9. Being consistent in steps 1 through 8.
10. Helping the client use props, a "reality board," and other aids.

A "reality board" consists of a large bulletin board giving accurate information as to time, place, date, weather, and, in some settings, the next meal. Most people using a reality orientation approach develop their own boards. The board should be placed at eye level for the elderly, including those in wheelchairs. It should be placed in a conspicuous location and be referred to during reality orientation sessions. "Answers" can be covered by pieces of paper or plastic that slide over them. A final reminder is that the information on the board needs to be updated regularly. The day of the week and date should be changed at the beginning of the work day, not later on.

Although reality orientation is ideally done throughout the day, many practitioners use *reality orientation classes,* a small daily group meeting in which the focus is reinforcement of day, date, time, place, and person. Classes ("advanced" or "basic") meet for thirty minutes. Along with basic information, the group can also work on names, word games, spelling, or any other activity that challenges the client to think, remember, and convey information. Care must be taken that tasks are neither too complicated nor too simple for clients.

The "advanced" classes use more complex materials and skills, such as reading, looking at maps, using flash cards, or playing word games.

Staff/Family Attitudes A critical aspect of reality orientation is involvement of all others in the social milieu of the client. Family, staff, and other helpers should use the same commmunication approaches as instructors in reality orientation classes (cf. Oberleder, 1969; Lamm & Folsom, 1965).

In addition, several attitudinal approaches are suggested for use with the client (cf. Oberleder, 1969; Lamm & Folsom, 1965). These approaches, collectively called *attitude therapy*, include the following:

> *Active friendliness*, to be used with withdrawn clients. Active friendliness requires constant warmth, attention, touch, and care.
>
> *Passive friendliness*, to be used with suspicious or fearful clients. Since these clients are likely to refuse active care, a more restrained approach is suggested.
>
> *Matter-of-fact attitude*, to be used with demanding or negative clients as an approach to help them take responsibility for their actions.
>
> *No-demand attitude*, to be used with angry or frantic clients. Clients are allowed to vent or express anger without any demands being put on them.

These simple guidelines are useful in helping staff and families interact with the older confused client.

Most theoretical writing about reality orientation emphasizes the need for "twenty-four-hour reality orientation." That is, the entire care-giving environment should be involved. However, involving staff and families in treatment is not a simple matter. Most of the principles of reality orientation came from the collaborative efforts of aides and staff, which meant that aides were integrally involved in the program. Too often reality orientation is taught to staff members as a rigid set of rules, which defeats the purpose of creating a sense of involvement in client care.

Evaluation Reality orientation can be thought of as being either curative or adaptive. That is, it can be used to "reverse" confusion or to maintain the individual at his or her highest level of cognitive functioning. The reversal of confusion may be considered curative only in cases where there is no underlying physical cause (e.g., senile dementia of the Alzheimer's type). Its focus is on cognitive processes; the targeted group is those persons who have cognitive loss.

The strengths of reality orientation are its specificity and the simplicity of its techniques. One potential weakness is that it can be applied mechanistically or be used in lieu of a total treatment plan for the client. The scientific validity of reality orientation has been debated, despite a fairly large number of studies that give some endorsement to its efficacy in orienting the elderly (e.g., Barnes, 1974; Citrin & Dixon, 1977; Zepelin, Wolfe, & Norris, 1981; Voelkel, 1978; Götestam, 1979). The research suggests that there are clear improvements in learning and remembering from reality orientation (Schonfield, 1980), but not necessarily in areas such as life satisfaction or other behavioral measures (MacDonald & Settin, 1978). Also, reality orientation, because of its explicit and simple procedures, can be taught to all levels of staff and family members fairly easily. Finally, reality orientation enjoys a certain widespread use, especially in nursing home settings.

However, there are also equally valid criticisms (Schonfield, 1981; Zarit, 1980; Götestam, 1980). One set of criticisms concerns the cognitive focus of reality orientation. There is little likelihood that addressing cognitive deficits will significantly delay deterioration of brain tissue. In addition, it is obvious that different processes are needed for different aspects of orientation. For example, "remembering" where one is (place) may involve recalling a name or associating it to the room in which a class is being held, whereas remembering one's own name is recalling an "unchanging" and presumedly well-learned piece of information more intertwined with one's sense of personal identity. It is not clear in reality orientation how relatively important each of these types of orienting response is, nor are specific methods presented for each type.

A second criticism has to do with the "focus" of reality orientation. Its behavioral matter-of-fact focus may overlook important symbolic meanings in "disoriented" responses. The older woman who keeps asking for her mother may be indirectly expressing a need for care that will not be addressed by telling the client her mother has been dead for twenty-years.

There are other criticisms of reality orientation. Virtually all studies have been done in institutional settings, which frequently are unstimulating and have staff who do not act therapeutically. It may be that any structural activity that gives staff a meaningful way to interact with clients would produce similar results. Despite its widespread use and simple procedures, staff do not fully understand it or use it consistently. Turnover and ineffective training are two reasons; lack of meaningful involvement in implementation is another. Reality orientation has also been criticized as being "too narrow" for managing the problems of OBS clients; a wider range of approaches is needed.

Given the research and criticisms, the status of Reality Orientation can best be summarized as follows: The idea of consistently reinforcing oriented responses seems valid and useful. However, care must be taken to ensure cooperation from others in the environment and more needs to be done to develop a complete plan for helping OBS clients cope with their circumstances.

Social Skills and Assertion Training

Many of the principles, techniques, and approaches used in behavioral interventions have focused on socialization skills in the aged (e.g., Hoyer et al., 1974; Berger & Rose, 1977). The key to their success lies in specifying the type and content of skills to be used, having the client practice specific aspects of the skill with feedback from a therapist or other persons, and then having the client try the new skill in a social situation. As was mentioned earlier, in institutional settings the types of skills may include verbalization, starting a conversation or otherwise engaging in social interaction. However, the form of social skills training most commonly used in the community, assertion training, may have limited utility in institutional settings, since the desired outcome (assertive behavior) may be poorly understood and be negatively rewarded by staff.

One of the more popular forms of social skills training in community settings is *assertion training*. The goals of assertion training are three-fold: improving ability to obtain material and social rewards; decreasing interpersonal stress; and improving self-perception (Rimm & Masters, 1974; MacDonald, 1975). Assertion can be defined as behavior that "(1) has both verbal and nonverbal components, (2) occurs in an interpersonal context; (3) is an expression of one's needs, wishes, feelings, or rights; (4) is performed in such a way as to respect the rights and feelings of others and (5) promotes the likelihood that others will respond (positvely) to the person's feelings, needs, wishes, and/or rights" (Edinberg, 1975, p. 9).

Assertion is differentiated from aggression—not respecting the rights of others and attempting to dominate them—and from nonassertiveness (passivity)—self-negation or inhibition in stating one's preferences or wishes (cf. Alberti & Emmons, 1970). There are several "types" of assertive response, such as saying no to an unreasonable request, accepting a compliment, confronting a salesperson or repairperson, giving negative feedback, or even initiating a conversation. Also, assertion is situation-specific; that is, an older person may be unassertive in one situation but assertive in another (Edinberg, Karoly, & Gleser, 1977). In addition, successful assertive behavior means that the client can maintain assertion even if the other person in a situation is unwilling to cooperate or is otherwise obstructive to the client's achieving his or her goals.

There have been a few reports of the effectiveness of assertion with the elderly, each suggesting that techniques can be adapted for individual clients (e.g., Wheeler, 1980; Corby, 1975). The principles and techniques described below, which have been used with the elderly (Edinberg, 1975), do not differ substantially from those used with other populations.

Techniques in Assertion Training with the Aged The Senior's Assertion *Manual* (SAM) (Edinberg, 1975) uses the following approach for an eight-session group training program. Each session has a group exercise, followed by individual practice on predetermined situations in sessions 2 through 5, or individual's situations in sessions 6 through 8. The group exercises are: introducing oneself to the group, discrimination training (learning why one is unassertive in specific situations), eye contact and nonverbal aspects, voice loudness, agreeing with a compliment and saying no to unreasonable requests, asking for repetition of unclear statements, self-evaluation training, and giving (as well as receiving) positive feedback.

The specific situations that all clients practice are situations in which it is appropriate for older adults to be assertive (Edinberg, Karoly, & Gleser, 1977). The situations are:

1. You are in a grocery store. You have just paid for seven dollars worth of groceries with a ten dollar bill. The clerk should give you three dollars change, but only gives you two. What do you say or do?
2. You have just received a medical checkup at a doctor's office. As you are getting dressed, the doctor comes in. He says, "Well, you might have some high blood pressure." What do you say or do?
3. You receive a phone call from a man who says he is with the banking commission. He asks you to take money from your account to catch a teller who is a crook. He will come by, pick up the money, and, when the crook is caught, give you a $300 reward. What do you say to him when he asks, "When can I come by for the money?"
4. You are at home one night. The phone rings. It is a family member who lives nearby. You are delighted to hear from him or her. You also know you are low on food and need someone to help you shop. When the relative asks, "Is there anything you need from us?" what do you do or say?

The techniques used for practicing situations are as follows:

1. Internal rehearsal (imagining oneself performing the scene)
2. Modeling (Bandura, 1969) (leader demonstrates)
3. Verbal rehearsal (saying response out loud)
4. Covert rehearsal (talking to oneself)
5. Performance (leader or other can "probe," test)
6. Feedback from others
7. Repetition of steps 2 through 6 if necessary

An additional step is to clarify the situation carefully. Is it one in which assertion is appropriate? How can the client continue to be assertive if the "other" does not relent or acknowledge the client's concerns?

Case: Mrs. Gomez, a Cuban-born woman, is sixty-five years old. She had been having serious difficulties caring for her husband, who had many problems, including not being able to swallow food. He would spend some time in the hospital and then come home, demanding that his wife wait on him every minute, even though it was not indicated by his medical situation. Mrs. Gomez discussed the problem in a group working on problems in being assertive. Both she and other members agreed she had a right to some time of her own. She practiced how to tell her husband that she needed to go to the senior center and subsequently reported that she did so with positive results: She was able to take more time for herself.

Evaluation   The goal of assertion training is adaptive, as is the goal for other social skills training. Its focus is on socialization, and to a lesser degree, cognition and affect as they relate to current defects in social skills. The targeted group is persons who are "unassertive," that is, who lack the ability to speak up for what they want or need in certain situations. Applications of social skills training in institutional settings should be carefully constructed so that the targeted goals are supported in the environment. The strengths of social skills training is its proven efficacy and focus on areas that can be considered as needs of many older adults both within and outside of institutions. The weaknesses are similar to those of other behavioral approaches, that targeted behavior may not be the most important to the client and that internal aspects are implictly considered peripheral.

COGNITIVE APPROACHES

Cognitive therapies focus on internal thoughts that lead to abnormal or unpleasant behavior. There has been a merging of cognitive and behavioral approaches in the last decade to create the so-called cognitive-behavioral approach. At the same time, little has been written of attempts to apply these approaches to the elderly (Storandt, 1983), although in a few instances these techniques have been reported as being effective (e.g., Haley, 1983a; Steuer, 1982; Gallagher and Thompson, 1983).

Cognitive psychology has uncovered certain general processes by which a client may "create" unpleasant thoughts or behavior. These include (Craighead, Kazdin, & Mahoney, 1976):

Attribution: the processes by which cause is linked to events
Placebo and demand characteristics: responding to a situation with an expectation of success or failure *or* responding to certain aspects of a situation due to subtle suggestion by authority figures
Problem solving: examining how clients attempt to solve their difficulties
Mediation: usually verbal internal thoughts that influence the response to the external environment

Any of these processsses may be "faulty"—that is, used to distort reality. Cognitive approaches are designed to help clients uncover faulty thinking in these areas and substitute thoughts and processes that are both more accurate and less distressing.

Of the three approaches outlined below, the work of Ellis and Beck have received the most attention.

Rational-Emotive Therapy (RET)

Albert Ellis and his colleagues developed one of the earliest cognitive approaches, rational-emotive therapy (e.g., Ellis, 1962, 1981a; Ellis & Harper, 1973). This therapy presupposes that "emotional" reactions are caused by both conscious and unconscious thoughts, judgments, or interpretations. When certain negative and "self-defeating" emotional states are experienced, such as guilt, depression, or anxiety, certain *irrational beliefs* exist; they can be verbalized but will not change unless the person holding the beliefs directly acts and thinks "against" them. However, many feeling states are sensible and not based on irrational beliefs; they are to be felt fully. By emphasizing both acting and thinking RET is, according to Ellis, a truly cognitive-behavioral approach.

The core irrational beliefs held by persons that lead to their discomfort in life are:[1]

> The idea that it is a dire necessity for an adult to be loved by everyone for everything he or she does
> The idea that certain acts are awful or wicked, and that people who perform such acts should be severely punished
> The idea that it is horrible when things are not the way one would like them to be
> The idea that human misery is externally caused and is forced on one by outside people and events
> The idea that if something is or may be dangerous or fearsome, one should be terribly upset about it
> The idea that it is easier to avoid than to face life difficulties and self-responsibilities
> The idea that one needs something other or stronger or greater than oneself on which to rely
> The idea that one should be thoroughly competent, intelligent, and achieving in all possible respects
> The idea that because something once strongly affected one's life, it should indefinitely affect it
> The idea that one must have certain and perfect control over things
> The idea that human happiness can be achieved by inertia and inaction
> The idea that one has virtually no control over one's emotions and that one cannot help feeling certain things

The RET therapist actively uncovers or detects irrational beliefs with the client. Often, the terms *should, ought, must,* or other absolutes are keys that an irrational belief is held. For example, the older client who says, "Children should respect their parents," is not simply stating a generational norm but may also have an irrational belief.

Along with uncovering irrational beliefs, a rational-emotive approach educates clients (insight) and uses specific techniques for changing irrational beliefs. Client education consists of explaining the so-called ABCs of disturbed behavior, a shorthand description of the model of emotion and cognition discussed above: A represents *activating experiences* (or events) that trigger B, beliefs about activating experiences, which can be rational or irrational, which lead to C, *consequences* (behavior) based on the beliefs. If the beliefs are rational, behavior will be adaptive. If beliefs are irrational, behavior will be maladaptive.

The main techniques are (Ellis, 1981b):

---

[1] Adapted from Ellis & Harper, 1973, with permission of Wilshire Books and Prentice-Hall publishers.

1. *Detecting irrational beliefs.* This means noting "shoulds" and "musts" when they occur in the client's discussion as well as uncovering other irrational beliefs noted above.

2. *Distinguishing rational from irrational beliefs.* Beliefs that express wishes, hopes, or concerns without an absolute operationalization are rational (e.g., "I am afraid of becoming a widow.") Beliefs that are absolutistic and expressed as concrete needs are irrational (e.g., "I cannot live without my husband, I am so depressed").

3. *Disputing irrational beliefs.* RET therapists actively dispute their clients' beliefs. A "scientific method" is used, uncovering the "reality" of the evidence to support the belief. Also, clients are continually reminded that they are *choosing* their beliefs and subsequent feeling state. Disputation is usually done in a questioning format using questions such as: "What evidence is there that X is true?" "What evidence is there that X is false?" "Can you rationally support your belief that you are worthless?" "What are the *worst* things that will *actually* happen to you if you do not get what you think you should (or do get what you think you should not)?" "What good things can you make happen if you do not get what you think you must?" "Why is it *awful* (depressing, horrible) that X takes place?".

4. *Pointing out the disadvantages of disturbed behavior.* Some people think it is good or correct to feel guilty or depressed. RET argues that these states and underlying beliefs almost always have harmful consequences.

5. *Pointing out that horrible consequences are more often than not only inconvenient.* One overgeneralized response to negative circumstances is "awfulizing," or making consequences worse than they are. RET challenges this response.

6. *Challenging "symptoms about symptoms."* At times the ABC cycle develops an additional BC cycle (e.g., "*I should not feel* frustrated over a loss, hence I am inadequate if I do so"). The beliefs about feelings can also be detected and challenged.

RET also uses imagery (picturing scenes) to imagine the worst consequences of events to uncover beliefs as well as role playing, desensitization, homework, actively practicing "rational statements," and other techniques. Although Ellis uses a confrontational style that is not suited to all mental health practitioners, the idea of challenging irrational beliefs may be an effective approach as part of a mental health practitioner's repertoire. At least one study (Keller, Croake, & Brooking, 1975) shows that older adults involved in a class in which RET concepts were discussed and role-played had both a significant increase in rational thinking and decrease in anxiety compared to controls.

> *Case*: Ellis (1981b) reports on the case of a fifty-five-year old man who was both depressed about his brothers' early deaths due to heart attacks and his own high blood pressure and potential heart problems. Ellis began by challenging the man's symptoms about symptoms, asking him how he felt about being anxious: "So you're anxious about your anxiety?" Ellis then focused on the awfulizing about the brothers' death: "It's terrible for them to have died so young . . . and it would be awful for me to die so young . . ." (Ellis, 1981b, p. 165). He reports that when the client became aware of his anxiety about anxiety, he was able to dispute the "awfulizing" beliefs that caused the secondary anxiety with a subsequent decrease in both secondary and primary anxiety.

Cognitive Therapy for Depression

Beck (1967, 1976) has developed both a theory and a series of cognitive methods for treating depression. His approach is quite likely to be effective with the aged (Steuer, 1982; Gallagher & Thompson, 1983). Since most depression in old age is "reactive"—brought on by actual losses—and Beck's therapy is designed for reactive depression, it is likely to be useful (Storandt, 1983). However, inasmuch as depression is "real," related to actual health problems, as a result of physiological changes due to illness, it may not be effective.

Beck suggests that people make five logical errors that can lead to depression: *arbitrary inference, selective inference, overgeneralization, magnification,* and *personalization. Arbitrary inference* refers to drawing incorrect conclusions, ones that are actually the opposite of what the evidence suggests. An older nursing home resident, for example, might think an aide hates her because the aide spends only ten minutes with her, even though the aide carefully spends more time with her than with other residents. *Selective abstraction* refers to focusing on only one detail of a complex situation without tending to its context. *Overgeneralization* refers to drawing conclusions (usually about self or self-worth) based on one incident. For example, an older male might think he is becoming impotent because of one failure to achieve erection. *Magnification* refers to catastrophizing, or assuming the worst possible consequence of actions or performance. *Personalization* refers to linking external events to self when, in actuality, no such link exists.

These five errors are found within negative views of the self, the present, and the future (a "primary triad"). Negative views of the self include attributing one's unworthiness to a moral, mental, or physical deficit. Negative views of the present include expecting failure and thinking the world is basically against oneself. Negative views of the future include seeing one's current despair going on forever.

Treatment of Depression Beck and others (e.g., Burns, 1980) have developed many techniques for treating depression. The three steps basic to these techniques are: (1) examining life history to both uncover and demonstrate to the client that current depressed thoughts were learned, (2) teaching the client to uncover self-statements that lead to depression, to distance self from these statements, and to examine them objectively and, (3) changing the client's general attitudes or world view arising from the "primary triad." In addressing both specific depressing conditions and "higher-order" or more general attitudes, Beck's approach is similar to Ellis's in that direct symptoms and "symptoms about symptoms" are considered "fair game" for the mental health practitioner.

A series of related techniques have been developed for treating depression. They include:

Writing down depressing thoughts on one side of a piece of paper
Deciding how much one feels depressed on a ten-point scale, and then rewriting them more "rationally" on the other side of a piece of paper, changing

categorical statements (should, ought, always) to more realistic statements (Burns, 1980)

Assigning homework that is pleasurable and increases the client's sense of mastery and self-worth

Learning to make realistic or self-enhancing statements *to oneself* when one is depressed; such statements are incompatible with current depressed thoughts (Meichenbaum, 1977).

These techniques can be used with individuals or in groups (cf. Sherman, 1979).

Neurolinguistic Programming

One of the more innovative forms of treatment to be developed in the last ten years is neurolinguistic programming (Bandler & Grinder, 1975, 1979; Grinder & Bandler, 1976). Neither its concepts nor its techniques have been rigorously tested to date. The following description is not meant to substitute for training in the approach.

Neurolinguistic programming (NLP$_{tm}$) has its roots in logic, psycholinguistics, cognitive psychology, and anthropology (particularly work in nonverbal behavior). The concepts behind NLP$_{tm}$ are that individuals experience their world in combinations of channels—visual, auditory, kinesthetic, gustatory, and olfactory. Sensory experience, language, and thought can also be organized in channel sequence. For instance, the individual who says "in my *view*" or "I *see* what you mean" is using visual language. The individual who thinks in pictures is using visual images, one who "talks to himself" is using auditory images. A client's world is thus represented as a series of images, metaphors, words, or feelings that can be analyzed through use of language, body language, and even eye movements, which theoretically reflect channels used in thinking.

The methods of NLP$_{tm}$ include using hypnotic trance, linguistically challenging certain irrational components of statements, training people to use several channels for thinking and expression, and symbolically "reframing" parts of components of the client's personality. In an adaptation from classical conditioning, imagery, feelings, and key words are used to create links to desired feelings (e.g., relaxation, confidence).

Case: Mrs. Smith, an eighty-two-year-old adult day-care client, was severely impaired. She was often disoriented to person, place, and time, and was "unable" to follow through on tasks such as winding yarn into a ball. One day she asked a worker, "What do I do next?" Rather than giving the client the next piece of string, the worker asked: "What do you *see* (visual) yourself doing next?" but got no response. She then asked, "What can you *tell* (auditory) yourself to do next?" and again got no response. Then, "What do you *feel* (kinesthetic) you should do next?" At this point the client picked up the next piece of string to be wound. After several trials it became apparent that instructions with "feeling" words elicited more desired behavior and communication from the client than instructions with only visual or auditory phrases.

Problem Solving

One of the deficits frequently found in all age groups is an inability to find workable solutions to problems. In several instances in Section I of this text, it was suggested that clients can be taught more effective problem solving skills. Several approaches are used to teach people how to identify and solve problems. Most are based on identifying the problem, setting goals, developing a solution, implementing the solution, and evaluating the outcome. In addition, individuals can evaluate the relative strengths and weaknesses of a given solution by listing them and assigning them weights, a process called force field analysis (cf. Brammer, 1979).

A recommended series of steps to follow and teach to clients is (Bradley & Edinberg, 1982):

1. *The problem is presented.* Initially, problems will be raised or suggested by the client.
2. *The problem is defined and/or refined.* Most problems raised by clients are pieces or partially thought out statements about troublesome situations. They are often phrased negatively (e.g., "I am depressed" or "I can't do anything about him/her"). The definition step requires diligent inquiry into all aspects of the problem. How much of it is the client's doing? How much of it is other persons'? How much of it is due to circumstances or situational constraints? What else may be going on? (This step is similar to the assessment phase of intervention described in Chapter 8).
3. *The problem is stated in one sentence as a positive statement.* This step is important both to cut down on vagueness about the problem and to reframe it as having possible alleviation. In a psychological sense, negative statements (e.g., "I can't do anything about him") are unsolvable, whereas positive ones ("I need to find a way to get him to listen to me") more easily lead to solutions, cure, or improvement.
4. *A piece of the problem is selected on which the client will work.* Many problems, even when stated positively, are global and difficult to solve in days, weeks, or even months. At this point, some breaking down of the problem into manageable pieces is suggested.
5. *Specific criteria are developed to determine if the problem or manageable piece has, in fact, been solved.* Criteria should be observable and specified in terms of frequency, length of time they need to occur, and for how long a period of time they should occur so that the client knows the problem is solved. For example, the elderly spouse who wants her husband to "love her" should decide exactly what he should do to show her he loves her, how often he needs to show her, and for how long he must do so for her to believe that, in fact, he does love her. This step has important significance for the client in that it forces the operationalization of what otherwise are vague and "unresolvable" feelings or perceptions.
6. *Ideas for achieving resolution of the problem are then brainstormed.* At this point any and every possibility for solving the problem should be put forth.

Remind the client that this is the time for ideas to flow freely, but not the time to evaluate them. Humorous and "silly" solutions are useful in that they can free the client from disabling affect, even though the solutions may be ineffective in their humorous form. Suggestions from the practitioner can be part of the list of possible solutions, as long as it is the client who performs the next step.

7. *Ideas from step 6 are chosen, thrown out, or combined into a strategy that will best solve the problem.* Out of the list of suggestions, some will have merit, some will be totally inappropriate, and some will have partial value. Time should be taken to put together the best "package" to solve the problem and any underlying concerns. The client needs to agree to implement the package.

8. *The strategy is implemented.* There should be a time limit on implementation (a day, a week) and a definite starting and stopping point for evaluation of the impact of the strategy.

9. *The strategy is evaluated by the criteria developed in step 5.* If successful, the client can "go on to bigger and better problems." If unsuccessful, choices can be made to redefine the problem, change criteria for resolution, come up with a new strategy, or "give up."

Evaluation of Cognitive Approaches

Goals   The goals of cognitive methods can be curative or adaptive, they can be used in treating conditions, such as depression, or helping persons adapt to conditions and circumstances that are "unchangeable," such as death of a spouse.

Focus   Cognitive methods focus on cognition, ways of thinking that lead to unproductive behavior or distressed affect.

Targeted Group   Targeted groups include people suffering from a range of affective problems, including depression, reactions to stressful circumstances, and, possibly, delusional belief systems. A prerequisite is that the client be able to think in a systematic manner.

Strengths and Weaknesses   The strengths of cognitive methods lie in their explictness of approach and theory, the range of techniques that have been developed, the range of adaptive situations to which they can be applied, and their proven efficacy with all age groups.

The weaknesses are those of any approach that focuses on one area of the individual's functioning as the "key" to his or her behavior. Inasmuch as dynamics, self-esteem, or situational constraints determine the individual's behavior, cognitive approaches will not result in behavioral change. Also, the person using these approaches has to make a judgment on the client's ability to handle their application, a task that is not always easily accomplished. Drawbacks notwithstanding, cognitive approaches may hold some of the greatest potential for the treatment of adaptive problems of the aged.

SUMMARY AND CONCLUSIONS

Behavioral and cognitive approaches are based on several assumptions about mental distress—that principles of learning determine formation and cure of mental problems; that overt behavior and/or thought processes, rather than subjective feelings or personality dynamics, are the correct focus of treatment; and that by changing maladaptive behavior and thought, the individual is "cured."

The major approaches in behavioral therapy are classical conditioning and operant conditioning. In each approach it is important to identify the problem behavior and determine what maintains or reinforces it. Then, through techniques such as relaxation, systematic desensitization, or reinforcement of desired behavior, changes can be made in a client's behavior to improve functioning. A wide range of conditions, including health problems, loss of walking, and disorientation to person, place, and time, have been treated in the elderly using these principles.

Cognitive approaches address irrational or maladaptive thought processes. The work of Ellis, Beck, and Bandler and Grinder are three examples of approaches that should be considered with the elderly. Although it is not always considered a mental health intervention, a knowledge of effective problem-solving methods can be helpful to older persons.

Behavioral techniques are powerful. They can be used in institutional settings to improve the quality of life, or conversely, they can be used to increase compliance to norms that benefit the staff more than the residents. Because of the power of these methods, the importance of using care in assessment (choosing the "right" problem) and care in guaranteeing clients' rights to refuse treatment and participate in goal setting cannot be overstated.

11

Humanistic and Creative-Expressive Approaches

THEORETICAL PERSPECTIVE

Each school or approach to mental health interventions has its own flavor, sense, or particular emphasis. Psychodynamic approaches focus on inner conflicts. Behavioral approaches focus on observable behavior and cognitive processes. Humanistic approaches take a particular philosophical view of people, one that says that it is in the nature of all human beings to have a natural tendency to grow, develop, or "actualize." This view is in part based on existential philosophy. Psychopathology, suffering, and other forms of human distress are, to this way of thinking, impediments that merely need to be removed so the natural positive tendencies of people will emerge and people will be able to handle life's problems in an integrated manner.

Humanistic psychology developed as a reaction to a perceived narrowness of dynamic and behavioral psychology. The humanistic viewpoint is that human behavior cannot be reduced to concepts such as drives, conflicts or learning. Rather, humanistic psychology focuses on "unique" human characteristics, such as love, compassion, creativity, meaningfulness, or values (Shaffer, 1978). Thus, humanistic approaches can be considered a voice of hope, concern, and compassion, the one approach that focuses on obtaining highest level of functioning rather than simply addressing the banishment of pathology.

The methods and ideas contained in humanistic approaches are varied and drawn from many sources. They incorporate non-Western approaches such as yoga, meditation, or Buddhist religious principles and theoretical and philosophical writings such as the work of May (1953), Maslow (1968, 1970), and Laing (1968). They draw on a wide range of therapeutic approaches, including client-centered therapy (Rogers, 1942, 1961, 1977); Gestalt therapy (e.g., Perls, 1969a, 1969b; Fagan & Shepherd, 1970); massage; bodywork; certain applications of dance, movement, art, and music therapies; and group work, including encounter groups and sensitivity training.

The humanistic perspective is not universally accepted, although many mental health professionals would argue that they subscribe to some techniques, views, or beliefs that can be found in its domain. Others may dismiss this approach as being unscientific or too vague to be of any real use in promoting change where psychopathology or severe problems such as dementia exist.

This chapter addresses certain principles behind humanistic approaches in working with the aged: Roger's client-centered therapy, Gestalt techniques, specific applications and programs for the elderly, and creative-expressive approaches.

HUMANISTIC APPROACHES

Principles and Concepts

Self-Actualization   Self-actualization is variously considered a goal of living (e.g., Rogers, 1951) or a state of being that is occasionally achieved. Self-actualization is, in essence, functioning at the height of one's creative, intellectual, and affective ability. Maslow (1968, 1970) defined several characteristics of "self-actualizing" individuals, including acceptance of others, acceptance of self, the capacity for deep and meaningful relationships, creativity, spontaneity, autonomy, inner-directedness, and an open approach to life and living. He also found that people who had these characteristics would occasionally have "peak experiences," or times when they were at the height of their personal powers, when a sense of wholeness and harmony with the world was experienced.

While many mental health professionals would argue that these attributes are not appropriate treatment goals and/or they are too vague to be useful, the utility of self-actualization is, at a minimum, that it challenges the limits mental health practitioners may subliminally set for their clients. In many settings, professionals have substantial power and control over clients' lives and functioning. Given certain tasks of aging, such as putting one's life in order, coping with death and losses, or handling subtle agism in society, the mental health practitioner may be the only health professional who provides opportunities or promotes activities that allow clients to live "fully."

Congruence   Much like self-actualization, congruence is a desired state of being. Congruence can be defined as being "genuine" or "real," as being "authentic," spontaneous, and without pretentions or phoniness (Rogers, 1977). Congruence can also be operationalized as a state in which words, tone of voice, body language, and other aspects of communication are consistent (Satir, 1972). Congruence does not necessarily imply that everything is shared or that a sense of privacy cannot exist. It does, however, address the issue of how feelings, cognitions, and behavior are tied together. It is also a concept that is often used to address behavior of the therapist or helper. The client will be helped most if the mental health practitioner is congruent in her or his interactions with the client.

Sense of Self   Several terms in humanistic therapies focus on a sense of self. The two most common are *self-worth* and *self-awareness*. Self-worth (e.g., Satir, 1972) refers to how a person values himself or herself. A low valuing of self leads to depression or unadaptive behavior. By having or obtaining positive (high) self-worth, the individual theoretically can eliminate depression, anxiety, and subsequent behavior problems.

Self-awareness is the individual's conscious understanding of self. Awareness leads to understanding how one denies certain feelings, to accepting one's limitations while appreciating self, to discovering how one allows oneself to be defined or validated by others, and to discovering that one has choices in reacting to the environment, to others, and even to one's own thoughts and reactions. Self-awareness is thus an important process in facilitating individual change.

These three concepts are imbedded in Roger's client-centered approach and, to a lesser degree, in Gestalt therapy, two of the most prevalent humanistic approaches.

Client-Centered Therapy and Approaches

Client-centered therapy is most closely associated with Carl Rogers (1942, 1961, 1977). The goal of client-centered treatment is to enable an individual to grow on her or his own. The mental health practitioner using a client-centered approach focuses less on specific problems and solutions, and more on "the person" as a means of helping the person understand and be able to manage his or her affairs.

For a therapist-client relationship successfully to lead to client growth, three conditions must occur: *congruence, unconditional positive regard and acceptance,* and *accurate empathic understanding.* Congruence has been discussed earlier.

Unconditional positive regard and acceptance refers to a profound sense of caring and concern for the client that exists independently of any action the client takes. The mental health practitioner conveys this attitude of acceptance through words and behavior, neither judging nor evaluating the client's behavior.

Unconditional positive regard does not mean the mental health practitioner approves all of a client's behavior or reactions; rather, he or she accepts the behavior or reactions as the client's best attempt at self-understanding at that moment in time.

Also, mental health practitioners are not expected to have positive regard at all times. The degree of positive regard may vary.

Finally, research in the area strongly suggests that having positive regard for clients is a key to therapeutic success, although it may not be enough in and of itself (see Chapter 8). The mental health practitioner who dislikes clients, who cannot accept their behavior, or who moralistically "preaches" to them is in all likelihood not working effectively.

Accurate empathic understanding means that the mental health practitioner understands what the client is experiencing and communicates this back to the client. Ideally, the mental health practitioner, by experiencing the inner world of the client, can help the client find better words to describe experience.

Empathy is more than cognitive understanding. It also includes not becoming overwhelmed by the client's feelings. Rather, empathy involves getting "in with" the client without losing one's objectiveness and own sense of identity.

Through the mutual exploration of the client's inner life, the client will begin to experience feelings, solve problems, and "develop." The "power" in the relationship is given to the client in that both client and mental health practitioner are seen as equals. The client makes decisions, the helper is "nondirective." Finally, the client becomes congruent and able to experience feelings and develops a higher degree of self-actualization.

Extensions of Client-Centered Therapy

Extensions of Roger's work have been proposed (e.g., Carkhuff, 1969; Egan, 1975; Ivey and Authier, 1978). These extensions are concerned more with skills than with philosophy, and have introduced several additional approaches.

Advanced Accurate Empathy   As the mental health practitioner begins to understand the client's world, she or he can move to *"advanced accurate empathy,"* in which techniques are used to deepen exploration of self and gain insight (Egan, 1975).

Self-Disclosure   Active disclosing of the mental health practitioner's views and reactions to the client is termed self-disclosure (cf. Jourard, 1971; Egan, 1975). Its purpose is to model and aid the client in establishing equality with the mental health practitioner, not to hinder or intimidate the client. Self-disclosure can help the client learn about trust or dependency. Skill and sensitivity are needed to gauge accurately when and how to use self-disclosure.

Confrontation and Concreteness   Both of these skills are more directive than the others discussed. *Confrontation* refers to focusing the discussion on inconsistencies (but not attacking the client) in a therapeutic manner. *Concreteness* refers to helping the client be specific about feelings, actions, or thoughts and is, in part, related to cognitive therapeutic approaches.

Active Listening   Gordon (1970) focuses attention on skills necessary to convey acceptance. Professionals may respond to clients by subtly commuicating what Gordon calls twelve roadblocks to communication:

1. Ordering, directing or commanding
2. Warning, admonishing, threatening
3. Exhorting, preaching, moralizing
4. Advising, giving solutions
5. Lecturing, teaching, giving logical arguments
6. Judging, criticizing, disagreeing, blaming
7. Praising, agreeing
8. Ridiculing
9. Interpreting, analyzing, diagnosing
10. Reassuring, sympathizing (talking people out of their feelings)
11. Probing for motives
12. Withdrawing by distraction or humor

Active listening, in contrast, attends to the feeling messages of others and to one's own reactions at a feeling level. Although it was developed as a focus for parents and children, it is useful in the counseling process with the aged and can be taught to older persons, relatives, and caregivers. The following case illustrates the successful application of client-centered approaches.

> *Case*: Mr. Brown, a seventy-eight-year-old man in a nursing home, refused to leave his room for any activities. When staff asked him to go to recreation or social events, he would tell them "Go away." Although wheelchair-bound, Mr. Brown was in good health. A counselor was assigned to Mr. Brown. After several attempts to get him out, the counselor finally said, "You know, if I were here in a wheelchair but otherwise all right, I might not want to go to activities with a lot of sick older people. I was wondering what you were feeling." Mr. Brown looked at her and replied, "I feel useless. There is nothing for me to do here, just a lot of sick people." The counselor than began to question and explore Mr. Brown's feelings of uselessness, his underlying embarrassment at being in a wheelchair, and his resentment at having to be on a floor with more severely impaired residents. He was willing to discuss his feelings, and as he did so, his hostile reaction to other staff decreased. When the opportunity arose for Mr. Brown to move to a floor with residents at a higher cognitive level, he gladly changed rooms.

As Corey (1982) has pointed out, the therapist's genuineness is critical for success in the client-centered approach. She or he needs to be able to maintain her or his own identity while being nondirective and "with" the client. Client-centered therapy is not passive nor is it as simple as reflecting feelings. Part of its misuse may come from an oversimplified application of its principles.

One final note is that many problems faced by the elderly may require more direct interventions of the nature suggested by Egan, Ivey, and Authier. Still, given the lack of meaningful relationships and roles for many elderly, the client-centered approach can provide needed emotional support.

Evaluation   Client-centered approaches can be considered as potentially curative, adaptive, and/or enriching the client's life, depending on one's theoretical viewpoint. From the humanistic perspective, enriching (bringing one beyond a "minimum" level of distress) and curing problems are synonymous. It is the process of putting individuals in touch with their reactions and subsequent loss in self-esteem that is important. Similarly, adapting to situations is synonymous with being able to experience one's full existing powers. One resoultion to this question of goal is to consider client-centered approaches (1) useful in establishing relationships that could lead to curing certain problems by introducing other techniques, (2) an important step in helping clients sort out their own feelings and reactions to life events, and (3) a central component in enrichment programs.

Client-centered approaches focus on attitudes and values about self. Cognition, affect, and behavior are of much less significance. The targeted groups can vary. Although the "ideal" client is one who has the mental capacity for insight into self-worth, many of the adaptive tasks of aging can benefit from concern, compassion, and care, even if the client is failing. We should not overlook the benefits of raising self-esteem in clients with severe cognitive deficits, even though the results may seem to be of short duration.

The strengths of these approaches are their utility in developing helping relationships, their value in raising self-esteem, and proven efficacy as a general approach to therapy. Their weaknesses are the lack of specificity in certain concepts (how does one know, for example, when one is being "congruent"?), a related lack of research on its validity in improving specific conditions (one can argue that the more specific the presenting problem is, the more other forms of intervention are called for), and the possibility that this approach will be the only one used when other methods would be effective in handling specific cognitive or behavioral problems that are not considered important in client-centered therapy.

Gestalt Therapy

Like client-centered therapy, Gestalt therapy is most closely associated with one person, in this instance Fredrich (Fritz) Perls (1969a, 1969b), although others have made substantial contributions to its development (cf. Fagan & Shepherd, 1970; Polster & Polster, 1973; Kempler, 1973). Also, like client-centered therapy, a Gestalt approach is directed toward the integration of personality. Clients are assumed to have the capacity to make their own interpretations of behavior, and there is a de-emphasis on interpretation by the mental health practitioner.

Gestalt therapy differs from client-centered therapy in its emphasis on the "here and now" as well as the techniques and stylistic approaches employed in its approach. The "here and now" refers to this actual moment in time and one's current experience, not views of the past, not views of the future, and not one's observations or comments about the present. By forcing the client to live in the here and now, and its implied intensification of feelings, the client will begin to finish "unfinished business," discover internal conflicts (polarities or dichotomies with a "top dog," usually a blaming, parental part, and underdog, a "powerless," victimized part), be able to fully experience living, and be congruent. The past and the future are a part of Gestalt therapy in that the feelings one has about past experience and expectations can be explored.

Along with its emphasis on the "here and now," Gestalt therapy also has several other guidelines or rules (Levitsky & Perls, 1970). They include:

I and Thou. Focusing on the interactive nature of communication
"It" language and "I" language. Focusing on ownership of one's behavior, for example, substituting "I am trembling" for "it (the hand) is trembling"
Using current awareness. Having the client focus on what she or he is currently aware of (bodily sensations, how feelings are experienced)
No gossiping. Having the client talk directly to others rather than "about" them. For example, "My husband never said goodbye" is turned to a direct discussion with an empty chair.

These guidelines are used to reinforce current awareness and feelings, to move the client away from overintellectualization and towards new insight and integration.

Gestalt Techniques

Perhaps more than any other therapy, Gestalt is known for its dramatic techniques, many of which have been adopted by therapists who are not necessarily advocates of a pure Gestalt approach. These techniques have been called "games" in that they have a playful aspect and a "goal." Several of the techniques are described below (Levitsky & Perls, 1970).

Games of Dialogue   This technique is one of a series that focuses on integrating the personality. It is often used when there is a "top dog-underdog" conflict. The client first identifies exactly what the two parts are, one being moralistically dominant, the other being a passive victim. The client sits in a chair and becomes the top dog (dominant), talking to an empty chair in which the underdog (victim) is "sitting." After fully experiencing the feelings of top dog, the client switches chairs to become the underdog. The switching of parts and dialogue can continue for several exchanges. This is in essence a self-played role play in which the client more fully experiences each part of a conflict while verbalizing his or her feelings. The mental health practitioner can prompt as well. The goal is integration of the polarity, not its elimination. By accepting the polarity rather than denying its existence, the client will achieve better internal harmony.

For the elderly this technique can be used not only to integrate polarities but also to "make peace" with family members who are deceased or geographically removed.

Staying With the Feeling   This is essentially an approach to help a client fully experience uncomfortable feelings. Often, clients will express an unpleasant feeling in passing, but then move on to a different topic. The mental health practitioner's task is to ask the client to "stay with the feeling," to confront it, to explore it, and to experience it fully. The goal is to gain better understanding and uncover blocks to real experience, not simply to feel the discomfort.

Reversals   At times clients act in such a manner as to be the "opposite" of an impulse or wish. This process is similar to reaction formation in psychoanalytical theory. Thus, the client who is always sugary sweet may have a repressed hostile part, the client who is cerebral may have a lusty, feeling part that is repressed. Gestalt therapists will ask clients to become the opposite part and act it out to give the client a better sense of the repressed part, with the goal of integrating it into conscious experience.

Exaggeration   Certain verbal and body language cues (e.g., shaking, voice tone, speed of speech, rocking, fist clenching) can be considered partial expression of feelings by a personality "part." In Gestalt work the client may be encouraged to exaggerate the voice tone or body language, or even to restate a particular statement louder and louder. The purpose is to help the client "feel the feeling."

Playing the Projection   Clients who express their feelings as perceptions about the world (e.g., "Everyone is out to get me;" or "This place is so depressing") can be encouraged to "become" the projection—to play the person "out to get them" or a depressed person. This is done to test to what degree the statement is, in fact, an internal conflict.

Unfinished Business   Whenever clients indicate that they have "unfinished business," that is, they feel resentment or a sense of incompleteness in relationships, they are encouraged to complete it in fantasy or reality.

"May I Feed You a Sentence?"   This technique calls for the mental health practitioner to give the client a sentence to "try on for size" to express a particular thought, attitude, or emotional reaction. Although interpretive in nature, in this process the client will benefit most by saying the sentence and experiencing her or his reaction to saying it.

Dream-Work   Gestalt therapy uses dream interpretation in a "here and now" manner (cf. Perls, 1970). When clients report dreams, they are directed in turn to "play" all people and obects in the dream. Dreams, according to Perls, are "messages of yourself to yourself" (1970, p. 27). Not unlike Freud, Perls claims that all aspects of dreams are important, especially the "voids," or what is being avoided in the dream. However, the Gestalt approach does not include interpreting the dream. By intensifying the client's experience through playing the dream, the client will make his or her own interpretation and integration of dream material.

Case: A widow of fourteen years complained of depression and crying whenever she thought of her husband. She would periodically go to her husband's grave and yell at him, telling him how much she missed him, how she was unable to go out socially as a single woman, and how angry she was. The mental health practitioner asked her (without having her change chairs) to pretend to be her husband and tell her his reaction to her problems. She said he would say "I want you to go out, I do not want you to spend this time crying over me, go, have a good time." The mental health practitioner asked if she believed him. She said yes. While this one incident was not the only part of the work with the client, it is an example of unfinished business being worked on through dialogue.

Application with the Aged:
Some Considerations

The Gestalt approach has several distinct advantages in working with the aged. The focus on "here and now" can be a powerful means of instilling hope. Also, the emphasis on unfinished business fits nicely with such concepts as life review and reminiscence. Many older persons have regrets, goodbyes that were never said, and what can be considered important unfinished business with people who are dead. The use of dialogue, role plays, and other "dramatic" techniques can aid older clients in reaching some closure on these relationships.

Finally, the empahsis on noninterpretation respects the client's ability to make his or her own judgment and interpretation at her or his own speed. Telling clients, "You have to decide what it means," implies that the client is capable of deciding on the meaning of an experience and will do so. In that sense, Gestalt approaches force older clients out of the "patient" role.

However, there are several potential drawbacks to the use of Gestalt techniques, particularly when they are not integrated into an overall intervention strategy (cf. Corey, 1982). First is the relative de-emphasis on cognitive aspects. Reflection, thought, and observations are generally discounted, although they are certainly part of human experience. Similarly, by avoiding interpretation, the mental health practitioner may miss useful and appropriate opportunities to help the client make meaning out of experience.

The abundance and powerfulness of the techniques in Gestalt therapy can be unduly seductive. They, rather than the client, can become the focus of therapy and actually hinder therapeutic progress. In addition, because the exercises or games of Gestalt are powerful, novel, and purposefully left without interpretation, clients need to be prepared for the experience. Preparation should include developing trust, explaining what role-plays and experiential exercises are, discussing the reactions that might be encountered, and having ample time for talking about the exercise after it takes place.

As a final note, Perls (1970) mentions several aspects of Gestalt work for the therapist that have special application to countertransference in work with the elderly. Specifically, Perls suggests that the mental health practitioner "listen to himself (or herself)," tend carefully to feelings of boredom or frustration, and be "your own therapist" much as the client is expected to provide his or her own interpretation of feelings and reactions to exercises.

Mental health practitioners often complain that older clients ramble, tell the same stories over and over, or otherwise block progress. A Gestalt approach to these reactions would encourage the mental health practitioner to fully experience his or her feelings of restlessness, frustration, or boredom, to withdraw into the fantasy of what the feelings mean, and, having resolved his or her own reactions, be able to attend to the client and what the client is communicating by rambling.

Evaluation   The goal of Gestalt therapy may be considered curative in that conflicts are transformed and emotional distress eliminated, or enriching in that a client or group member can experience the "here and now" on the "fullness of human experience." The focus is both on affect (feeling the feelings) and attitude/ values—being in touch with one's "whole" self. The groups most likely to benefit from such an approach are those who can "play" (engage in fantasy work without unnecessary distress) and those who have an interest in learning about why they act as they do. The techniques are dramatic; conflicts and feelings are likely to be heightened by the experiences. Such techniques may be particularly beneficial in situations where feelings are not easily expressed. However, it is not clear what risks are incurred by enhancing feelings of internal distress. This is not to say that Gestalt techniques should be avoided. Rather, the individual and others in the social environment (including the staff of a nursing home) should be prepared for strong expression of affect in sessions and possibly after sessions are over.

The strengths of the approach are the emphasis on the here and now, the power of the techniques to elicit strong feeling and raise the individual's awareness of inner conflicts, and the possibility for eliminating distressful conflict. The weaknesses are the lack of scientific validation of the approach with the elderly, the potential for misuse of techniques, and the lack of emphasis on cognition and reflection. Many older persons need either to handle deficits (cognition) or to work on issues related to putting one's life in order (reflection). The use of Gestalt techniques can be powerful, they have certain limitations; suggesting that the mental health practitioner consider integrating aspects of this approach with other approaches in work with the elderly.

Programs Using Humanistic Approaches

Several types of workshops, courses, or group work with the aged using humanistic approaches have been discussed in the existing literature. The two examples that follow have certain similarities. They focus on growth rather than pathology; they have been designed to include both "well" and "ill," not only "ill" elderly; and they focus on experience rather than interpretation. Both use group methods as a primary form of "treatment" and neither has been designated as "mental health treatment." The projects are the SAGE Project (Dychtwald, 1978; Luce, 1979) and the Ventura County Creative Aging Workshops (Reinhart & Sargent, 1980).

The SAGE Project

The SAGE (Senior Actualization and Growth Experience) project is a growth program designed specifically for the elderly (Dychtwald, 1978; Luce, 1979). In 1974 Luce, Dychtwald, and Gerrard, three therapists, ran the first such group.

It consisted of fifteen clients with whom they worked both individually and in group settings. The purpose of the group was to "vitalize the minds, bodies, and spirits of its older participants" (Dychtwald, 1978, p. 71). The techniques varied, in part determined by the leaders' skills. They included massage, deep relaxation, sensory awareness, meditation, application of Gestalt techniques, communication skills, biofeedback, autogenic training, and other therapeutic modalities aimed at development of both mind and body.

The SAGE project used Gestalt principles to handle death and mourning, and these principles are also applicable in other settings. One technique is to have an empty chair in a session to represent the dead group member. Other group members are asked to imagine the part of themselves the person represented. One by one, group members leave the circle, and remaining members continue to imagine the part represented by the person leaving the group. As the group becomes smaller, the feelings of grief and loss intensify. Other related exercises include writing one's own obituary and writing down answers to questions such as: "What are my concerns about dying?" "How will others feel when I am gone?" "Who will take care of my unfinished business?" (Luce, 1979).

The SAGE project also focused on skills, abilities, and potential of participants. One unique aspect of the program was that seniors were encouraged to become co-leaders of similar groups after receiving "core" group training. SAGE groups have been run in community and institutional settings, with exercises being adapted to the physical and cognitive abilities of group members.

Case: Dychtwald (1978) describes a case of a seventy-three-year-old "post-cancer case with high blood pressure" who reported that at a party she ate the "wrong things," went home, and had a tachycardia attack. She then used deep relaxation and yoga breathing and was able to control the attack. She also used the SAGE group to work through "old" grief about losing several family members, some of the repressed grief coming up in a breathing exercise. Her final comment was, "No one ever had a chance at age seventy-three to live a new life as I have" (Dychtwald, 1978, p. 70).

The only formal evaluation of SAGE groups is reported by Lieberman and Gourash (1979). The main impact of the groups seems to have been on improved self-esteem, lessened depression, and to a lesser degree, decreased anxiety about health. Based on this study, the SAGE program seems to have measurable benefits, although the degree of change or growth does not necessarily mean that clients become "self-actualized."

The Ventura County Creative Aging Workshop

Reinhart and Sargent (1980) describe a direct application of humanistic philosophy and techniques in work with community aged. The program grew out of a recognition that only 2 percent of the clients at a particular community mental health center were over age 65, and that other approaches were needed to reach the elderly. The center developed a series of public workshops on common emotional problems of old age, including coping with death and dying, being alone, physical health, and senior survival.

The workshops emphasized sharing experiences and feelings as well as delineating issues. The workshops were given twice, once for a Spanish-speaking population. Although the value of a one-day workshop is difficult to assess, hundreds of elderly turned out to discuss the topics openly, evaluations were positive, and the percentage of elderly receiving services in Ventura County doubled in a year, suggesting that this type of approach has value to older people and may better link them to mental health services.

Evaluation of Humanistic Approaches

Goals   The goals most frequently associated with humanistic approaches are enrichment and adaptation, although it can be argued that, by becoming congruent or having peak experiences, individuals are cured of their problems. The purpose behind humanistic approaches is to help people function at the peak of their abilities, which is, in the framework of this text, a goal of enrichment.

Focus   There is some variance in focus among the humanistic approaches. Client-centered and Gestalt therapies, the two approaches discussed in this text, focus on attitudes/values (self-worth) and affect ("feeling the feelings"). Cognition and behavior are of minor significance.

Targeted Groups   In general, humanistic approaches seem best suited for people interested in gaining better understanding of their behavior. The power of the helping relationship is also quite useful for helping isolates, be they living alone or socially insulated from others in a residential or institutional setting. Similarly, putting people "in touch" with feelings may be quite needed in an antiseptic environment. Clients with severe cognitive deficits should, to some degree, be able to experience feelings and verbalize them. Gestalt and client-centered approaches may be quite useful as a form of stimulation if used judiciously.

Strengths and Weaknesses   Humanistic approaches are a reminder that one possible goal of intervention is to have people function at their full capacity. They tie concern for other people to methods of relating and treating emotonal distress. They are well suited to certain parts of adaptation—to death, to widowhood, to retirement. They emphasize the "whole" person and can thus be related to the multiple problems facing the aged.

One of the weaknesses of humanistic approaches is a certain lack of clarity in principles, use of techniques, or how to resolve feelings or conflicts that may arise when the strategies are used. The scientific validity of these approaches when used to "cure" problems is limited.

Humanistic approaches are powerful and have utility in examining one's affect and sense of self-worth. They also require a high degree of skill and sensitivity on the part of the practitioner. Skill is best gained in supervised settings, where the practitioner can be observed directly or, if necessary, on video or audio tape.

CREATIVE-EXPRESSIVE APPROACHES

Creative-expressive therapies include art, movement-dance and music treatment approaches. Each is predicated on both the intrinsic value of the art form used as well as its value as a vehicle to reach deep levels of problems and feelings. The medium becomes a way for clients to express themselves and socialize. The three examples that follow, art therapy, movement-dance therapy, and music therapy, are evaluated together as they have many aspects in common.

Art Therapy

Art therapy is a therapeutic modality in which emotional expression and group interaction is encouraged through use of artistic media, such as collage, drawing, and painting. Art therapists receive special training in this work, but aspects can be used by mental health practitioners in many settings. Wolcott (1978), a seventy-nine-year-old art therapist, decribed how she conducted art therapy in a nusring home, using collage, scribble drawing, "sausage figures," drawing other group members, drawing animals, drawing landscapes, and eventually working up to a year-long study group with group-designed projects. Wolcott's approach focuses more on developing "creative process" than on solving or symbolizing personal problems, but it does show how growth can take place in institutional settings. Art therapy approaches have also been suggested as a way to reorient clients (Dewdney, 1973) or be used in life review (Zieger, 1976).

Many mental health practitioners have little professional or personal experience in the use of art forms, but they should realize that artistic expression may, for some clients, be a key to unlocking feelings and problems or relieving isolation. Also, the value of creativity should not be overlooked or underestimated in limited environments or for clients with severe deficits.

Movement-Dance Therapy

Therapeutic movement, or dance therapy, is a relatively new field in which rhythmic movement is used to help clients express themselves and communicate with others (Caplow-Lindner, Harpaz, & Samberg, 1979). Dance therapists can integrate the use of space, types of movements, and interaction between clients in movement sessions to assess and help clients change behavior.

Movement therapy has several specific advantages for geriatric clients. First, it is generally nonstrenuous but still emphasizes movement and physical well-being. Second, it can be done in groups of quite varied sizes. Third, in institutional settings there are few opportunities to express or vent negative or strong emotions verbally and physically. Movement groups can help clients vent, channel, and change these behaviors (Sandel, 1975, 1978a).

One of the longest ongoing programs was started by Sandel in Connecticut (Sandel, 1978). Working with severely impaired clients, Sandel has been able to create cohesion in the group and has included aspects of reminiscence as well as verbalization, vocalization, venting of feelings, and socialization (Sandel, 1978b).

Movement sessions are fairly consistent. For example, in one session clients sit in a circle and begin with warmups for various parts of the body. The leader starts with a specific movement (pulling a cloth in a tug of war); vocalization (grunting) can be added, along with rhythmic verbalizations ("I want it, I want it"). At this point, the leader focuses on what clients want in their own lives and how they ask or fight for it.

Exercises emphasize touch-physical contact between clients, such as holding hands in a circle or "passing" a squeeze around. Physical contact can have a powerful "organizing effect." Clients who seem apathetic, disoriented, or removed may become oriented and alert, even if it is only for a few seconds (Sandel, 1978a).

Other specific concerns and suggestions for organizing movement sessions are given in *Therapeutic Dance/Movement Expressive Activities for Older Adults* (Caplow-Lindner, et al., 1979). The authors suggest ways to handle sensory loss and physical impairment; they also attend to the "nuts and bolts" of running movement sessions, including warmup exercises, exercises for expression, group interaction exercises, specific instructions for recorded music accompaniment, and types of musical instruments that can be used in sessions.

In considering the use of movement in group work with the elderly, the mental health practitioner should address the following issues: For what purpose is movement being used? How comfortable is the mental health practitioner with his or her own body? Are the movement exercises appropriate for clients' physical conditions? Is the mental health practitioner prepared for affect that may arise around sexuality or aggression, two topics ordinarily discouraged in institutional settings but ones that are likely to arise in expressive movement groups?

Music Therapy

Music therapy includes such diverse activities as vocalizing, group singing, music appreciation (discussing musical theory), rhythm bands, using music for relaxation and meditation, or discussing feelings raised by a particular melody or lyric. Musical activities are particularly useful in that they include verbal and physical aspects (e.g., singing, humming, moving or tapping toes), and provide a socially acceptable way for older people to interact in groups.

Hennessey (1978) reviews several benefits of music therapy: It creates a sense of group cohesion; subtly affects physiological functioning; facilitates reminiscence with songs linked to an era or specific historical event, such as World War I; creates opportunities for socialization; possibly helps in treatment of short-term memory loss; and serves as an adjunct for therapeutic movement. Music can provide a sense of ritual, as when the same songs are used to introduce or end a group session. It can also open a "new" area for risk taking: Some older adults need to be encouraged to sing. Their feelings of self-consciousness about "not being able to carry a tune," though deeply ingrained, can be overcome.

Moore (1978) presents several guidelines for the use of music therapy with the aged:

Mood is affected by music; however, some songs may have a paradoxical effect—"cheerful" songs, for example, might deepen depression.

Tempo (how fast the song goes) is very important; rhythm and volume are slightly less important.

Familiar music is powerful in "reaching" many clients. Participating in a familiar song can create cohesion and active interaction in a group and can facilitate reminiscence.

In designing listening activities, use good equipment, keep bass high, and do not overdo selections. Silence is also useful.

Selections of music should tap into ethnic, cultural, and cohort values. However, the values of "pop" tunes should not be overlooked. One movement group in a nursing home, for example, requested and used "When I'm sixty-four" by the Beatles as a warmup tune.

Participation in music groups can take several forms, such as listening, humming, tapping feet or hands in rhythm to music, clapping, singing, moving, and playing instruments. The leader needs to make it safe for a client to participate.

The leader does not have to be a musician to incorporate music therapy into treatment. However, if the leader has no sense of rhythm or cannot carry a tune, an assistant (either a professional staff member, a student, an aide, or a client) may be needed to help "get things going."

Music can be integrated into other treatment modalities (Needler & Baer, 1982; Sandel, 1978a). A "theme" song, music for meditation, or music to end sessions can give a sense of continuity to a group and provide an easy way for members to begin socializing. While the focus of treatment may not specifically include socialization or aesthetic appreciation, it can be argued that in many institutional settings there is such a cultural and interpersonal vacuum that any use of the arts has some intrinsic value.

Evaluation of Creative-Expressive Modalities

Goals The goals of creative-expressive interventions are primarily enrichment, although in settings with limited opportunity for artistic and self-expression (as in many institutional settings) they can be viewed as adaptive.

Focus The focus of creative-expressive interventions can vary: At times they will be a source of socialization; at others, a way to discover and experience affect. It can also be argued that the process of being creative and participating in artistic modalities has a positive influence on self-worth. Finally, movement therapy has an obvious side effect of potentially enhancing physical health.

Targeted Groups Creative-expressive interventions can be tailored to any level of functioning. However, it should be recognized that some individuals will be unwilling to participate in "arts and crafts" because they find it either demeaning or unfamiliar. There is a fine line between encouraging a client in an institution to participate in a new experience and providing undue pressure to "go along" with an authority figure. Persons who may potentially benefit from such experiences have the right to refuse to participate.

Strengths and Weaknesses One strength of creative-expressive approaches is their novelty. They will not be seen as "therapy" and allow participants to assume a positive role. They are also concrete—something is "accomplished," even if it is simply successfully remembering the words to a song. The three modalities described above as well as others, such as poetry therapy or having client's stories taped and transcribed, can be useful in different approaches, such as reminiscence and life review.

Creative-expressive approaches can be used with persons having a wide range of artistic, verbal, mental, and physical abilities. They provide possibilities for therapeutic interaction generally not available in other treatment modalities. They are also fun and provide golden opportunities for socialization.

One weakness of creative-expressive approaches is their lack of experimental validation as a mental health intervention with the aged. In a time of limited resources, it can be difficult to argue for their use as opposed to other treatment forms that more directly address psychological concerns and have more proven value. Nor is it always clear how the creative process influences well-being or how the practitioner without extensive background in a particular medium may use it effectively, although it is suggested that the use of these modalities be incorporated into the mental health practitioner's "bag of tricks." Finally, the modalities, while having the qualities of innovativeness and tapping into potential sources of strength, may not be effective as curative measures and may only be adjunctive in helping older persons adapt to losses.

SUMMARY AND CONCLUSIONS

Humanistic approaches are predicated on the assumption that the goal of intervention is the attainment of one's highest level of functioning as a whole person. Client-centered therapy and Gestalt therapy are two humanistic approaches that address how individuals live and how they feel about themselves. Several programs have been developed for the elderly using humanistic approaches. Humanistic approaches have value in that they focus on the therapeutic relationship and increase individuals' awareness of the "here and now." They are powerful in eliciting strong emotions and highlighting conflicts in the individual client's life. It is not clear, however, what their scientific validity is, nor is it clear what role they can play in the treatment of specific pathological conditions, such as organic brain syndrome.

Creative-expressive therapies use artistic modalities such as art, movement, dance, and music to give clients a means of artistic expression and the opportunity for exploration of feelings. They are nontraditional in that participants are not considered "patients." They are fun and have an implicit value in that socialization occurs when they are used in groups. Several types of programs use the arts as a treatment or adjunct with older pesons. These modalities may be useful as enrichment and adaptive activities in institutional settings, although their scientific validity is questionable and other forms of treatment should be considered for the range of problems likely to be found in an institutional setting.

Although the validity of humanistic and creative-expressive approaches is questionable, there is a richness in their range of approaches and areas of concentration. This richness should not be overlooked by the mental health practitioner who wishes to improve the functioning of clients in varied settings.

12

Group Approaches

THEORETICAL PERSPECTIVE

One of the decisions facing the mental health practitioner in many settings is how to serve a large number of clients in a limited amount of time. Also, in many settings, clients seem to need to improve socialization and social skills, due to both client condition and an influence of the setting. One response to these conditions has been the use of group treatments and activities in nursing homes, mental hospitals, and senior centers.

Groups are more than the sum of their individual members. A significant literature and set of theories have been developed both to describe group functioning and to aid the group leader in understanding the relative contribution of individual problems and "group dynamics" to the immediate concerns and behavior of group members (cf. Reddy & Lippert, 1980). A complete review of group theory is beyond the scope of this text, but a working knowledge of theories of group development is recommended for the mental health practitioner who will work with groups. Relevant theories can be found in works by Bion (1961), Whitaker and Lieberman (1964), Bennis and Sheppard (1956), and Tuckman (1965).

One of the distinctions authors make in group work literature is between group work and group psychotherapy (Burnside, 1978). *Group work* is a fairly general term, covering everything from discussion groups to encounter or growth groups. *Group therapy* refers to working with groups who have defined psychiatric problems to alleviate their problems. This distinction becomes a bit blurred when one realizes that behavioral and humanistic schools dispute or do not accept the traditional classification of "psychiatric problems." For purposes of this chapter, group intervention will cover any type of group that has psychological goals. Thus, discussion groups and most health, education, or community organization activities are not considered, but growth groups, therapeutic groups, or focused groups such as remotivation groups are.

CONSIDERATIONS IN GROUP INTERVENTIONS WITH THE ELDERLY

Rationale for Group Interventions

There are a variety of reasons that suggest using group interventions with the aged (cf. Burnside, 1978; Yalom, 1970; Bradley & Edinberg, 1982). They include:

Cohesion Cohesion has been defined as "the attractiveness of a group for its members" (Yalom, 1970, p. 37). While cohesion is not necessarily "curative," it can have great value for older clients. Particularly in long-term care, groups may be the only positive social identification older clients have.

Mutual Emotional Support Another reason for group work is that members can provide meaningful emotional support for each other. This is perhaps most true when the leader is substantially younger than the clients or is from an ethnic, cultural, or socioeconomic group other than that of the clients. Some clients will feel that the leader cannot truly "understand" how things are. Empathy from another person of the same age and ethnic group will be more acceptable (cf. Gonzalez del Valle & Usher, 1982). Also, for groups in which participants already associate, mutual support can occur at times other than when the group is meeting.

Therapeutic Value The group process has certain therapeutic values that are potentially useful for older adults. That is, certain conflicts and problems are best solved in a group. One example is provided by Alcoholics Anonymous, which relies on large group meetings as its major rehabilitative structure.

The Group as a Laboratory Groups are both "real world" and "non-real world." The real world aspect is that other people are present who can comment, react, and observe the client as well as give emotional support. However, because of its nature, a group can focus on aspects of living not usually discussed in real world settings, such as feelings, personal conflicts, or specific feedback (positive or negative criticism, observations about other group members). Clients can also "try out" new roles or new types of behavior either in simulation (role playing) or "for real" (e.g., the client who "for the first time" is joking around in group sessions). The group can be a safe place to try new behavior.

Relationships   One serious deficit faced by the elderly is the lack of opportunity to develop close relationships. Widowhood, having to care for a sick spouse, or living in a nursing home are only three of many situations with limited possibilities for interpersonal intimacy faced by substantial numbers of elderly. Groups can provide a needed opportunity for meaningful friendships to develop.

Interpersonal Learning   The group setting offers an opportunity for members to learn from each other. Older adults' experiences and wisdom can be shared. The value of teaching each other fits well with the value of maintaining independence and gives the participant a nonpatient role.

Options for Participation   Groups provide the opportunity to participate at different levels. Some people prefer to participate actively in groups more than others. Some prefer to observe, a characteristic that may be more prevalent among the elderly than in other age groups. Observational learning (Bandura, 1969) can take place easily in a group. Also, a person can play a variety of roles in the group, including gatekeeper, joker, leader's helper, and voice of reason.

Status   In some settings, being a member of the group can become a status symbol. This has been seen in nursing homes (e.g., Burnside, 1978), but may also be true in other settings in that a professional or staff member is spending time with a "select few."

Socialization   Especially for isolated clients, the socialization offered in groups is valuable. In other situations, it is a subsidiary goal and benefit.

Cost Effectiveness   Despite their needs for larger space, groups are generally less expensive to run and administer than individual sessions.

Impact on Systems   This last advantage cannot be overstated. In many institutions, staff, families and administration inadvertently "give up" on the clients. By using facility space, by scheduling regular meetings, and by making other demands on staff for an activity that is designed to promote change, the group can subtly and directly influence how staff and others treat group members and other clients in the system. Older clients can even use the group to help combat "institutional agism" (Settin, 1982). A successful group will arouse interest and potential support from other elderly as well as staff, be it in a senior center or nursing home. The group leader will also enjoy some increased status as well, which can be quite useful in promoting changes in care.

Cautions in Group Interventions

There are some serious cautions to be considered in implementing group approaches with the elderly. They are:

Inadequate Leader Preparation   Although there are few formal criteria for conducting group therapy or group work, many professionals concur in that working with groups is often more difficult than working with individuals. The mental health practitioner has to attend to all group members, their interaction, and group dynamics to appreciate the life of a group at a given moment. Too often, group leaders do not have the following basic background in groups: participation as a member in a group with strangers, coleading a group with a more experienced leader, leading a group with supervision, and having a sound knowledge of theory, stages of group development, and group literature. While group work with the aged is "safe" in that older people are less likely to "fall apart" or "open up" dramatically in most group settings than younger clients (Burnside, 1978), the question of preparation should still be a concern.

Inadequate Screening and Selection   Screening in groups for the aged should be considered as carefully as screening for other age groups (e.g., Reddy, 1972). Specifically, clients need to give consent to participate, which implies that they know and understand the nature and goals of the group, and they should not have physical or emotional difficulties that would make participation difficult. Clients for groups with a particular focus such as assertion or socialization should have needs in those areas. One other aspect of screening to be considered, especially in settings where people know each other, is existing cliques or subgroupings being incorporated into the group, which can create "insiders" and "outsiders."

Heterogeneity of Members   Are different levels of ability in cognitive, verbal, and activities of daily living skills (including incontinence) being mixed? If so, will some group members be so advanced that they become bored while others are so far "behind" that they find the group meaningless? People with varied levels of functioning can benefit from group experience, but their differences need to be considered in designing a group.

In noninstitutional settings (day care, senior centers), the same problems arise. Ideally, a good understanding of group goals and other appropriate screening will result in group members who, on the whole, are suited for the group.

Domination By Some Members   For a variety of reasons, certain members may dominate sessions at the expense of others, either by talking most frequently or by being the most "needy." This can be a particular problem with clients who talk "off the topic" or tell complicated and long stories. Interpretation and confrontation can be used by the leader, but some capacity for insight on the part of the client is necessary. Other possible strategies include giving the problem member a specific role (e.g., one gentleman in a day care setting who was a monopolizer and would sing throughout group sessions was given the task of suggesting songs at various points in group sessions), asking for others to "take a turn," counseling monopolizers out of the group, or letting the group deal with the monopolizer.

Group Versus Individual Sessions Some clients would receive more benefit from individual sessions. Some clients will be unwilling to discuss personal matters in front of peers or even relative strangers. Some will be inhibited and only observe others. Finally, some will have problems or concerns that are not shared by other group members.

Negative Status Although being a group member may bring positive status, groups can also be given negative status by staff or even other older adults. Negative status may not be obvious to a leader, but group members will know and be a source of information if it occurs.

Conformity Members of a group may feel pressure to conform to social or institutional norms (Hartford, 1980). The power of the group experience is potentially destructive as well as constructive. It is possible that groups may be used to foster dependency, stifle complaints, or even subtly coerce members into accepting unethical or illegal care by others.

Development of Dependency Dependency relationships may develop that will not be worked through. Group leaders may have impact on older clients in such a way as to create a dependency that is not fully resolved by the time a group ends. The mental health practitioner needs to consider how time-limited groups can terminate without leaving clients with the feeling that this is just "another of many losses." This suggests allowing time for group members to work through their dependency on the leader for validation of behavior.

Issues in Group Interventions

Although many aspects of group interventions with the aged are similar to those with other age groups, several special considerations merit careful concern for the aged.

Role of the Practitioner

The therapist working in a group has a different role and uses different techniques from the therapist engaged in individual treatment (cf. Yalom, 1970). In group work, the influence of the therapist is much more indirect; the major curative factors are enacted by other group members. The two major tasks of the therapist are to maintain the group (be aware of potential dropouts or signs of the group's disolving) and provide the impetus for creating a "group culture"—through implicitly reinforcing and modeling useful norms such as listening, focusing on appropriate content, and reinforcing interpersonal sharing and insight. Interpretation of individual behavior is less important.

The group therapist is a process commentator, a person who helps the group understand what is happening here and now, both between individuals and in the total group. The key issues are for the therapist to recognize the processes underlying group behavior, to time an intervention so that it has maximum impact, and to word it so that defensiveness is decreased. Interpersonal interaction and intensity are then increased, leading to group cohesiveness.

Goals and Objectives of the Group

Groups can be thought of as having one or more of the four general goals used to describe therapeutic interventions in this text: they may be curative, adaptive, enriching, or preventive. They may also have one or more focuses: behavior, atttudes/values, cognition, affect, or socialization.

Most groups have explicit objectives that provide a purpose for the group's existence. With the elderly, objectives may be quite circumscribed, such as improving ability to remember the day, date, and time in a reality orientation group in an institution. At times objectives will be much broader, such as improving communication ability in a "sensitivity group" run at a senior center or congregate housing site. The objectives of the group should be directly communicated to prospective members as part of screening.

In addition, the leader needs to determine if the group goals fit client needs and, in addition, if the goals are too limiting. For example, in long-term care it may be assumed that "nothing can be done" for "severely regressed patients," so that entertainment or arts and crafts are used when in fact more "demanding" group activities would be beneficial. Objectives should be neither too low or too high for clients' capacities.

Screening

Screening refers to the selection process for group membership. As was mentioned earlier, it can be poorly done, resulting in a group that is not ready, prepared, or able to function within the structure of the objectives. There are three key issues in screening. The client must give *informed consent*: Prospective members should understand what will happen and agree to participate—not easily done in institutional settings where degree of impairment and tendency to comply may interfere. The group should be *appropriate* for the client: The client's abilities, deficits, and problems should be appropriate for the type of group, and the group should not interfere with other treatment being received. A final issue is the *mix of people*: Are there obvious conflicts that will occur? Are the levels of functioning compatible? (They do not have to be the same.) Are physical disabilities, including incontinence, able to be accommodated?

Group Size

Group size is in part a function of leader skills, goals of the group, and cognitive level of the clients. For example, some literature suggests that reality orientation groups be kept as small as four to six clients. Some other types of groups have had well over ten clients on a regular basis. The question of how to include or exclude in a specific setting becomes complicated. In one adult cay care center, for example, the author ran a group for six months with all seventeen clients, as there was no space for a small group to meet.

Contract

Along with giving informed consent, clients should have an explicit understanding of what is expected from them as members, including type of participation, how often the group meets, and what kind of evaluation or data collection (if any) is part of the group. It is useful for this to be put in writing in the form of a contract.

Confidentiality

An important part of the implicit understanding of the contract in any group is confidentiality; that is, what is said or shared in a group should not become gossip or a general topic of discussion outside of the group. This is important for creating a sense of safety and cohesion among group members.

This point should be reiterated frequently in the initial stages of the group, as members will be questioned by others (peers, family, and/or staff, depending on the setting) and may need help in finding appropriate ways of describing the group without betraying confidentiality. The mental health practitioner also needs to decide how and where group information should be shared. Too often, there is little sense of privacy in institutions and senior centers. A needed sense of privacy can be enhanced by confidentiality in group sessions.

Integration of the Group Into the Setting

Integrating the group into the organizational setting is a two-way street; that is, aspects of the group will be altered by organizational needs and the organization has to accommodate the presence of the group.

Cooperation from the organization includes the following:

Publicizing the group
Identifying possible members
Having staff "talk it up"
Having staff understand what the group is about and not deride it
Providing transport (if clients cannot walk)
Providing appropriate space that is private and accessible
Listing the group in schedules of activities
Helping staff reinforce changes in client behavior
Giving staff release time to colead groups or assist in screening

Each of these aspects represents a use of time, energy, and/or money and should be considered before implementing any group.

The group may have to accommodate the organization in many ways: The scheduling of meetings should not conflict with the organization's activities, *especially* meals (meeting an hour before a meal is a good idea). The number of clients may be more or less than optimum, the number of meetings per week or total number of meetings may be less than optimum, and the physical space may have to change or not be totally private. Moreover, certain types of clients may have to be taken in, even though they may present problems for the group or leader.

The integration into the organization is negotiated at many levels. Most of the changes will come from the host organization. The mental health practitioner should appreciate the demands placed on the organizational system and be willing to preplan and work with the system to implement a successful group in its context.

Crisis Situations

Several crises can occur in group work with the elderly that may require intervention from the leader in her or his role in maintaining the group. Burnside (1978) mentions death of members, staff strikes, and other major environmental changes, as well as small changes such as a slight illness or change of place or time the group meets, as crises that, if not openly discussed, may lead to tardiness, absenteeism, and dissolution of the group. Because of some cohort tendencies not to "confront" anyone about these issues, the group leader needs to be particularly sensitive to these issues and be able to focus discussion on them in a productive way.

Termination

One of the expected transition points in any group is its ending or termination. Groups are often designed with a specific time framework, which theoretically makes the reality of their end more obvious than in individual treatment (Yalom, 1970). Also, group members can provide support for each other in discussing and going through the process of "giving up" the group. The leader also has to work on his or her own wishes and concerns as part of the termination process, which is much like that in individual treatment.

With the elderly, two other considerations frequently have impact on termination. One is the likelihood that the group represents an unusual and positive source of identity, one that may not be replaced after the group ends. Group members may have strong emotional reactions to the ending, especially in impoverished social environments. However, such reactions may not be easily expressed and the leader will have to make a concentrated effort to uncover and discuss them.

The second consideration is that groups are frequently run in settings where participants know and see each other outside of the group. This can be viewed as a positive force in aiding termination, as the contact and assumed identity from being a group member may be reinforced after the group ends its meetings.

Work With Impaired Elderly

Although over thirty years old, the work of Linden (1953, 1954, 1955) stands as classic in terms of group therapy with severely impaired elderly (Burnside, 1978). Not only did Linden pioneer the use of a cotherapist, but he also developed a series of useful principles based on his work with older institutionalized women. Some of Linden's principles are:

> Changes in behavior can take place, although the rate may be slower than for other groups.
> The institutional atmosphere contributes to clients' behavior and feelings of hopelessness.
> Mood, altertness, memory, and orientation are important areas to be continually evaluated in the group.
> So-called senility can be the result of how the environment (staff) treats the older person and how the older person treats himself or herself.

These four concepts are useful in guiding the group leader in work with impaired elderly. In addition, the following guidelines are suggested:

> Use communication principles presented in Chapter 5.
> Keep the size of the group small (four to six members).
> Structure activities that are both challenging and can be successfully accomplished.
> Hold the group in a quiet place with few distractions.

APPROACHES TO GROUP INTERVENTION WITH THE ELDERLY: SOME EXAMPLES

It is reflective of the state of the art that the type and variety of groups (many of which have been used with the aged) is quite diverse, if not bewildering. All groups have commonalities in terms of process and development; however, their goals, methods, and type of leadership is quite varied. For purposes of this text, group interventions will be categorized both by their goals—curative, adaptive, enrichment, preventive—and focus—cognition, emotion, attitudes/values, behavior, and socialization. The following section reviews some approaches that have been used with the elderly.

Curative Approaches:
Psychotherapeutic Groups

Traditional psychodynamic therapy in groups is not usually used with the aged. Rather, the focus of therapy groups with the aged is more on enhancing verbalization, creating support, or improving social functioning (e.g., Feil, 1967; Wolff, 1967). Insight—a "full" understanding of the unconscious motivations that lead to one's group and related outside-the-group behavior—is generally not a goal of therapy groups with the aged, but is used in a more limited fashion.

The few studies of the effects of group therapy on the aged continually support the contention that older persons with defined mental health problems can be helped in group treatment (see Hartford, 1980). There does, however, seem to be a tendency to focus on current life events and circumstances as the basis for insight. When insight into the past is a goal, reminiscence and life review are two commonly used procedures in therapeutic groups with the aged (cf. Ingersoll & Silverman, 1978; Ebersole, 1978b). The techniques for these two procedures are presented in Chapter 9 and will not be repeated here.

Adaptive Approach:
Groups Focusing on Cognitive Loss

Reality Orientation and Sensory Awareness

Reality orientation (discussed in Chapter 10) is often used in groups in adult day care and institutional settings. The leader's role is directive. However, the style of direction should be supportive and encouraging. Loss or confusion should not be emphasized. Rather, correct orientation should be rewarded.

Specific logistical concerns include having clients at similar levels of functioning, having the group meet at the same time of day and in the same place, and ensuring that props (scrap books, jigsaw puzzles, symbols of holidays) are easily recognized and understood by clients.

Reality orientation groups are most effective if the principles are integrated into care by others (staff, family) and if the environment is "worth" the client's being oriented. One reason for withdrawing is that the social environment is sterile and uninteresting. To orient people to an unhuman and uninteresting environment is of questionable value.

A final point in reality orientation is that *sensory awareness* is a suggested and at times a necessary adjunct. It can be argued that sensory impairment due to lack of stimulation leads to or enhances cognitive deficits. By stimulating clients in all five senses, the group leader can enhance orientation. Food, objects with varied colors, objects of obvious textures, objects with distinct sounds, and objects with tastes and smells that can be discerned by all group members can be passed around, experienced, and discussed. Basic sensory awareness can be incorporated into aspects of nursing care (e.g., a bath or a meal) on an individual basis. It can also be expanded into fairly complex group activities in body awareness and perceptual activity (cf. Ross & Burdick, 1981).

Remotivation and Resocialization

Remotivation and resocialization groups are two related types of group work that are often considered sequentially to follow reality orientation. That is, clients in remotivation groups are somewhat oriented to person, place, and time, although remotivation has been used with clients who are unresponsive or who have memory loss and a variety of other problems (e.g., Brudno & Seltzer, 1968; Needier & Baer, 1982).

Goals of remotivation include making clients aware of current surroundings, giving clients opportunities for socialization, practicing memory and cognitive skills, and enhancing verbal abilities. Like reality orientation, the group also serves as a way of building self-esteem and focuses on treating clients with dignity.

Remotivation sessions are fairly structured. There are five steps in a given session (Robinson, undated):

1.   Creating a climate of acceptance. This is initial communication and orientation of the group to the day's session. As each session has a "focus" (e.g., foods, the season, holidays), the initial activity serves to both break the ice and create attention toward the theme. Each client is greeted "individually," and comments are directed to how the client looks. Touch (handshakes, hugs) is encouraged.

2.   Building a bridge to reality. The subject for the day is then introduced. A variety of methods can be used. The subject should be meaningful to the clients. The initial presentation should focus on a concrete object—a picture, the date (if a holiday), a type of clothing (if the topic is a season), or a song relevant to the topic (cf. Dennis, 1978; Needler & Baer, 1982; Schell, 1975).

3.   Sharing the world we live in. The topic is developed by using a structured discussion guide (the questions can even be written down ahead of time), as well as props and visual aids. This step serves to broaden the topic as well as focus on specific aspects. For example, if the topic is Thanksgiving, questions can be asked about what foods are eaten, who gets together, parades, and how a Thanksgiving meal is prepared.

4.   Appreciating the work of the world. At this stage, topics are expanded to include emotional reactions or advanced concepts. For example, people might discuss how they will spend Thanksgiving or Thanksgiving's history.

5.   Developing a climate of appreciation. Sessions end with the leader thanking all members for attending. A sense of mutal appreciation is fostered by acknowledging attendance and participation.

Other general guidelines for remotivation groups are to ask questions that elicit more than one-word answers and to create an atmosphere in which it is "expected" that clients can respond. The choice of topics and how to develop them are limited only by the resourcefulness of the group leader.

There may be a time when clients are too advanced for as highly structured an experience as remotivation groups. Several authors have described *resocialization groups* as a less structured discussion format to maintain cognitive functioning as well as focus on relationships and feelings. Reminiscence has also been used in such groups. Resocialization is considered a "third step" in reorienting confused or withdrawn clients.

Although remotivation and resocialization are not new approaches, their scientific value is questionable (Dennis, 1976; Storandt, 1983). Often, the groups are led by non-mental health professionals, who may be unaware of group dynamics or how the group experience benefits its members. On the other side of the coin, however, is the benefit individual leaders see the clients who have limited cognitive and social skills and do seem to enjoy, anticipate, and participate fully in this structured experience.

Adaptive Approach: Groups Focusing on Transition to Nursing Homes

Dye and Richards (1980) have developed a method of group work designed to help members adapt to nursing homes. As tested by Dye and Erber (1981), putting new admissions into groups to discuss feelings, adaptation, and problem solving in the nursing home environment seemed to result in less anxiety and a greater sense of internal control over the environment in a short time. The concept of using groups to enable older people to adapt better to a new environment is intriguing and should be pursued further.

Curative or Adaptative Approach: Milieu Therapy

Originally conceived by Jones (1953), milieu therapy consists of organizing a ward or other group setting so that the entire environment operates as a "therapeutic community" to provide support and help to all of its members. Through encouragement of interactions between clients as well as with staff, along with appropriate activities, a sense of community and support is developed outside of "formal" therapy meetings (Almond, 1974). Often, there are group meetings as well as "community meetings" for all clients and staff.

Milieu therapy has not been rigorously tested as a modality for the elderly. One drawback to its use is that some older clients may not have adequate verbal skills for this type of treatment (Götestam, 1980). However, many clients with higher level functioning who are in adult day care, intermediate long-term care, and other settings could benefit from such an approach. Several questions need to be considered in "creating" a therapeutic community with elderly clients: Does the concept have value? (This question can only be answered through experimental studies, which are currently lacking.) Is the program truly a therapy of milieu? Are clients encouraged to have meaningful interactions, are activities optimally designed to provide emotional support, and are staff actively encouraging supportive interactions with clients? Is there a sense of support and community? Merely labeling a program "milieu therapy" does not make it so. Similarly, providing entertainment or pleasant activities do not in themselves create a therapeutic community.

The mental health practitioner needs to be skilled in group work as well as capable of being therapeutically aware the entire time she or he is in the milieu. Some clients will need particular guidance and support in interacting with others; it should be given without the mental health practitioner's abandoning an emphasis on the client's mastery over her or his environment. The spirit of therapeutic and supportive interactions needs to be reinforced and periodically assessed in therapeutic community settings, which is not an easy task. However, despite the lack of empirical evidence, the development of therapeutic milieux for the elderly in many settings may hold promise in the future.

Adaptive Approach:
Groups Focusing on Social Skills

Assertion Groups The use of assertion training with the elderly in groups, while not widespread, is growing (cf. Wheeler, 1980; Corby, 1975; Edinberg, 1975). Although assertion training can be done in either individual or group settings, groups offer peer support and modeling of new behavior that can provide the impetus for older people to speak up for what they need. Assertion training should be considered for use primarily in community settings unless staff in institutions are prepared to handle and respect the "assertive" resident. (See Chapter 10 for a description of assertion training.)

Other Behavioral Groups Several other types of behavioral groups have been run for older clients with specific goals such as increasing verbalization (Hoyer et al., 1974). "Structured learning therapy," which uses modeling, role playing, feedback, and transfer to other situations, has been successfully used in groups to teach institutionalized clients such skills as how to start a conversation or cope with difficult social situations (Lopez et al., 1980; Berger & Rose, 1977). Structured learning therapy has several facilitative aspects: "concreteness, a supportive atmosphere, high degree of structure and predictability, and a multi-channel (auditory and visual) presentation of materials" (Lopez et al., 1980, p. 404).

Enrichment Approach:
Groups Focusing on Development of "Self"

Humanistic and creative-expressive group approaches are, by their nature, more global in terms of goals than almost any other approaches to group work with the aged. The best known program in this area is SAGE, which was described in Chapter 11. Each of the approaches in Chapter 11 can be considered to have its own group work approach. However, therapists often combine several in their own approaches, including creative-expressive modalities.

The key concepts in humanistic group work are a focus on the here and now; an emphasis on current experience rather than reflections on the experience; working to uncover meaningful feelings or wishes; and working for one's growth and development rather than eradicating mental illness. Humanistic groups frequently focus on interpersonal interaction, staging or structuring exercises to promote growth, particularly in Gestalt groups; and they emphasize feedback and comments to members from the other members as to their reactions and observations about their behavior.

Lieberman (1980) has identified nine types of events that promote change or reduce blocks to change in growth groups:

The ability to express positive and negative feelings about group members and events.
The experiencing of strong and negative feelings, even if not expressed
Observing others having meaningful emotional experiences
The instillation of hope
Gaining perspective on one's problems by exchange of ideas and solutions
Self-disclosure, that is, appreciating that others have similar problems and sharing personal information or feelings that are not usually shared
Experimenting with new behavior and receiving feedback from others
Observing others model constructive behavior the client wishes to obtain
Achieving some insight into one's own behavior or problems. As Lieberman, Yalom, and Miles (1973) pointed out, it is critical to have *both* self-disclosure and insight for change to occur in growth groups.

These events may be considered yardsticks by which the leader can determine how successfully the group is going. The focus of a humanistic group might include changing self-defeating behavior, promoting psychological health, developing humanized relationships, promoting interpersonal effectiveness, and self-actualization (Johnson & Johnson, 1982). Because humanistic approaches emphasize holism (an integration of body, mind, and spirit), they pay more attention to nonverbal behavior, bodily reactions, and physical awareness than other approaches.

The relatively free nature of growth groups and the emphasis on expression and experience of feelings means that the leader needs to be able to handle strong reactions, be directive, but also be able to provide a sense of safety in the group.

Also, it should be pointed out that the use of exercises (some were presented in Chapter 11) can be overdone. Rogers (1977), in fact, suggests that most exercises arise from a desire by the leader to control the group.

Humanistic Groups and the Elderly

Several issues arise in considering the use of growth groups with older clients: The first is whether older adults are likely to benefit from these groups. The literature on humanistic groups for the elderly is limited, although the few existing studies are encouraging (e.g., Lieberman & Gourash, 1979). The lack of work in this area may be due to an assumption by gerontologists and growth-group leaders that older people cannot benefit rather than to any facts on the matter (Storandt, 1983).

What aspects of growth groups will be different for older people than for younger aged persons? Certainly, age-related changes would suggest using slower pacing of experiences for learning and adapting exercises for physical impairments, particularly as nonverbal communication and body awareness are two important aspects of growth groups. Also, it seems that the current cohort of elderly is somewhat reticent about expressing feelings or giving feedback in groups. At the same time, growth groups may offer needed stimulation and enrichment in otherwise impoverished social environments.

Another related aspect is that growth groups for the aged are likely to take place in settings where participants know each other, such as nursing homes or senior centers. One of the goals of such groups may be to improve existing relationships. This implies that there are likely to be aftereffects of feedback and expression of strong feelings by group members, not only in terms of "gossip," but also in clients' interaction between group meetings. Leaders and staff of programs or facilities should attempt to channel this in positive ways, including discussing "outside the group" interactions in group sessions and setting up specific contracts for handling related incidents that occur at times the group does not meet.

Some mental health practitioners and health professionals also expresss a concern that older people should not experience strong feelings because they are too "fragile" or "frail." One cannot, for example, imagine encounter groups being very successful with cognitively impaired older adults. However, to assume that older adults by virtue of their age or their general medical status (e.g., being in a nursing home) cannot benefit from humanistic groups may represent a bias rather than a rational assessment of the elderly or the treatment modality.

Should humanistic groups be considered mental health interventions with the aged? This is an extremely important question for reimbursement, programmatic, and ethical reasons. Many settings, including mental health centers, nursing homes, and hospitals, have limited resources to spend on interventions with the aged. Questions such as: "Are growth groups more appropriate to meet mental health needs of institutionalized elderly than behavioral programs to decrease incontinence and increase socialization?" are continually going to be asked in the next decade as choices about interventions are made.

On one hand, humanistic groups might be viewed as an "untested" luxury; only useful to help people feel good or relate to each other. On the other hand, such groups have hope, dignity, and humanization as important focuses, concerns that are lacking in many settings.

EVALUATION OF GROUP APPROACHES

Goals Group approaches can be used for varied goals in treatment of the elderly. Curative, adaptive, and enrichment goals can be met through group methods.

Focus Similarly, groups can focus on one or more areas of functioning, including cognition, behavior, affect, attitudes/values, and socialization. With the elderly, the implicit socialization and identity from being a group member is particularly valuable.

Targeted Population Groups have been designed and implemented for older persons with all degrees of impairments, concerns, and abilities. Certain modalities—

for example, reality orientation, remotivation, behavioral social skill training, and creative-expressive approaches—show promise for older adults with severe cognitive and physical disabilities.

Strengths and Weaknesses   Although the strengths and weaknesses of group approaches were discussed at several points in this chapter, they can be summarized as follows: The strengths of group approaches are their flexibility and applicability to many problems facing older adults, their implicit creation of social interaction and positive identity, their efficacy (many persons served) and, in certain cases, their proven scientific value.

The weaknesses are a certain lack of clarity in applying group principles, the potential problems (e.g., inadequate leader training, scapegoating, reinforcement of unhealthy norms in the setting), and, for many approaches such as reality orientation and humanistic groups, some uncertainty about their scientific validity. Despite these weaknesses, groups are likely to continue to be a major intervention modality in many settings for years to come because sufficient staff to provide one-to-one treatment will be lacking.

SUMMARY AND CONCLUSIONS

Group treatment approaches are commonly used with the elderly in many settings. Cohesion, a sense of identity, large numbers of clients, and socialization are among the reasons for using group approaches. At the same time, certain dangers should not be overlooked: inadequate leader preparation, the potential for destructive behavior such as scapegoating, or the reinforcement of inappropriate social norms (conformity). The practitioner's role in the group is facilitative, although in certain specific groups, a more directive stance is needed.

Groups have to handle many issues, including contracts, confidentiality, crisis situations, and termination. The goals and focuses of groups can be as varied as that of any other treatment approach. Thus, the goals of group approaches used with the elderly have included cure, adaptation, and enrichment.

The flexibility and widespread use of groups is encouraging. The lack of scientific validation in some areas will be a source of debate for some years to come.

13

Family Approaches

THEORETICAL PERSPECTIVE

Even though most family therapists would argue that they belong to one of the major "schools" of psychotherapy, family approaches to the treatment of mental health problems are substantially different from psychodynamic, behavioral, or humanistic approaches. The major difference is that, in family therapy, the entire family is the appropriate and necessary focus of treatment. Most family approaches implicitly reject the idea that pathology rests with the individual, arguing instead that while one person may exhibit symptoms of psychological distress (this person is often referred to as the "identified patient"), his or her behavior is symptomatic of distress experienced by all members of the family. Thus "pathology" is really a state of distress or breakdown in the family's functioning.

What Is the Family?

One of the first questions in approaching mental health problems of the aged from a family perspective is how to define *the family*. The family can be considered all persons in three generations, including the identified older patient, spouse, brothers or sisters, children, and their nuclear families. However, some older persons have close, familylike relationships with others not included in the family, such as persons sharing living quarters, friends, or even staff in a nursing home. For practical purposes, the family can be defined as all blood or marital relatives in a three-generation range (four if the client's parents are alive) and all others that have kinshiplike relations with the identified patient, including staff, neighbors, and friends.

The Family as a System

The theroretical underpinnings of most family therapy approaches lies in general systems theory, which was developed as a way of unifying how all science is conceptualized (cf. Bertalanffy, 1966). A basic premise is that each family is an interdependent system, with patterned sequences of behavior that follow certain "rules" or principles governing all systems. One can begin to appreciate the tenets of a systems approach through the following axioms:

1. The total system is more than the sum of its parts.
2. To understand the individual requires an understanding of the total system and its relationships.
3. Relationships and behavior are interactive; that is, all events are part of a sequence, a response is also a stimulus for another response from other family members. To think of any family member's behavior as simply a response is inaccurate.
4. To change individual behavior, the system's patterns, styles, or motivation must also be altered, as systems work to maintain themselves at a current level of functioning (homeostasis).

To illustrate the difference between individual and systems approaches, consider two descriptions of individual behavior:

1. A man wearing a white pinstriped outfit with a visored hat and a large glove on one hand stands in a field for ten minutes facing in one direction. All of a sudden he runs to his left, catches a small white ball in the glove, and throws it back.
2. A woman dressed in shorts, shirt, and shoes with cleats stands on a field for ten minutes. All of a sudden, she tenses slightly, stoops, and catches a large white ball. She then stands up and kicks it in the air.

While certain aspects of these two people's functioning can meaningfully be examined, their behavior is much more comprehensible if we are given the following information about their "systems": that the man is playing centerfield in a baseball game and that the woman is a soccer goalie. Also, if we knew nothing about the particular sport, we would need to know who the other players are, what their functions (their "roles") are, the objectives or goals of the game, and the rules of the game both in terms of what can and cannot be done. To increase our understanding still further, we would need to know some expected or possible patterns or plays, such as a sacrifice fly or double play in baseball or a corner kick and header in soccer. We could then begin to appreciate momentum, team spirit, and conflicts between team members off the field that affect their performance during the game.

The above observations are similar to those that can be made for any family system. We need to know who the family is and what roles each member plays (e.g., parent, child, "general," follower, martyr, tyrant, supporter, nurturer, and so forth). We need to know the "goals" of the family (what the family seemingly is working toward). One assumption is that functional families work toward growth, development, and protection of their members, but that dysfunctional families act as if their goals were to lead to distress or destruction of family members. We also need to know rules of the family—implicit standards that are adhered to or violated with subsequent penalties or sanctions—and the family's patterns of communication or behavior.

Also, just as coaches, players, and students of sports argue about the relative importance of different aspects of the game, students and experts in the field of family therapy see different aspects of family functioning as being critical and use a variety of techniques and approaches to help families function in a better manner. Jones (1980), for example, identified seven major schools of family therapy, each differing in its values, focus, theory, and techniques. The range of approaches is too great to summarize adequately in this text. The practitioner should be aware that an extensive family therapy literature exists and is worth studying as appropriate background for work with the families of the aged.

A RATIONALE FOR THE USE
OF FAMILY INTERVENTIONS
WITH THE AGED

The unique perspective of family therapy approaches give them certain advantages in handling the multisystem and adaptive problems of the elderly. Family approaches have three major advantages that also constitute a rationale for their use with the aged:

A Nonpathological Perspective   The family systems view is nonpathological. That is, it focuses on making the sytem as functional as possible rather than identifying and curing pathology. Whereas much of the emotional discomfort suffered by the elderly is adaptive, there is a natural fit between this type of approach and older persons' identified problems.

Focus on the Support System   Unlike any other treatment approach, family therapy approaches make the likely support system of the elderly the primary focus of assessment and intervention. Given the role the family plays in the care of the aged, such a focus is potentially quite useful.

Access to Issues Not Easily Accomplished in Other Treatment Modalities
This last area includes attention to communication and power relationships, as well as relating family behavior to a series of conceptual schemes designed to give the

"missing pieces" on how (or why) the family behaves as it does with the older relative. Any practitioner who has worked with families of the elderly knows that there are communication patterns, specific power relationships, and what can be called undercurrents (dynamics) that are related to how family members interact "in behalf" of the older relative. The many family therapy approaches attempt to uncover and alter disharmonious patterns. (See Herr and Weakland's approach described later in this chapter as one example.)

Why Family Approaches Are Not Widely Used With the Elderly

From a theoretical point of view, family approaches have much to offer to older persons, family members, and mental health practitioners. Yet in the aggregate, family therapy does not seem to be a treatment of preference for use by older persons and those who provide mental health services to them. The following reasons or forces act to work against the use of family interventions with older persons and their families, even when such interventions are warranted.

Individual Orientation to Psychopathology Most mental health practitioners are trained in an individual orientation to psychopathology. Also, persons who choose to work with the elderly have, in a sense, identified themselves with a generation of a given family and may have to reconsider their "professional" identity to work with family units.

Medical Orientation to Care of the Elderly Virtually all subsidized third-party payments for care of the elderly are based on a medical model of care. This orientation is particularly incompatible with a family and systems perspective about pathology. Payments for services are made on the basis of contact with patients, not with families. Diagnoses are made on the basis of *DSM-III* categories, not a description of system or communication patterns.

Reimbursement Mental health services are poorly reimbursed under current funding and legislation. Families may need more than forty- or fifty-minute sessions to get "air time" for all persons. While family interventions are therefore more time costly, one counterargument is that problems in one generation are prevented from being passed on to following generations and that a family approach is, in fact, efficient in the long run.

The Nature and Occurrence of Certain Mental Health Problems in the Aged Many problems of the aged are such that they are viewed as the client's rather than the "family's." For example, dementia, delirium, or reactions to change such as retirement or spousal illness are not likely to be viewed by either older persons and their families as a family problem. While family members may admit these events have impact on the family system, the onset and certain aspects of these problems may not seem to have much to do with the rest of the family.

Role of the Older Client in Family and Legal Systems   Family therapy was developed for use with identified psychiatric patients, many of whom were children. Most older persons with mental health problems are not labeled as "mental patients," but have family roles of mother, father, uncle, or aunt, a position of implied leadership and past child rearing. The older person may not want other family members "drawn in" to treatment or may resist any implicit suggestion that the family he or she raised has "problems."

Reinforcement of Other Implied Barriers to Family Interventions   Nursing homes, mental institutions, adult day care settings, and other service agencies reflect the first four barriers to family treatment—that is, in such settings there is often an indidvidual orientation to treatment, a medical basis for client selection, a reimbursement schedule based on individual pathology, and an orientation to client (versus family) problems. Several other aspects of these settings make treating family units difficult. One is the lack of suitable space for a mental health practitioner to meet privately with a family. In addition, there is delegation of caretaking responsibilities to these systems that, while decreasing family stress, does nothing to help the family "work through" or adapt in a healthy way to the changed status of the older client.

Logistics   Geographic mobility, increased numbers of women working, and work schedules make getting the family unit of an older person together difficult. Times when families can get together (vacation, holidays, or evenings) are precisely those times most mental health professionals prefer not to work.

Bias Against Older Clients' and Families' Capacity to Change   A belief related to agism is that older people and their families have such a long history of maladaptive behavior or coping responses that any attempt to alter these dynamics is doomed to fail. In reality there is no evidence to suggest that older persons and their families are less susceptible to change than "younger" families.

These barriers are not sound reasons for avoiding family interventions with older person's family systems. Rather, they are a description of the status quo, one that perhaps should be changed. The following sources of stress for the elderly suggest, in fact, that family interventions should be used with older persons and their families.

SOURCES OF STRESS OR CHANGE
ON OLDER PERSONS' FAMILIES

Several types of expected changes in older families are likely to have an effect on family systems.

Illness and Disability

Important potential changes or forces are set in motion in family systems when one adult member becomes ill. For example, family "rules" or values about how to be sick and how to take care of a sick member become an important aspect of the family's functioning. A healthy spouse, for example, may become a silently suffering caregiver, and a subsequent illness by the caregiving person may lead to chaos in the rest of the family.

One current trend is that "young old" are caring for "old-old" parents (Olson & Cahn, 1980). Hospitalization and transitions between hospital and home are likely stress points.

Identification
of Organic Brain Syndrome (Dementia)

The onset of organic brain syndrome creates significant changes and stresses for family systems. The older client may require time and resources from a family system that has other priorities, such as child rearing. Family members may react with denial ("There's nothing wrong, really"), withdrawal, or resentment when faced with the need to care for a failing older relative. The realities of care, especially in advanced stages of dementia, are quite demanding and can include feeding, bathing, and changing clothes frequently if incontinence occurs. The impact of dementia will be felt in other existing conflicts in families, including those between spouses, between parents and children, and between home and work.

The family system may also be torn between a loyalty to the previously functioning older adult (e.g., respecting the person's privacy, letting him or her make family decisions) versus a need to take a more active role in these areas. In addition, the family may, at some level, be mourning the loss of the identified patient's functioning as well as be adapting to the changes.

A final consideration is that in the course of dementia, the identified patient becomes a dysfunctional family member. The roles that person played in the family (e.g., father, mother, and peacekeeper, general, nurturer) become vacant. Some adjustment may take place to create a new balance or homeostasis in the family's communication system. Mental health intervention can focus on guiding the family system to adapt to continuous changes, to manage behavioral problems associated with dementia (Haley, 1983a), to recognize and grieve the loss, and to identify where its labeling inhibits client and system functioning (see Chapter 6).

A role not usually considered but possibly called for in cases of senile brain disease is that of facilitator, opening new possibilities for communication:

Case: A family therapist was interviewing a woman in her eighties with Alzheimer's disease and her fifty-five-year-old son. The woman was quite disoriented and sat silently through much of the session, responding to questions with one- or two-word answers. The son complained about the difficulties in caring for his failing mother, who had "never given him much" through the years. As they got up to leave, the woman turned to the therapist and said quite clearly, "I am sorry for the pain I have caused my son over the years."

Role Reversal

A dynamic frequently found with the aged is "parenting the parent," or a role reversal in which a child becomes a major source of emotional support for an older parent. This is often the case in illness, dementia, or death of a parent's spouse. From a family therapy viewpoint, several issues may emerge that can benefit from mental health intervention. First is strengthening the degree of differentiation of self the "parent" of the parent has: Can this person handle the role change without bringing in prior grievances or unresolved differences? Another issue is "triangulation." Is a third person drawn in as a "victim" as the role reversal goes on? Guilt and anger are two affective expressions of these "problems." Intervention would take the form of discussing how to differentiate self from parent and, if triangulation took place, working on ways to decrease the negative influence with all three people (cf. Bowen, 1971).

Conflicting family loyalties or values may emerge in role reversal. For example, one value may be to take care of the sick, a competing value may be to respect one's elders. In addition, the change in roles can lead to some blurring of boundaries (who has to be involved with whom and on what basis) or ambiguity in family rules, either of which may create a sense of tension and dysfunction in the family (cf. Satir, 1972; Minuchin, 1974).

In Chapter 2, the need for a sense of reciprocity in exchanges between generations was suggested as a goal of intervention in situations with role reversal difficulties. Working toward understanding and appreciation of the other's position is also a suggested goal.

Divorce

There are growing numbers of divorces among people over age sixty. Many times, an older husband leaves a "younger" wife, who is then left with no access to the husband's pension and social security benefits. The divorcee is also in the unenviable position of having "been left."

In the divorce of an older couple, family members may be torn between loyalty to each parent or may coalesce around taking sides in a dispute. The older woman who is "left for a younger woman" may well be viewed as a victim and receive substantial emotional support from others, although the resulting family behavior patterns are likely to be a continuation of previous patterns and can inhibit growth as well as provide support. New patterns may have to emerge or be developed as the family system attempts to adapt to the change in status of its elder members.

Death

Death of a family member leaves a void in the family's interactional system that needs to be filled. Whatever roles were played by the now dead older person will become filled by other family members.

How this is done will depend on the family's traditions, loyalties, rules, and adaptability of the family. At times, invisible loyalties and rules may lead to an uncomfortable resolution, such as when the family becomes the sole source of support, entertainment, and socialization for a widow because it "feels obligated" to do so rather than the caring being an issue that is resolved for the benefit of all family members (see Chapter 4 for guidelines in working with survivors).

Moving In

Having an older relative living under the same roof as younger family members brings with it two structural issues for family functioning. The first is how the work load in the house becomes divided. Certain subsystems ("adults" and "chore-doers") have a new member with certain rights and potential responsibilities that need to be negotiated.

The second issue is that unresolved or "old" family conflicts are likely to be rekindled by having the parents and their adult children in contact "twenty-four hours a day." While painful at times, this is also an opportunity for family members to "make peace" as adults and to detriangulate from each other. For all of these reasons, the transition from "independent" to "family" living is likely to be one of stress and one that can benefit from mental health intervention, although it is certainly not necessary in all instances (see Herr and Weakland's approach, discussed in this chapter, for a suggested way of approaching this problem).

Institutionalization

One of the greatest sources of family concern, guilt, resentment, and unresolved feelings is the issue of institutionalization. Surface questions that are often raised include ones about appropriateness ("Are we doing the right thing?"), cost ("Should we pay to have Mom as a private patient?"), and finding the right place ("How good is this place?"). If the issue is nursing home placement of a "deinstitutionalized" mental patient, the family may assume a need that is not felt by the patient (Hyer, Collins, & Blazer, 1983; O'Farrell et al., 1983), with resulting stress in relationships. The idea of institutionalization may also represent an implicit message that the family does not love the parent "enough" to care, even though the family members go to considerable expense and devote substantial time and energy to the relative after institutionalization.

One way to aid the institutionalization is to implement programs such as the one reported by Dye and Richards (1980). The National Institute of Mental Health sponsored a project in which family groups, including new residents and family members, were given the opportunity to meet and discuss their feelings and reactions to the institutionalization process. The goal of this project was to create better understanding and appreciation of the daily problems faced by residents and relatives. The first four discussion sessions focused on exploring feelings about the placement and feelings about the loss of roles experienced by the client, how the client can maintain contact with friends in the community, and anticipated "perceptions" of what the nursing home would be like. Later sessions were directed towards problem solving and coping with the "daily living" issues for both family and residents—such as how to give care without doing too much, or how to be an advocate without being a "complainer." The idea of a family group including residents was useful in working with families on the issue of institutionalization.

ABUSE AND THE ELDERLY

One of the greatest tragedies in families is the existence of abuse, a condition where one family member psychologically or physically harms another member. While child abuse has been intensely studied in the last decade, only recently has the question of elder abuse become a concern for mental health practitioners.

Definition of Abuse, Neglect, and Abandonment

Abuse is a multifaceted problem, including concerns for legal rights, psychological well being, and physical safety. *Abuse* refers to intentionally inflicting pain (either physical or mental) on an older person. This can be accomplished through inflicting physical injury, mental anguish, or inappropriate confinement as well as by actively depriving the older person of services needed to maintain his or her physical and mental health. *Neglect* refers to failure to carry out care-giving responsibilities. *Exploitation* refers to illegally using an older person's estate or resources for personal profit. *Abandonment* refers to deserting or neglecting to fulfill legal obligations and duties to the older person (Wolf, Strugnell, & Godkin, 1982). Abuse can be *physical* (including beating, withholding food, not providing adequate supervision) or *psychological* (including threats, verbal assaults, or other non-physical infliction of pain). Neglect can be either *active*, with willful attempts to inflict suffering, or *passive*, where there is a failure or refusal to provide expected care but no intentional attempt to create distress for the older person (Wolf, Strugnell, & Godkin, 1982).

Several states have laws requiring that abuse of the elderly be reported: Connecticut, for example, has an ombudsman system with designated ombudsmen in each area of the state to investigate abuse, neglect, and abandonment of the aged.

Aspects of Abuse

Several studies have attempted to find correlates of abuse. However, the numbers of persons surveyed were small, the definitions of abuse and neglect varied, and because data depended on professionals' reports, all conclusions are based only on cases receiving help from organized services (Wolf, Strugnell, & Godkin, 1982).

With these reservations in mind, the following factors and "facts" have been identified as correlates of the existence of elder abuse and neglect. The abused person is likely to be older (over seventy-five), a Caucasian female, living either in a private home or dwelling, having more than one impairment, making the person dependent on the abuser for care (Block & Sinnott, 1979; Falcioni, 1982). It has been estimated that 4 percent of the elderly population are subjected to abuse. Even when older persons are abused several times, they are reluctant to report it as they may either fear the "unknown" (possible institutionalization) or be reluctant to acknowledge that they have failed as parents (Beck & Ferguson, 1981; Harbin & Madden, 1979).

The person performing abuse (the abuser) is likely to be a family member or other significant caregiver. Studies as to whether males or females are more likely to be abusers have reported different results. Substance abuse, lack of communication skills, a history of retardation and psychiatric problems, and a history of personal abuse have also been found among abusers (Rathbone-McCuan, 1980; Falcioni, 1982).

Abuse may take place slightly more frequently in middle-class than in lower-class families. The form of abuse found to be predominant (psychological versus physical) has varied from study to study.

Intervention Guidelines

Most existing studies give suggestions for intervention, although the efficacy of any type of intervention has yet to be proven in cases of abuse. One of the problems is determining the goal of intervention. Is it to preserve "rights," protect individuals from harm, improve psychological health, improve morale, or to decrease stressors (substance abuse, burden of care)?

The suggestions given for interventions in cases of abuse include initially obtaining accurate information and creating a trusting relationship, then providing counseling and supportive services to decrease impact of stressors and make it possible to remove the victim from an endangering situation and make referral to social service agencies. Steuer and Austin (1980) also suggest decreasing the abuser's guilt, giving accurate information as to the older adult's condition, and training the abuser in needed social skills.

A number of questions need to be answered in designing effective therapeutic interventions in cases of abuse: What are the communication and behavioral patterns in the given family that lead to abusive behavior? To what degree can the family system learn to work together to prevent further abuse? How can stressors, including the burdens of care, be better managed by the family systems through better negotiations? To what degree is abuse influenced by changes in subsystems and boundary management? If there is a history of abuse in the family, how can the pattern be broken to prevent abusive behavior in future generations? Finally, how can indirect methods, including support groups, help this problem?

AN INTERVENTION STRATEGY FOR THE AGED:
HERR AND WEAKLAND'S APPROACH

The major work on family therapy with the elderly is that of Herr and Weakland (1979). Their approach aims at solving specific problems and, as such, is a specific short-term strategy. They argue that realistic constraints (including ones mentioned earlier in this chapter) will make their approach applicable in the frequent crises that mental health practitioners have to handle with older people and their families, many of which were reviewed earlier. Their approach to practice consists of eight steps.

Establishing Initial Contact

In making the initial contact, it is the mental health practitioner's job to translate whatever he or she is told or presented with into family systems thinking. The mental health practitioner is likely to be the only one who will think "beyond" the depressed or organic older client. Specific guidelines include being available and letting clients and families know you actively encourage them to be part of treatment, that they may talk about their feelings and not just the problem. Also, by defining the issues as "family problems," family members can be encouraged to participate as problems solvers or helpers rather than as "patients." Clients must also have an "equal opportunity" to share negative feelings and expectations about failure.

Inquiry and Definition

A key aspect of inquiry and definition is to find out specifically and concretely (e.g., how often, when, where, how it is expressed) what the problem is, how it is a problem, and to whom. Very often, mental health practitioners will accept a seemingly specific description (e.g., "I'm depressed" or "she's depressed") that actually needs more concreteness before any changes can be made in the problem situation. For example, persons who say they are depressed are usually depressed about something, even if that is a "trigger" and depression is more pervasive.

The mental health practitioner also needs to shift the family's focus from that of one person's being "the problem" to the family system's having a problem. The practitioner should be prepared to be persistent without being offensive, using reflection and paraphrasing to ensure that communication is understood. Also, many messages and communication about the family's role and function are likely to be unclear, as certain family members will not want others to hear what others have to say or will not want others in the room when certain matters are being discussed.

Inquiry into current solutions allows the practitioner to find out what has already been done to solve the problem as well as to acknowledge the family's commitment to the older member in question.

Inquiry Into Current Solutions

Ideally, the mental health practitioner focuses on one problem at a time, finding out both what has been helpful and what has not been helpful, being careful to pay attention to and respect solutions that did not work. At this point the mental health practitioner also has to be careful to avoid sharing both "emerging" thoughts about the family system and solutions. However, it is important to recognize and acknowledge that the problem is difficult.

Finding Minimally Acceptable Goals

In finding minimally acceptable goals, the mental health practitioner attempts to create consensus on what concrete "observable" behavior will suggest distinct improvement. This is a multipurpose step. First, it reinforces the idea that something can be done, even if it is not an ideal or complete solution. Second, it continues to move the family system from global and vaguely defined problems to specific goals that can be achieved. Finally, the goals give some realistic limits and a contract to the nature of the counseling sessions.

The mental health practitioner's approach is to work for realistic and achievable goals. The goals the family sets may turn out to be somewhat unrelated to the initial problem. The mental health practitioner will continually be asking the family for the smallest acceptable change for which it will work, deflating global statements and abstractions. For example, "What can we do about mother's dementia?" may be worked down to "We need to make sure her apartment is relatively safe for her over the next two months and then reassess." Earlier solutions may be recalled, reused, or refined and used, but they must carefully be assessed. As this work goes on, Herr and Weakland caution about the dangers of undue optimism on the part of the mental health practitioner, as there may be a tendency to move the family to develop overly ambitious goals. Also, because a large amount of information is exchanged in this phase, the family can usually benefit from a review of the process, including a summary of attempted solutions and each family member's role and stake in finding a solution.

Understanding System Dynamics

After a minimal goal has been set, the mental health practitioner should take time alone to form a picture of the family system. This can be done by terminating the session, or, if logistics require continuing, calling a "recess" to think about all of the information that has been presented.

The first question the mental health practitioner should ask herself or himself is: Does the family still need counseling? Assuming more aid is needed, Herr and Weakland suggest the following framework:

1. Determining the system, including nonkin, or out-of-town family members
2. Determining how the mental health practitioner is a part of the family subsystem, including determining who is involved in the family system, who the allies and adversaries are
3. Determining family rules, including an assessment of both flexible and inflexible rules
4. Determining if there is still an identified patient
5. Determining how indirect and direct power are used, including an assessment of "games" and ploys such as unconsciously using illness to gain control.

6. Determining how the family has avoided solving the problem, including an assessment of "solutions" that maintain the problem and a prediction of how the family might act if the problem were solved, as "solved" problems could unconsciously create other stresses for the family.

Given all of these considerations, it is of little wonder that Herr and Weakland suggest that the mental health practitioner take time alone to consider them.

Review and Planning

After the initial session and periodically during the course of treatment, the mental health practitioner needs to make temporary assessments of goals, individuals' openness to change, and individuals' involvement in the problem. The mental health practitioner also needs to assess what seems critical in maintaining the problem and how she or he can avoid reinforcing it.

Further Interviews and Interventions

Herr and Weakland use the term "mobilize" to describe how the mental health practitioner gets the family's cooperation in implementing new solutions to improve problem situations. Herr and Weakland emphasize the importance of understanding the family's "language" (cf. Bandler, Grinder, & Satir, 1976) or how the family views the world. If the mental health practitioner cannot "make sense" to the family, any help will be rejected.

Assuming some degree of trust and acceptance of interventions by the family, change is initiated by *reframing,* a two-step process. First, the mental health practitioner must assess what the family needs and then make a suggestion that is compatible with the family's frame of reference about how to change. It is critical that the family's value system be respected. Simply telling the family they are wrong is ineffective.

At times, however, the client family's neurotic behavior is such that "respecting" their beliefs makes change virtually impossible. Herr and Weakland suggest *complex reframing* in these cases. This includes pointing out to certain family members how their behavior actually gets them opposite results from those they wish, such as telling an "explosive" son that his attempts to keep control actually result in others controlling him. The concepts and skills implied for complex reframing have been discussed by Haley (1963), Bandler and Grinder (1975), Grinder and Bandler (1976), and Bandler, Grinder, and Satir (1976).

Homework assignments (or experiments) with specific instructions are often given to help the family begin to change or to gather information about symptoms. *Symptom prescription,* that is, encouraging clients to do more of whatever maintains problems, can be used judiciously when the family seems unable to gain insight into how it behaves. The argument for symptom prescription is that any change, even increasing dysfunction, allows opportunity for change. Also, symptoms can be "given up" slowly to give families a sense of control over their behavior.

The mental health practitioner has an obligation at this point to pace the rate of change, making sure she or he does not go too fast. Families need time to adjust to change and to develop new patterns of behavior or even topics of discussion. Some family members (often the most anxious ones) will unwittingly reverse the process to get to "familiar territory," the dysfunctional interaction pattern. Some families will have an uneven progress, moving two steps forward and one step backwards.

Termination

Herr and Weakland emphasize that how the therapeutic relationship is terminated will have long-term effects on family functioning. There are three aspects of termination: wrapping up, giving credit, and getting out.

Wrapping up means that the mental health practitioner decides it is time to finish working with the family. This may be difficult because of the practitioner's problems in saying goodbye, it may be an implicit statement of the limitations of the changes made, or it may, at some level, reflect a need to be indispensable to the family.

Giving credit means that the family is encouraged to feel a sense of accomplishment over changes that have been made and is given responsibility for both positive and negative changes. One of the points that may arise here (or earlier in family work) is self-depreciation: The family, now realizing it has responsibility for its behavior, feels guilty because they held on to their dysfunctional system for so long. The mental health practitioner should provide reassurance and give the family credit for having been able to find the strength to challenge these patterns.

A final sense of credit is that due the mental health practitioner. However, he or she should not seek this credit from the family. Colleagues, supervisors, or published accounts are ways the mental health provider can take credit without taking responsibility away from the family.

As a final step in termination, the mental health practitioner should anticipate how things may go astray in the future. This is done by both identifying and discouraging sabotage—conscious or unconscious—of desired changes. Families should be aware that one success does not guarantee that all future problems will be solved. Also, it can be pointed out in a caring manner how individual family members may subvert progress in the future.

Herr and Weakland's approach is clear and well presented, with ample case examples. It is not, as the authors note, the only approach nor necessarily the best in all cases. Several other authors, including Headley (1977), Haley (1983a), Maxey (1981), Richman (1978), and Blazer (1982) have addressed general issues, work with families of confused elderly, marital couples work, and family therapy where depression is the primary symptom. If the orientation and benefits of family therapy approaches can be realized by families, practitioners, and service delivery systems, more attention will likely be paid to this underutilized approach and more research and meaningful differentation of appropriate strategies will be found. Because family interventions are designed to eliminate transfer of ineffective behavioral patterns between generations, family approaches for problems of the elderly may be an untapped source that could help prevent mental health problems for the rest of the population, a claim that cannot be made for any other treatment approach.

EVALUATION OF FAMILY APPROACHES

Goals   The goal of family interventions is to make the family system as functional as possible. This can be considered curative, adaptive, enriching, or even preventive depending in part on one's view of pathology. With the elderly most family interventions can be considered adaptive.

Focus   The focus of family approaches is on the total functioning of the family unit, including aspects of cognition, affect, attitudes/values, behavior, and two previously unmentioned categories: communication and relationships. Although the focus will vary among specific family therapy approaches, the emphasis on relationships and communication is fairly constant.

Targeted Population   There is no specific targeted population for family therapy approaches. We do not yet know what type of family is most likely to benefit from this type of approach.

Strengths and Weaknesses   The strengths of family therapy approaches are that they focus on the functioning and relationships of the older person and the person's support systems, they offer a preventive and adaptive perspective, they are a nonpathological approach to treatment, and they provide both frameworks and techniques not contained in other approaches.

Their weaknesses lie in a lack of clarity of technique in certain systems, little scientific validation of their effectiveness with the aged, and the many barriers that make the use of family approaches difficult to implement.

SUMMARY AND CONCLUSIONS

Family approaches with the aged differ quite significantly from other approaches discussed in this text. The major difference arises from considering the family unit to be the source of distress and the focus of intervention. Thus, concerns about communication, relationships, and the support system of the older adult receive needed attention in these approaches. There are many reasons family approaches are not widely used with the elderly, including orientation of practitioners, a medical orientation to care of the elderly, and reimbursement procedures. However, many expected life changes such as illness, death, and increasing dependence on others may make several types of family approach more attractive to practitioners working with the elderly in the future. One specific problem-solving approach used with the aged and families, that of Herr and Weakland, was reviewed. Although it is not the only way to treat families, it provides a good example of how theories of family intervention can be applied in the practice setting.

14

Indirect Approaches pets, plants, and environmental manipulation

RATIONALE FOR INDIRECT APPROACHES

This chapter focuses on what can be called indirect approaches, intervention that is aimed at altering aspects of the older person's environment for the purpose of improving the person's mental status, mental health, well-being, or independence.

There are several reasons to consider using indirect approaches. First, research evidence suggests that specific aspects of the environment affect one's well-being and psychological state. To ignore these relationships is to limit unnecessarily the mental health practitioner's ability to enhance quality of life for her or his clients.

Also, taken in a different framework (a behavioral approach), environmental and indirect approaches create new reinforcement possibilities for clients. These approaches can encourage and maintain appropriate or desired behavior (including independence) or can help decrease or eliminate undesired behavior. Moreover, many clients can be reached through indirect methods, although the ways in which they are reached and the resultant impact may differ from that of direct approaches. Perhaps more important, indirect approaches are useful as an adjunct to other forms of mental health intervention, in that they help certain clients maintain or develop emotional attachments.

However, indirect approaches have certain drawbacks or limitations that have made them relative newcomers in the field of mental health care of the elderly.

First, with a few exceptions (primarily in the area of specific environmental changes), most studies on the impact of indirect methods are inconclusive. One unanswered question is to what degree the results are due to the specific form of intervention (pets, plants) and to what degree they are due to the underlying psychological processes (increasing independence or control over environment) that lead to desired changes. A related question is whether the changes are long-lasting (Schulz & Hanusa, 1978).

A second drawback is that these approaches are not ordinarily a part of the clinical training or skills of the mental health practitioner. In some settings indirect approaches may also be viewed as an inappropriate use of time for a counselor, social worker, nurse, or psychologist.

Finally, there is a subtle resistance to indirect approaches that becomes evident through such comments as "Why give older patients plants or pets? They can't take care of themselves." Somehow the idea of nursing homes or even senior housing as places where people take care of plants and pets or actively use and interact with their environment seems to go against conventional wisdom; it does not match preconceptions about how life "should be" for older clients who need economic support or who are sick, frail, or failing. Many indirect approaches involve aspects of life that are not antiseptic or serene (dogs have fleas, plants have dirt, things can get messy); certain environmental aids are not necessarily "pleasing" to the eye or ear of younger persons. However, these aids may be exactly what is needed to make settings for the elderly more interesting, stimulating, humane and supportive of independence. It may be that conventional thinking (and related staff or family behavior) needs to be changed.

This chapter reviews three potential areas for indirect interventions: pets, plants, and environmental manipulations.

PETS AND PLANTS

Pets and Animals as Therapeutic Aids

The Value of Pets

Most people have either owned or had contact with pets. Owning and caring for a pet is one way to take on responsibility as well as to give and receive affection. Pets are also a source of stimulation as they can initiate their own activity. Finally, and perhaps most important, there is opportunity for a "special" relationship to develop between pet owner and pet.

Having a pet is also of psychological value. This is evident from the reaction of "joyousness" that has been observed in nursing home residents when pets are introduced into their settings. Pets can also meet needs for status or companionship (Brickel, 1980-1981), giving their owners a role in which affection is allowed, in which another living organism is dependent on them, and in which they are not defined as sick, poor, a "patient," helpless, and otherwise dysfunctional. And because pets can need an organized routine in their care, they can be instrumental in encouraging improved functioning in their owners.

Caring for pets is often a continuation of a previously held role with positive memories. Pets can provide an opportunity for reminiscence about fond events and times and for reviewing positive aspects of one's history. Finally, pets can be viewed as enhancing self-esteem or even facilitating development of relationships with other people (Brickel 1980-1981).

Use of Pets with the Elderly

"Pet therapy" or "pet-facilitated psychotherapy" (Corson, Corson, Gwynne, & Arnold, 1977) refers to the use of a pet as a companion for a client with a psychiatric problem. However, in using pets with the elderly, a somewhat broader focus is needed. Pets can potentially serve to ameliorate the impact of loss, institutionalization, or other traumatic experiences that do not necessarily imply mental illness in the person.

Pets as Companions Pets have been used as companions in a variety of settings (Brickel, 1979; Lago, Knight, & Connell, 1982). Interestingly enough, there seems to be implicit administrative resistance to pets as companions in both institutional and community settings. Several states have succeeded in passing legislation to allow pets in public housing for the elderly, but in many instances pets other than fish are not allowed, even though potential health problems can be handled and potential gains from introducing pets may outweigh risks (Stauffer, 1982; Nussman & Burt, 1982). If a companion program is developed, involvement of organizations such as the Society for the Prevention of Cruelty to Animals or local humane societies is recommended to ensure the rights of the animals are adequately protected.

The following considerations apply in placing pets as companions (Stauffer, 1982).

1. Pets should be suited to the physical environment in which they are placed.
2. Consideration has to be given to whether young and older animals are most appropriate as well as to which type of animal is preferable.
3. Giving due consideration to differences among breeds of cats and dogs as well as to an individual animal's "personality" may make for better pet placement.
4. Companion programs should have contingency plans to allow the client to keep the pet as long as possible, for example, providing help with pet care when the client is sick.
5. When a pet is placed in a nursing home, one person (staff or resident) should be responsible for its care. There should be one place for the pet to sleep and eat. Regularly scheduled exercise and feeding will help the pet to adapt to its environment.

Animals can also be used in other ways to provide companionship for the elderly. A pet can be "owned" by a floor or facility, pets of staff members can be brought in for visits, and organized events like pet shows can be held (e.g., Heaman & Moore, 1982).

Also, the care of animals does not have to be limited to those that are domesticated, but can include activities such as maintaining bird feeders (e.g., Banziger & Roush, 1983).

Pets as Aids in Therapy   A somewhat different approach is to use pets to "bring out" clients for whom other forms of treatment are not working and clients who are withdrawn or isolated (e.g., Corson & Corson, 1977; Corson, Corson, & Gwynne, 1975; Mugford & M'Comisky, 1975). Clients who are virtually uncommunicative in other situations can be seen to stroke, pet, or talk to pets brought in for a weekly visit. One way to facilitate the process is for the therapist to be the one who brings in the pet for visits. The pet then is a natural topic for conversation with the therapist. It is likely that, in therapy, the benefits of pets themselves are not much different from those of pets used as companions. The difference lies in how the relationship between client and animal is handled by the therapist, with the pet serving as a source of discussion and a link to reminiscence, life review, or specific problems. This, in turn, suggests that pets, by themselves, should not be considered a substitute for human contact and other forms of therapeutic intervention.

Benefits of Pet-Facilitated Therapy

Several studies have been made of the value of pets. However, care must be taken to not overgeneralize results, since most have methodological problems, such as sampling (often very specific groups of clients are used). It is also hard to separate the intrinsic value of the pet from the effects of added attention paid to the client or the values of responsibility, stimulation, and introducing a predictable and enjoyable event into an otherwise dull and uninteresting environment.

A range of positive outcomes of contact between elderly and pets have been reported. Although the evidence is sparse, pets have been associated with improvement in morale, health, and longevity (Katchner, 1982). Other benefits include changes in self-attitude (Mugford & M'Comisky, 1975), providing a "bridge to reality," and improvements in life satisfaction, sociability, happiness, habits related to activities of daily living, attendance at social functions, and general quality of life (e.g., Banziger & Roush, 1983).

Several other relevant approaches with animals could be developed, such as using pets with terminally ill clients, using nocturnal animals (those who are active in the evenings) for pets when the client is up at night, or even a "sooth room" where pets could be available for petting or care in institutions (Brickel, 1980-1981). In community settings, pet ownership may also provide impetus for participating in a group that meets to discuss pet care.

The Loss of a Pet

One of the facts of life of pet ownership is that pets die due to limited life span, disease, and accidents. Grief and suffering over the loss of a pet is intense.

Older clients may be reticent to discuss their reaction to the loss of a pet because they feel they would be ridiculed (Katchner, 1982). Well-intentioned practitioners may avoid using pets because of the potential for loss.

However, there are still several reasons to use pets, even if there is likelihood of their death. Protecting clients from the possibility of feeling a loss implies a degree of emotional fragility that may not be present and denies the client the joys of attachment. While the loss of a pet can cause distress, it can also be the vehicle for meaningful interaction with the therapist about the loss or coping with one's own mortality. By prohibiting pets in many settings, workers are inadvertently stripping the individual of a useful role and source of satisfaction in life.

The Use of Plants

The use of plants—so-called plant theory—has value for older clients, both because of the intrinsic value of plants in the environment and because older people can become involved in the care and maintenance of plants. Plants can also be considered a way of reaching hard-to-reach clients in institutions.

The Intrinsic Value of Plants

Plants are living organisms. They grow, change, and predictably respond to environmental factors—watering, feeding, light and heat, possibly even talking. Plants also are a source of visual, olfactory, and kinesthetic stimulation. Finally, there is a certain satisfaction in putting one's hands in dirt.

Plants provide an opportunity for ownership and responsibility without onerous burdens of care. They also can give one a degree of control and over the environment and are predictable in their needs and growth. When plants are of a group project, such as caring for a flower or vegetable garden, clients have opportunities for involvement, planning, seeing plans implemented, and being part of a group (cf. Relf, 1978). As is the case with pets, owning a plant or working in a garden is often a positive previously held role. As such it can trigger memories or be a link to the past, either of which can enhance self-esteem.

Plants also allow for some expression of creativity in their care, and they provide a mechanism for practicing concentration and planning (Hamill & Oliver, 1980). Finally, they can allow clients with physical limitations a way to express themselves and symbolically communicate with the environment.

Use of Plants with the Elderly

Many residents of senior housing projects keep plants. Plants are also becoming more common in long-term care, although certain plants are noxious or cause problems for clients with respiratory problems. Plants can also be an impetus for group projects, such as holding a plant show or even designing and building a greenhouse. Finally, plants and the interest they engender are a potential link to the community through garden clubs, service orgranization projects, or guest speakers. There is an implied equality among plant owners that can make the interaction with "outsiders" more of an equal exchange than is the case with other types of visits. This in turn can provide needed roles with positive status and resultant self-esteem.

Benefits of Plants

The few studies evaluating the benefits of plants have been done more to test the impact of psychological variables such as responsibility (e.g., Langer & Rodin, 1976; Rodin & Langer, 1977) than the value of plants themselves. However, Relf (1978) reports that residents show a great deal of interest in plants, asking many questions and generating meaningful discussion on the topic. One could expect life satisfaction, morale, and enhanced interaction with the environment to be aided by appropriate introduction of plants.

Evaluation of Pets and Plants as Indirect Intervention

Goals The goals of using pets and plants can either be adaptive or preventive. Most of their potential benefits would be to help older persons either maintain a sense of identity and a positive role or, theoretically, to prevent further erosion of self-worth through the responsibility of caring for a pet or plant and the joy of interaction with a pet.

Focus Interventions using pets and plants often focus on socialization. It also can be argued that the preservation of identity and a positive role also places the focus on attitudes and values, that is, improving self-worth.

Targeted Population Most pet and plant therapy programs are targeted to elderly who can be considered impoverished in their social interactions, both in the community and institution. Pets have been used successfully with clients suffering from severe cognitive and physical losses. The range of possible targeted groups is quite large and includes persons at the lowest levels of functional ability.

Strengths and Weaknesses The scientific validity of using pets and plants as a therapeutic approach is somewhat questionable for previously mentioned reasons: It is not clear whether the form of intervention (pets or plants) leads to change or whether other aspects of the intervention (attention, having a regular positive activity, or having a sense of control over the environment) are responsible. Existing evidence also suggests that benefits of pets and plants are greatly enhanced by how they are introduced into the environoment. Possible influences include the older person's having a choice in the decision to own a pet or plant, taking responsibility for the pet or plant, having control over when events (feeding, care) take place, and having these positive events take place on a predictable schedule.

In addition, it may be that control and predictability of pleasant events are critical in the success of indirect approaches (Schulz & Hanusa, 1978). For example, in assessing the impact of visitors (another indirect approach that provides emotional support), Schulz (1976) found that either giving nursing home residents control over the timing of visits or letting them know when visits would take place led to positive "zest" and health status compared to residents who had unanticipated visits or no visits at all.

There is considerable flexibility in how pets and plants can be introduced and used in the home, senior housing, and institutional settings. The methods are clear, and with some attention to sanitary details there is little likelihood of harm. These approaches can provide nonthreatening ways for older adults to have meaningful interaction with their environment in a manner that either draws on past positive roles or develops new ones. Although not a substitute for direct intervention in most older person's problems, pets and plants can be integrated into many older person's lives.

However, there are potential drawbacks. One is the issue of how to handle the death of a pet. Another concerns long-term effects of these interventions. While some studies (e.g., Rodin & Langer, 1977) indicate that short-term improvements hold over time, Schulz and Hanusa (1978) found the reverse to be true. Also, discontinuance of the program supporting pet- or plant-facilitated therapy raises still another issue. What happens if the pet or plant remains but the counselor, group meetings, or other organizing aspects stop? This does not mean that programs should be avoided because they can create long-term problems, but rather than their benefits and the key aspects of successful implementation (responsibility, control) have to be integrated with other aspects of care to ensure likelihood of long-term benefits.

ENVIRONMENTAL INTERVENTIONS

The environment can be defined as the milieu and/or context in which we live. It can include aspects of the world such as geography, air quality, neighborhood, type of housing, quality of housing, specific features of buildings such as stairways, design of toilets, or the amount and quality of light in a room. Although a growing number of gerontologists are studying the relationships between older people and their environments, most mental health professionals are unaware of how the environment can have impact on the behavior and self-concept of older persons and, more important, what types of environmental interventions can improve self-concept, independence, and overall quality of life.

Why Tend to Environment?

Beyond the general idea that one should know about all aspects of aging to be an effective practitioner with the elderly, the following are pertinent reasons to study environmental interventions:

1.   The environment is "there;" it is part of all persons' functioning.

2.   As individuals age and face increasing physical decline or disease, aspects of the environment that once had little or no impact on them may take on tremendous importance and become barriers to functioning.

3. The environment is potentially a rich and uptapped source of ways to improve morale, mental functioning, and quality of life. Mishara (1979), for example, found that enriching an environment with activities, staff, interaction, and trips was more effective than instituting a token economy in improving orientation in older institutional residents.

4. Once interventions or changes are made, the positive impact extends to many clients.

Conceptualizing the Environment and the Individual

It is possible to conceptualize the environment in several ways. One of the more important themes is consideration of the interaction between competence (an individual's capacities, including physical and psychological functioning) and "environmental press" (the demands of the environment that lead to adaptive or nonadaptive behavior) (Lawton & Nahemow, 1973). Clients' needs for environmental stimulation, challenges, and supports will vary according to their abilities and competence in physical, psychological, cognitive, and social areas of functioning. When the challenges of the environment in any of these areas are either overwhelming or unstimulating, the individual may respond with a general form of maladaptive behavior, such as being depressed or withdrawn.

For instance, we may agree that a sense of independence is quite important to all older people, but the form and manner in which it is realized must be varied to accommodate the physical, mental, and social competence of the individual older adult. Independence for a woman confined to a wheelchair may mean having her room arranged so that she can use the bathroom without help. In contrast, independence for an ambulatory resident of senior housing may mean having access to public transportation. The purpose of environmental manipulation, then, is an attempt to maximize certain aspects of the individual's functioning (e.g., pleasant stimulation, identity, self-concept) while providing necessary supports so that the degree of challenge in the environment matches the individual's specific set of competencies in several areas of functioning.

The following discussion of environmental attributes, the elderly, and potential interventions is presented with this purpose in mind, namely, to give the mental health practitioner specific ideas on how to make the environment in which clients live more conducive to positive self-image, independence, mastery, and other dimensions that underlie the principle of human dignity.

Windley and Scheidt (1980) distinguish between *attributes* of environment and *taxonomies*, or classifications, of environment. They discuss eleven attributes of environment that exist in all types of settings, can be linked to behavior, and are sensitive to interactions between people and environment:

1. *Sensory stimulation*—quality and intensity.
2. *Legibility*—organization and clarity.
3. *Comfort*—conditions contributing to a sense of physical comfort.
4. *Privacy*—how does the environment create a sense of personal privacy?

5. *Adaptability*—can the environment be easily changed if the client has new needs?
6. *Control*—includes decision making and sense of ownership.
7. *Sociality*—how environmental features promote social interaction.
8. *Accessibility*—includes ease of access and degree to which objects in the environment can be used or moved.
9. *Density*—crowding and proportion of elderly in the setting.
10. *Meaning*—both meaningfulness and emotional attachment to environment.
11. *Quality*—aesthetics.

These provide the framework for the following discussion of environmental considerations in the home and institution.

Sensory Stimulation

Visual Sense

As was mentioned in Chapter 3, visual changes that accompany aging include changes in the lens, muscular changes, and onset of certain eye diseases. Perhaps more important, it may well be that visual problems are correctable but have not been carefully assessed. Snyder, Pyrek, and Smith (1976), for example, found that 24 percent of the residents in a nursing home were legally blind and 35 percent had low visual acuity, yet 81 percent had no recorded eye care history since becoming residents of the nursing home. The authors also found a relationship between degree of visual impairment and degree of confusion as measured on a mental status exam.

Other research suggests that hallucinations may be related to amount of light and can be "induced" by glare or shadows (Phillips, 1981). Fluorescent light, especially when uncovered or nonfull spectrum, is visually discomforting and may enhance confusion.

Visual Deprivation   Older adults are often unwittingly subjected to partial visual deprivation—lack of adequate sight stimulation. Older persons need significantly more light than younger persons to see, read, and participate in visual activities. Insufficient light in apartments, nursing homes, or congregate rooms will subtly reinforce nonparticipation in social activities.

Other factors contributing to visual deprivation include medication, lack of visual contrast in the environment, and the effects of bed rest. Also, the visual field is restricted when one is lying on one's back or side with the head turned to talk to a visitor. A "side view" makes face-to-face contact difficult. Finally, the visual field is experienced differently from a permanent sitting position (e.g., in a wheelchair), if only because environments (including signs) are designed for people who are standing (Phillips, 1981).

Visual Overload and Accommodation   Several related aspects of environment can have negative consequences for older clients. One is *glare*. Glare can be produced by any shiny surface, including bedrails, metal tiles, wax-shined floors, fluorescent lights, wheelchairs, or even direct sunlight shining into dark rooms or corridors. Glare can be physically discomforting. Observers will see older persons avoiding rooms or areas with glare, including social rooms, although most would not know why they avoid these areas.

Glare can also create visual hallucinations, in which the contrast between glare and nonglare areas creates the illusion of steps, solid objects, or even animate objects. Some clients may interpret these visual illusions to mean they are losing mental acuity, with resultant anxiety. For all of these reasons, glare may inhibit the older person from venturing into the environment.

A related visual phenomenon occurs when the older person goes from a well lighted area (room) into a dark area (hallways). Older persons need time to accommodate to change in light. Sudden changes can produce hallucinations of steps, which in turn can lead to avoidance or stumbling.

Visual overload also affects recognition of others. With age changes, likelihood of disease, glare, and inadequate lighting, older clients in institutional settings will have difficulty identifying the multitude of personnel they encounter. Similarity of uniforms and different staff working different shifts do not help matters. Uncertainty about whom one is talking to can only reinforce uncommunicativeness and withdrawal.

Still another area of visual deprivation and overload has to do with color. With age changes in the lens, pastels may appear quite similar, as will dark shades of dark colors (Phillips, 1981; Newcomer & Caggiano, 1976). Even when colors are distinguishable, they may not appear the same as they did twenty years earlier, so clients may have difficulty identifying colors.

Interventions   The key interventions in this area are improving lighting conditions and giving clients time to accommodate to light-dark changes in both institutional and community settings. Full-spectrum fluorescent lights, decreased glare (no-shine waxes, fewer tiled areas), and the use of blinds or other light deflectors (transparent curtains) are useful. Observation of where clients avoid congregating may provide a good clue to light deficiencies. Dimmers can be used to vary the amount of light in multipurpose rooms allowing good light for activities such as sewing or dimmer light to set the mood for a dance or candlelight dinner.

Auditory Sense

The major functional changes in hearing that are expected with age are loss in capacity to hear high pitches, loss in speed with which words or sounds are understood, and some difficulty distinguishing relevant sounds or voices from background noises (Hatton, 1977; Phillips, 1981). Clients with hearing problems (often a "hidden" loss) can rapidly become socially isolated. Others in the environment may inadvertently reinforce nonuse of the auditory sense by using slang, mumbling, covering lips while talking, or chewing gum—in fact, routine caregiving is "easier" if one does not have to communicate with the client (Phillips, 1981).

Interventions   The first and foremost form of intervention is controlling background noise. Any sounds that are unexpected, that interfere with conversation, or that are intermittent or reverberating are environmental barriers to auditory communication (Newcomer & Caggiano, 1976). This includes Muzak, which is interfering, often high pitched, and without any visceral stimulation; public address systems in which sound is distorted and often somewhat unintelligible; and sounds in congregate rooms with poorly soundproofed walls. Usually only ceilings have soundproofing (despite the fact that few people talk to ceilings). Special television "hearing aids" have become available that compensate for an individual's high pitch loss without the need to turn up the volume in a communal area. Finally, clients, and particularly those with cognitive impairment, should be able to control sounds from a stereo or radio.

Kinesthetic, Olfactory, and Gustatory Senses

Although some change in kinesthetic function can be expected with age, many deficits arise as much from circumstances as individual changes. For example, in the physical environment of an institution most substances are hard, made of either plastic or metal. Similarly, most institutional food lacks taste, due to both sense changes in the elderly and food preparation methods. Personal physical contact is "procedural," not caring. Social norms about how and when to touch are restrictive for the elderly. To a lesser degree, the same problems occur in congregate housing.

Interventions   The tactile environment can be stimulating and a source of important information when other senses are impaired. Textures should vary to provide both stimulation and identity in the environment. This includes having objects that can be squeezed or manipulated and furniture that "feels" good. Finally, objects should be available so that the individual can decide when and how to touch them.

Spices and special foods can be used to enhance the living environment, even with patients who have dietary restrictions. Some loss of smell can in part be countered by adding more spices. Also, servings can be made visually attractive.

Improving Legibility of the Environment

Several concerns, including level of stimulation, are relevant to making the older person's environment clear and organized, although older clients may tacitly assume that their difficulties deciphering the environment are due to age.

Visual Environment   Several types of intervention have been suggested to organize visual aspects of the environment. One is to use color codes and/or recognizable names for different floors and wings of nursing homes and congregate housing, as well as different colors for bathrooms and door frames (Holmes et al.,

1979; Phillips, 1981). However, since clients are unlikely to have used color codes to "read" an environment in the past, they may not "catch on" without instruction.

Signs are rarely lettered or designed for the elderly, nor are they placed where they can be read by older ambulatory clients, much less by clients in wheelchairs. Optimal height for any sign is five feet off the ground (Holmes et al., 1979). Ideally, signs should use capital and lower-case letters, dark letters against a light background, and simple lettering. They should use words rather than symbolic pictures. Floor numbers should be clearly visible upon leaving an elevator or flight of stairs and should not be complicated. Graphic designs, for example, can be difficult to identify.

Persons' names and room numbers should be placed on doors of rooms in easy-to-read raised letters and numbers. Labeling personal belongings is particularly important in institutional settings, as personal items (e.g., dentures) can become lost and create subsequent distress.

Visual cues can also be used to indicate congregate and residence areas. For example, walls near congregate areas might have higher concentrations of pictures or wall hangings on than resident sections. Pictures related to the type of activity— for example, still lifes of food near the dining room and pictures of people interacting near recreation rooms—can also provide visual input to help the client organize the environment.

A final consideration is using the visual environment to orient clients. Clocks (digital clocks are not always useful), calendars, bulletin boards, and up-to-date activity boards should be part of all institutions and residences.

Auditory Environment   Even without cognitive impairment, it is likely that announcements over P. A. systems or in groups will be misheard or not understood by everyone "listening." Clients need a means to check out their interpretations of what they hear.

Auditory cues can provide help in organizing aspects of the enviornment, especially for visually handicapped clients. A combination of lights and bells can help older persons anticipate arriving elevators. Similarly, certain music, tones, or other auditory cues can be used on a P.A. system to designate activities or regularly occurring events.

Kinesthetic Environment   Objects with different uses should feel discernably different for visually handicapped clients. In home settings, varied handles and placement (front or back of a drawer, etc.) can provide the key to the use of an implement. Changes in floor surfaces can also be used to indicate that a person is approaching an elevator, stairs, or even a congregate area.

It should be noted that these alterations do not take the place of working with individual clients to determine what specific help they need in understanding their environment. Sometimes help is needed in breaking stimuli down into small and meaningful steps (e.g., using white tape to indicate the bathroom, adding signs to designate a client's dresser in a shared room, or teaching a client how to get his or her clothing and put it on).

Other Attributes of the Environment

Comfort

Needless to say, if areas in the environment are physically uncomfortable, clients will avoid them. Previously discussed sources of discomfort include background noise, fluorescent lighting, and glare. Temperature and air quality are also concerns (fresh air may be an unspoken wish in institutional settings).

An area of comfort usually overlooked is the types of furniture available to older adults. Chair heights, for example, should be varied so both tall and short persons can comfortably sit in a congregate room with feet on the floor. Chairs with seats that are too wide or too long back to front will result in sprawling. Similar problems occur in wheelchairs, most of which are too big for older women.

Privacy

Privacy, that is, a sense of some control over environmental input from others, is related to self-concept as well as autonomy (e.g., Windley & Scheidt, 1980; Westin, 1970). Also, Moos (1976) found that when personal space is unavailable, people withdraw from social interaction. Ways in which privacy can be encouraged are: giving clients control over visual input, such as putting light switches within arm's reach of beds, using physical room barriers (even curtain room dividers), decreasing hall noise, allowing clients to have their room doors closed, arranging room furniture so that people conversing can have a sense of private space, and setting aside areas or places where confidential conversations may take place.

Adaptability

Environmental adaptability is in part a matter of design. Ideally, rooms and congregate areas should be designed so that residents with varying degress of dependency and physical needs can be change features to fit their needs.

Control

Control and territoriality are often related to privacy. Windley and Schedit (1980), for example, conclude that certain defensive behavior from nursing home residents would decrease if they had control over a physical area where personal objects could be kept.

Control also has to do with choice, decision, and mastery of the environment. Clients can gain a sense of control when they make choices about what clothing to wear, what food to eat, and other aspects of daily life. The need for control may also mean that staff should not force social interaction (Newcomer & Caggiano, 1976).

Sociality

Given that both congregate housing and institutional settings are designed to promote socialization, it is often surprising to find fairly low levels of social interaction among residents (Tate, 1980). However, low levels of interaction should not be taken to mean lack of interest.

The impact of environment on sociality is probably greater than most mental health practitioners realize. One example is how the presence, absence, and placement of furniture affects interaction. Chairs strung out in long rows along dimly lit corridors inhibit interaction. Clients are more likely to socialize if they can congregate in "interesting" places, such as nurses' stations, lobbies, or rooms with views of traffic in and out of facilities or housing. Appropriate placement of chairs in these areas should be encouraged (Newcomer & Caggiano, 1976; Holmes et al., 1979). Similarly, long tables in a dining room discourage communication; smaller tables create a better atmosphere for communicating (Somer, 1970). A small coffee table near a window with a view of the employee parking lot may lead to informal meetings and gossip; chairs along walls in a recreation room with a "scenic" view may not.

One implicit barrier to sociality is the idea of *pseudofixed space* (Steele, 1973). That is, most people treat objects in the environment as immovable. Thus, if chairs are set against a wall (not a good position for face-to-face conversation), few people will move them. Grouping chairs is a useful way to encourage sociality; however, changing the arrangement in a common room may also infringe on territory (people tend to "own" their seat in a dining room). Staff also tend to rearrange furniture "back the way it was." Involving all levels of staff and clients in changes for sociality is important.

Finally, some clever planning and plotting of traffic flow can lead to creative ways of creating socialization. Some colleagues, for example, have suggested that activities be planned to take place outside of dining areas or recreation rooms while clients gather before a meal or planned activity.

Accessibility

Accessibility encompasses both the ease of getting between two points and the ease with which objects can be manipulated in the environment. Issues of getting from place to place focus on availability of ramps and elevators, as well as access to toilets and sinks. Object manipulation includes being able to open bottles, manage in a toilet or kitchen, or see objects in a room.

Seating and eating are two areas related to access. Because of likely physical changes, some older persons need help getting in and out of furniture; their chairs should have arms that extend to the ends of the chairs, firm seat ends, and seats that do not angle back (customary to inhibit urine from flowing to the floor in institutions).

Geri-chairs, however, often set the person in them apart from the environment, both physically and symbolically. Their height and the ease with which others can touch the client set geri-chairs apart from other furniture. Even with trays removed, chairs cannot always be placed close enough to tables to allow clients to feed themselves easily without a risk of spills. Subsequently, clients may cease to feed themselves, as this barrier to self-maintenance will, if not countered by higher tables or transfer to another chair, be insurmountable.

A similar problem exists with footrests on geri-chairs and wheelchairs. Their placement makes it difficult for the elderly to get in and out of the chairs, and as a consequence, they do less walking than their degree of impairment would dictate. A related problem is bed rails. Some, when down, are in a position where a person's feet will hit them as he or she gets out of bed.

Other concerns relating to access are somewhat more amenable to structural solutions. Ease of self-care and impetus for dressing may be enhanced by having mirrors available and at good heights for wheelchair or bedridden persons. Clients may need to be taught how to organize their environment to maximize access, including putting glasses and slippers near the bed, putting glasses on before going to the bathroom, using slippers on the floor as a guide for knowing where the bed is as one is backing in, having a light switch at the bedside, and using tools or aids to simplify use of cabinets and household implements (cf. May, Waggoner, & Hotte, 1974). Some attention should also be paid to likely impairments for clients in designing recreation and leisure activities (cf. Hammill & Oliver, 1980).

These interventions may seem simple and not in the specific province of a mental health practitioner. However, all persons in contact with the elderly should be aware of how to restructure the environment to prevent withdrawal, confusion, and loss of self-esteem.

Density

Because of previously mentioned physical changes in sight and hearing, certain clients will have difficulty communicating with several people in a room. Crowds may also increase anxiety or confusion. "Crowds" have to be considered potentially as being two or more persons, depending on the client's competency.

Meaning

The environment may have a very different meaning for clients than for family, facility staff, or mental health practitioners. Hyatt (1982) tells the story of an older nursing home resident who claimed that the physical therapy area was a "mental testing room." "They took me down there, pointed me at three stairs leading up to wall and told me to walk up the stairs. Any fool can tell you you don't walk up stairs into a wall so I refused and they let me go. I passed and never had to go back . . . you know, there are some pretty stupid people here. They bring them down here twice a week. They walk up the stairs, they walk down the stairs, and they never figure it out."

Clients who do not understand the significance of "events" like arts and crafts, recreation, physical therapy, or instructions may withdraw. Too often, providers assume this response is the result of a psychological or physiological condition rather than difficulty understanding the environment.

Quality

Quality refers to the aesthetic quality, or degree of beauty, in the environment. Aesthetic quality can be a difficult aspect of the environment upon which to agree and then to intervene. Definitions of beauty vary. Also, administration, workers, and residents are usually more concerned with functional aspects of environment, such as ease of maintenance or access, than with aesthetic quality. The two may be seen as antithetical (Windley & Scheidt, 1980). In addition, expected physical changes with age make certain pleasing uses of color or sound somewhat ineffective for older clients, such as the use of pastels in rooms. Finally, aesthetic quality is not a direct responsibility of any profession or specific job description in most settings for the elderly.

Nevertheless, improving the aesthetic quality of living arrangements for older adults has several benefits. An aesthetically pleasing and stimulating environment may have a corresponding effect on morale of both older persons and those who work with them. The presence of paintings or wall hangings with aesthetic value or aesthetically meaningful music (not Muzak) in specific places or sites can create stimulation and be used for discussion topics.

Evaluation of Environmental Interventions

Goals   The goals of environmental interventions are primarily adaptive and preventive: They are designed to provide support in numerous ways to compensate for specific losses and allow individual clients maximum flexibility and independence of functioning within the limits of their losses or disabilities.

Focus   The focus of environmental interventions varies, often emphasizing areas such as behavior and socialization. At the same time, certain interventions, such as decreasing glare, can be said to eliminate or prevent onset of problems in other areas (e.g., confusion, illusions). Also, by fostering independence and socialization, environmental interventions reinforce a positive self-concept and thus may address attitudes or values.

Targeted Population   Environmental interventions are potentially useful for all elderly, although the ones presented in this chapter focused on groups in which there was some noted degree of impairment. They have particular importance when the degree of impairment in one or more areas of functioning is great.

Strengths and Weaknesses   The major strengths of environmental interventions are their flexibility and breadth of application, their potential to affect the lives of many persons, the clarity with which most can be described, and their availability as an "untappped" resource in improving the functioning of older persons. The major weaknesses are a lack of "hard" data on the incremental gains of their implementation (e.g., what percentage of confusion disappears when the lighting is improved), a lack of knowledge and awareness of their impact by those who are in a position to implement these changes, and a sense that the environment is not exactly part of any particular discipline. Environmental interventions represent an area that has great untapped potential for research and development of new approaches in the future.

SUMMARY AND CONCLUSIONS

Indirect approaches include introducing pets and plants into the social milieu of the older person as well as altering specific aspects of the environment. The value of pets and plants has been documented, but they should be considered primarily for their value in socialization or as an adjunct for other forms of treatment.

While we can be somewhat sure that antiseptic, unstimulating, uncomfortable, unpleasant, and inaccessible environments limit client behavior, parameters for improving functioning are unclear. We also do not know to what degree altering the environment, introducing animals or plants, or having clients in control of their surroundings reverses confusion or slows decrements due to conditions such as Alzheimer's disease. It is possible that clients with the same condition will respond differently to indirect and environmental interventions because of unique differences in past experience, including roles, meaning of events, and style of adaption. Individual differences in other than diagnostically significant areas, such as speech, hearing, and vision, will also influence client response to these interventions. Not surprisingly, even armed with substantial knowledge, the mental health practitioner will still have to attend to the individual client, at times using an intelligent trial-and-error methodology to determine an optimal mix of environmental or indirect approaches.

15

Delivering Mental Health Services to the Elderly

INTRODUCTION

This chapter addresses five issues: the nature of the mental health system as it relates to the elderly; some general observations about the nature and functioning of human service organizations; the nature and characteristics of institutional settings serving the aged; the nature and characteristics of community agencies serving the aged; and alternatives to traditional services that are being developed—specifically the use of outreach, peer counselors, and work with support systems.

One major difficulty in appreciating the impact of these five overlapping issues is that they are experienced indirectly and are interpreted as personal issues by many mental health practitioners. For example, a mental health practitioner trying to develop a movement therapy program in a nursing home may find no administrative support, little interest from staff, and no easy way to be reimbursed for her or his time. An immediate response to the situation is to assume that the administration and staff do not care about mental health. This may be true to some degree, but other factors may be more important, such as the work load individuals have, how they perceive themselves, the degree to which the "new" service conflicts with organizational values and norms, and availability of resources to cover the costs of the program. If the practitioner can accurately assess the relative impact of these factors, she or he can also take steps to decrease or eliminate barriers and improve quality of service.

THE NATURE OF THE MENTAL HEALTH SYSTEM AND THE AGED

Older people are patently underserved by all forms of mental health service (Redick & Taube, 1980). Only 2 percent of patients in psychiatric clinics and no more than 6 percent of patients in community mental health centers are elderly (Kramer, Taube, & Redick, 1973; Gatz, Smyer, & Lawton, 1980). Less than 5 percent of psychiatrist's clients are elderly (Marmor, 1975). Well over half of all nursing home patients have symptoms of mental health problems, yet mental health services for this group are, in general, nonexistent. Programs that successfully reach the elderly are usually ones that bring in the least amount of fees, are costly in terms of outreach and coordination, and are therefore the first to be cut back when budgets become tight (e.g., Puterski, 1982). It can be argued that the nature of social and medical care of the elderly is such that the psychological needs of the neediest are overlooked (e.g., Estes, 1979).

Historically, mental health services to the elderly were provided in institutions such as state mental hospitals, where geriatric patients were persons with "chronic" conditions such as schizophrenia who had grown older in the institution. Their condition was often viewed as unchangeable, and they received medication rather than active treatment (Kramer, Taube, & Redick, 1973). Medication was used to control the more dramatic symptoms of mental disorders.

Two legislative events changed this picture: the Community Mental Health Centers Act of 1963 and the Social Security Amendments of 1965, which instituted Medicare. The Mental Health Centers Act provided some federal funds for states to develop community mental health centers (CMHCs). The act was amended several times, the fifth being in 1975, when services for the elderly were finally mandated. However, since then the percentage of elderly seen has not changed (Gatz, Smyer, & Lawton, 1980).

Medicare legislation led to the growth of the nursing home industry, as long-term and recuperative care could now be reimbursed. While the act's developers attempted to create supports to maintain older persons in their homes, the system inadvertently supported institutional solutions to problems that may not require institutionalization.

While there was a general trend in the 1960s for less institutional (state mental hospital) care for all age groups, older schizophrenics and persons with senile dementia remained in mental hospitals. However, in subsequent years, there was a trend to "return" elderly clients to their communities. "Communities," unfortunately, often meant a nursing home ill prepared to cope with behavioral problems presented by schizophrenic or severely impaired elderly. The transition from institution to community has historically not received close follow-up and coordination.

As a result of these trends custodial care of the elderly has risen proportionately, older persons have left or never entered the formal mental health system, and settings such as nursing homes have become the agencies to provide mental health care, even when they are ill-equipped to do so (Kahn, 1975).

Furthermore, older persons with mental health problems "fall within the bailiwick of both mental health programs and programs and services for the aged" (Gatz, Smyer, & Lawton, 1980, p. 7) and may be served by neither. Agencies that fall under the auspices of the Older Americans Act of 1965, including meal programs, certain social services programs, and programs funded by discretionary grants do not, as a rule, have close working relationships with mental health system services.

In addition, what has been called professionalism has served to keep barriers to service maintained. That is, providers of services have become increasingly competitive about being licensed and certified and have lobbied for legislative protection of their service areas (Sarason, 1977; Estes, 1979) as each "profession" attempts to stake out its area of expertise, even though all overlap in the area of human behavior. Professionalism has also influenced the lack of integration of many areas of human service delivery, including acceptance of common record keeping and professional review systems (e.g., Weed, 1969).

Within this context Gatz, Smyer, and Lawton (1980) suggested that the next decade will see the following in terms of the mental health system and the elderly:

1. An emphasis on community-based service
2. Decentralization of services
3. Emphasis on community support systems
4. Extending services to underserved populations and areas
5. Somewhat more emphasis on prevention

Indeed, legislation that would enable needed services was passed in 1980, and it had specific provisions for the aged. However, it was never enacted. Under the Reagan administration, the Omnibus Reconciliation Act of 1981 (PL 97-35) was passed, cutting federal funds for mental health services by 25 percent. Mental health program funding for the aged was then placed in direct competition with all types of programs under Block grant programs, the priorities for which are set by state and local governments. Thus, money previously targeted for elderly services or prevention became lost in general funding (cf. Puterski, 1982).

Mental health and aging services networks have not been particularly effective in educating and influencing policy makers, legislators, and local politicians to provide continuing services geared to the prevention and active treatment of mental health problems of the elderly. The issue of influence takes on increasingly more importance as the rest of human service care becomes even more politicized than it has been in the past.

SOME OBSERVATIONS
ABOUT HUMAN SERVICES ORGANIZATIONS
AND SERVICE TO THE ELDERLY

The delivery of service to the elderly usually take place within organizations. Any organization can be analyzed on several dimensions (e.g., structure, decision making, quality of service, client characteristics) (Katz & Kahn, 1966). While similar types of organizations, such as mental hospitals or nursing homes, have certain aspects in common, each individual organization is unique in many ways, including its atmosphere and the specifics of how individuals provide care for other individuals. Thus, all nursing homes are not the same.

The analysis of an organization's functioning usually includes an assessment of organizational dynamics. *Organizational dynamics* refers to underlying processes that affect organizational behavior. The processes are not obvious nor are they usually addressed consciously or directly by people working in an organization. Some major areas affected by organizational dynamics are goals, values, roles, leadership, norms, decision making, communication, and conflict resolution. All are important and are intertwined to give each organization its own identity, purpose, and atmosphere.

Formal Versus Informal Power Structures

One of the most important differentiations within the organization is between formal and informal structures. Both formal and informal structures in organizations exert influence on power, decision making, and information flow. Decisions, power, and information go through formal channels (e.g., meetings, memos) and informal channels (e.g., people talking over lunch, in the halls, on the way in and out of meetings). The "politics" of almost any system refers to influence exerted in an informal manner—that is, who is really key to decisions, who owes favors, and so forth.

Two important aspects of the informal system that are often overlooked in implementing new programs are "status by virtue of longevity" and the types of influence exerted by lower-level staff. Any human service organization has a fair amount of turnover, with new staff coming in on a regular basis. One result is that persons who stay on for extended periods of time gain special status. A nursing supervisor with twenty years on the job will have much more influence over staff "going along" with pet therapy than one with only a month on the job. Similarly, the administrative assistant who thinks his or her mental health center should not provide "social" service to the elderly and has been there ten years may inadvertently (or directly) create barriers to new or innovative services being offered. Conversely, the "old guard," if approached correctly, can become a strong ally for mental health services to the elderly.

A second consideration is the relative power of the lowest level of staff (usually aides, health aides, or outreach workers). Staff at the lowest level are usually least paid, least educated, and least trained, but they spend the most contact time with clients. This level of staff is rarely involved in decisions about clients. At times this means that they cannot write in charts. At other times they will be excluded from formal meetings about patient care plans. Yet these staff are critical in supporting mental health programming, both in reinforcing its goals and in providing treatment (cf. Dillon, 1978). Their comments to clients can effectively sabotage or support a program. It is highly recommended that the lowest level of staff be given more input, feedback, and responsibility in planning and decision making than is usually done.

Staff Issues

Issues among staff include status, pay, race, age, time on the job, and time in the profession. Although they may be essentially inoperative, these issues are part of all organizations. Staff are keenly aware of differences in status, control of resources, and salary; whether men treat other men differently than women (usually men have higher status in the organization) and how white supervisors treat minority aides (usually minority group members are in the lowest part of the hierarchy).

The interpersonal dynamics of staff are influenced by these issues. Despite a value in mental health practice for the client to share intimate problems, rare is the organization in which problems around status, race, pay, and "new" versus "old guard" workers are openly discussed.

Professionals' Motivations

A professional's motivations will influence how he or she deals with the aged and other professionals. In Chapter 8 several types of motivation for working with the elderly were discussed, such as trying to resolve one's family problems or identifying with a mentor who works with the elderly. In another vein, motives such as job security, advancement, or need for power may influence a person's clinical interventions as well as his or her behavior with other professionals in an agency. One of the facts of organizational life is that several motives may influence individuals' decisions or behavior in the organization.

In addition, the different professions may have a tendency to define needs of the elderly in terms of areas their profession can best handle. That is, psychologists are more likely to think of aging problems as psychological; physicians or nurses are likely to view problems as health-related. Social workers will conceptualize problems in ways that require social work service, and counselors in ways that require counseling (cf. Sarason, 1977). This tendency also works against collaboration, resource sharing, teamwork, a multidisciplinary view of problems of the elderly, and nontraditional approaches to treatment.

Cooperation Between and Within Agencies: Fact or Fiction?

All organizations in a service area have shared history and perceptions of each other that influence how they act toward each other. While services for the elderly may be new, they are often housed in pre-existing agencies. Life being what it is, however, rare is the agency so untarnished that all other systems view it as reputable, open, and excellent. The result of this natural and expected state is that information, communication, and referral between agencies is often complicated by interagency issues and varying levels of trust (cf. Sarason & Lorentz, 1979).

One result of this state of affairs is that cooperation between agencies is discussed, publicly acclaimed, and generally not accomplished. Agencies have an understandable concern with "turf" and control of resources. This is not to say that agencies do not value good care for clients, but rather that other pressures (including survival, balancing books, low trust) make cooperation difficult.

Within an agency or organization, the same holds true. How many times has it been proclaimed in staff meetings that "we're all one happy family," or "we're all on the same team," only to turn out that two services are competing for clients, there is a power struggle between two section heads, levels of staff do not trust each other, or there are personality conflicts? Again, cooperation can take place, and sometimes it does so quite easily, but it should be viewed as an achievable end rather than an assumed beginning point.

Implications for Mental Health Care
of the Elderly

This brief introduction to organizational issues in delivering mental health care to the aged leads to an inescapable conclusion: We cannot ignore the interaction between the caregiving system and the type of care given to the elderly. Be it by formal training, reading, or having "street skills," tending to organizational concerns is an area in which all practitioners should be sophisticated.

One of the major distinctions that should be made in considering delivery of mental health services is between institutional and noninstitutional care. Each is discussed separately below.

DELIVERING MENTAL HEALTH CARE
IN INSTITUTIONS

Ordinarily, institutional facilities include nursing homes and mental hospitals, both of which are designed to care for persons from a few weeks to an indefinite period of time.

Several general facts apply to these systems (cf. Redick & Taube, 1980). First, only a small proportion of older people needing mental health services utilize psychiatric services. Second, the number of elderly patients in public facilities has been decreasing substantially. For example, from 1965 to 1975 the number of elderly mental hospital patients decreased from 140,000 to 54,000. Also, the average length of stay in mental hospitals is fifty-three days for an elderly patient. This figure suggests that in the future nursing homes and community services will need to provide better follow-up and active treatment for the growing number of older persons with diagnosed and identified chronic mental health problems.

Finally, it is likely that the degree of family support, type of impairment, and previous history interact to create the need for institutionalization (Smyer, 1980; Shanas, 1979). While family support is most often needed with instrumental activities of daily living such as shopping and cleaning (Branch & Jette, 1983), it needs to be assessed to ensure that it is being used appropriately to postpone unneeded institutional care (O'Brien & Wagner, 1980).

Strengths and Weaknesses of Institutional and Long-Term Care

Strengths   Psychiatric hospitals, inpatient units of community mental health centers, general hospitals, and long-term care settings have certain features that can be considered potential advantages for mental health care of the elderly. First is that the client can be treated and observed twenty-four hours a day, giving mental health practitioners firsthand data.

Also, many services (social work, psychiatry, psychological evaluation, nursing, physical therapy, occupational therapy) can be made simultaneously available to clients. Because they are under one roof, service coordination and teamwork are likely to occur. Finally, clients may have more opportunities for social and other types of interpersonal interaction in an institution than in their home environment. The burden of care felt by relatives may be lessened, leading to stronger family ties (cf. Smith & Bengtson, 1979).

Weaknesses   At the same time, there are several potential disadvantages to institutional care. By being a twenty-four-hour-a-day caregiver, the institution implicitly becomes responsible for all social, spiritual, recreational, physical, and mental health aspects of a person's life. This is an expensive responsibility and one that is rarely carried out with enough differentiation to meet all individual needs.

Similarly, the social ecology of institutions is such that persons "confined" in institutions become prisonerlike. That is, they become increasingly dependent on staff for direction and care to a degree not warranted solely by the nature of their disorders (cf. Barton et al., 1980; Goffman, 1961).

Placement in (and out) of institutions means a transition to a new and unfamiliar environment. While not necessarily detrimental, the transition is a source of stress to the client, who can experience it at the time of the decision to institutionalize, on entry into the institution, or on moving to a more intensive level of care (Solomon, 1982). (See the following section for a discussion of the impact of institutionalization).

Other disadvantages are the high cost of institutional care, a medical-curative focus that does not include preparing the client to return and adapt to the home environment, the large percentage of client time spent in nontherapeutic activities, and finally, lack of access for and care of minority elderly (Bennett & Eisdorfer, 1975; Carter, 1982).

Nursing Homes:
Utilization and Institutionalization

At any moment in time, 5 percent of the elderly population is institution-alized, primarily in nursing homes (Butler & Lewis, 1982). While this figure is lower than most people estimate, the odds are actually one in four that an older person will spend some part of his or her life in an extended care facility (Kastenbaum & Candy, 1973).

What exactly is a nursing home? A variety of terms have been used to describe institutional settings for the elderly, including group homes, old age homes, veteran's homes, extended care facilities, long-term care facilities, skilled nursing facilities, intermediate care facilities, and of course, nursing homes. In part, the terms reflect the history of each setting, some starting as town-run homes for the aged and veterans, others being started to provide long-term medical care on a twenty-four-hour basis. One can also conceptualize the amount and sophistication of medical care given on a continuum starting on the lowest level—with group homes where room and board is provided—going to intermediate, and finally to skilled nursing care, where more complex medical and nursing services are needed. Specific requirements for each level of care are determined by each state. In terms of health care, nursing homes provide services at one or both of two levels, skilled and intermediate. Two-thirds of all nursing home dollars come from public sources. Nursing homes are also making an increasing demand on the nation's health dollars, rising from 1 percent of health costs in the 1960s to over 5 percent in the 1970s (Pegels, 1980).

Several generalities can be made about who is likely to be institutionalized, although there is no specific "type" of individual who will end up in an institution (Tobin & Lieberman, 1976). Upon entering a facility, one is likely to be white, female, and have adequate income (Robb, 1980). However, over time, the typical resident is likely to be female, white, and poor (Pegels, 1980). One reason for the change in economic status is the tremendous drain nursing home care places on an individual's finances. Minority group members may be excluded for any of the following reasons: racism, cost, unacceptableness of nursing homes to ethnic culture, unfamiliarity with how to get access to nursing homes, or possible avail-ability of social supports, although the latter has been questioned (e.g., Sue, 1977).

Nursing home residents are likely to have multiple chronic conditions that require care. Less than half can walk without assistance, more than half need help bathing, 40 percent have more than three chronic diseases. When one considers that the average age of a nursing home patient is seventy-nine years and that many are poor, in poor health, and widowed, it is not surprising that staff find questions of quality of life secondary to providing needed medical services, although this does not have to be the case (Jackson, 1980; Pegels, 1980).

In considering the nature and impact of nursing homes on mental health care, two related aspects emerge. One is that they are generally considered to be "last resort" by the elderly. The other is that there is little active mental health care provided in nursing homes. Psychiatric social work services provided in many facilities are insufficient to provide all needed treatment.

Why is the nursing home feared by the elderly and often considered as having a stigma in the community? No doubt some of this concern comes from a belief that to be in a nursing home means that death is pending, that the family and older client should "give up," that abuse and neglect occur. Perhaps related to the stigma is concern over the impact of institutionalization. Without question, the move from the community to an institution is stressful. The client must usually leave possessions, friends, and a familiar environment, and he or she becomes a "patient" on a full-time basis. The transition from home to nursing home has been evaluated by several authors. Some studies have found that the transition has led to higher mortality; other studies found no difference in mortality. Schulz and Brenner (1977) have analyzed the research and found that voluntary transition leads to a lower rate of mortality than involuntary transition does. They argue that the greater the sense of control and predictability the client has over his or her environment, the easier transition is. Two suggestions stemming from their work are that older clients be included in all decisions being made about nursing home placement, being present for discussions and interviews with nursing administrators and staff, and that "transition programs" be developed for clients before and after they become residents in a long-term care facility.

Issues in Long-Term Care Relating to Mental Health Services

Institutions are social systems that serve a particular purpose for society. That is, they care for people who cannot care for themselves. They also have their own set of organizational dynamics and issues that directly relate to the type and quality of care given to residents (Bennett & Eisdorfer, 1975).

Furthermore, long-term care institutions have conflicting goals (as do all organizations). The major conflicts from a mental health viewpoint are between providing quality service and keeping down costs; between actively treating problems and the institution's functioning as if it was designed simply to protect clients from harm; and between treating medical problems and meeting the range of basically nonmedical needs that may be predominant for a client (Bennett & Eisdorfer, 1975).

The following issues relate directly to the mental health practitioner's concerns in implementing mental health care in long-term care settings:

Conflicts Between the Facility's Structure and Needs of Clients Bennett and Eisdorfer (1975) point out that a tight hierarchical structure with narrowly and clearly defined tasks is ill suited to twenty-four-hour care, in which social, physical, recreational, and mental health needs must be met. Unfortunately, while staff may be keenly aware of psychological needs, they may be unable to provide appropriate support in psychosocial areas because of narrowly defined roles. An aide, for example, makes beds, gives baths, feeds clients, but does not provide "psychological" service. Also, staffing and staff-to-resident ratios are such that actively treating mental health problems is discouraged. The residents who create problems in management are the ones most likely to receive attention.

Staff Reactions to Mental Health Programs　Two mistaken beliefs in developing programming in long-term care settings are: (1) that staff are defensive and uninterested in client welfare and (2) that programming will be accepted with open arms. In fact, the response is likely to be somewhere between these two extremes. Programming may meet with skepticism rather than resistance from all levels of staff. After all, from a staff perspective they are working full-time to maintain clients. How can an "outsider" come in and make things better when staff are working hard just to keep things "as they are?" Staff may also have been exposed to mental health practitioners who have been ineffective, available for a short period of time, or were condescending and insensitive to staff's feelings.

Several guidelines for gaining the staff's trust include: giving a full explanation of what the program is; encouraging questions, feedback, and suggestions about the programming (staff can become the best consultants a mental health practitioner has); not being "all business" and recognizing that informal relations matter; and respecting others' "turf." Recreation and nursing staff, while potential allies for mental health programming, are two groups who will have knowledge and a sense of ownership over "psychological" functioning. Their knowledge and position should be respected.

Issues Between Shifts　One of the institutional "facts of life" is that there are three shifts of staff, and because demands for client care vary by time of day, each shift is quite different. Most programming, for example, takes place on the day shift—7:00 A.M. to 3:00 P.M. The evening shift—3:00 P.M. to 11:00 P.M.—is a "transition" time, when families can visit after work or school, dinner is served, and residents are put to bed. The night shift—11:00 P.M. to 7:00 A.M.—is the time of least activity, although specific problems such as day-night confusion are prevalent.

Not surprisingly, there is a potential for miscommunication and mistrust between shifts. One concern is who is responsible when a resident is not properly cared for. Some aides will cover their mistakes by improper reporting; others will blame the previous shift. Supervisors may be torn between loyalty to subordinates and loyalty to peers on other shifts.

The mental health practitioner should consider the following guidelines for "between-shift" issues: Get direct information from shift members rather than relying on second- or third-hand reports; make an effort to include some in-person training for all three shifts if in-service training is part of mental health programming; and be sure that the design of intervention allows shifts to show what they are accomplishing rather than what is not being done.

Effects of Mental Health Programs on Staff Workload   Mental health programs that lead to a higher degree of independence, more self-generated activities, or a higher degree of socialization for residents will mean more work for staff. Almost all staff would agree that these are admirable goals, yet the behavior of staff when such goals are beginning to be realized may subtly (or overtly) sabotage the program because clients are becoming "unruly" or more difficult to manage. Staff need to be prepared and systematically reinforced for changing their own behavior and supporting the changes in residents' behavior.

Family Involvement   Good family ties can be strengthened through appropriate institutionalization (Smith & Bengtson, 1979). Visiting may help adjustment and well-being (Greene & Monahan, 1982). Family members can also be critical in reinforcing mental health programs in the institution, but like staff, they will need specific information and opportunities to discuss their role with the practitioner or others in the long-term care system.

A Guide for Psychosocial Care

For lack of a better framework, the following five dimensions are suggested for planning psychosocial care of the elderly. With the exception of the last (dignity), all can easily be operationalized and measured. The acronym of these five dimensions is MIDMAED: Mastery over the environment, Identity, Decison making, Meaningfulness of Activity and Environment, and Dignity.

1. *Mastery over the environment.* This dimension refers to both capacity and opportunity to have a sense of control over the environment. Being able to care for oneself, knowing where one is and what the date is, being able to walk, and participating in recreational activities are all examples of mastery.

2. *Identity.* How much opportunity and environment support is there for the client to maintain a sense of personal identity? Activities such as reminiscence, life review, discussion of holidays, reality orientation, or even talking about personal items can give clients a sense of identity.

3. *Decision making.* One area related to mastery is decision making. Is the client making decisions? How can meaningful decision making be implemented? Making choices is an excellent way to stay connected to one's environment. Decision making can also be incorporated into structured activities, such as resident councils (Getzel, 1982).

4. *Meaningfulness of activity and environment.* Do activities have any meaning to the client? Can other activities be developed that would better fit the client's past roles and interests? If reality orientation techniques are to be used, why should people have to know the date or time if the environment is unchanging? Also, "complex" activities will have to be broken down into meaningful steps to develop or redevelop meaningfulness in the client's life. Finally, activities (recreation, social) should be linked to meaningful aspects of clients' lives.

5. *Dignity*. This dimension is important in considering how activities are presented or how activities of daily living are handled. Issues such as privacy and respect for the person are included in a dignified approach. Attitude therapy (see Chapter 10) can be subsumed under this aspect.

Each dimension can be easily operationalized and individualized, that is, set at the level of individual competency. For example, a client care plan may include (1) allowing Mrs. Jones ample time for toileting (dignity and mastery); (2) reminding her of her name and where she is (identity); (3) aiding her in self-feeding and self-bathing (mastery); (4) making sure she is allowed to choose her wardrobe (decision making); and (5) discussing current events with her, since she was a social studies teacher (meaningfulness).

The dimensions are such that staff can become actively involved in defining each for client care. This enables staff to aid in the process of care planning rather than only carrying out the orders of superiors. This alone should improve care given in many settings.

DELIVERING MENTAL HEALTH SERVICES IN COMMUNITY SETTINGS

Community services to the elderly represent a wide array of agencies and types of service, a range that can be characterized as patchwork, uncoordinated, of uneven quality, and of insufficient strength to meet existing needs. This does not mean that all community services are ineffective, do not serve individual clients well, or are not staffed by dedicated and well-trained individuals. There are simply not enough services to meet mental health needs of the aged (Knight, 1982; Estes, 1979).

Potential Strengths and Weaknesses of Community-Based Services

Strengths   One major advantage of community-based mental health services is that the individual is maintained in her or his home environment. Thus, theoretically, services can better be integrated with family and social networks than can institutional services.

Another advantage is the wide range of choice for types of services within the continuum of care. This, of course, assumes services exist in a given geographic area or neighborhood. Community-based services are also less expensive. The cost per client per day in institutions is generally higher than the cost of services provided in the home, especially if they are not needed on a twenty-four-hour basis. Still another advantage is that many resources and agencies can be involved in the care of one client. This can include family, friends, and social institutions such as the church.

Weaknesses The major weakness of community-based services is fragmentation of care. This includes lack of follow-up and the inavailability of appropriate services. When a range of services exist, they may work independently to the point where one client has workers from different agencies who barely know that other agencies are involved. Moreover, the amount of time a worker can give to each client (one or two hours a week) may not be enough to make substantial change in the individual or his or her living situation. A related problem is "drop-out." A client who does not show up for appointments or moves without notice may be dropped from service even though the need is there and unchanged.

The issue of "office versus home" visits warrants comment. An office is the mental health practitioner's "turf"; the home is the client's. Many practitioners are uncomfortable leaving their offices, traveling to a client's home and providing service in that setting. Practitioners complain that there is no privacy, it takes too long to go there, or the neighborhood is unsafe. These are undoubtedly valid complaints, but rarely are the advantages of home visits mentioned: service provided in the living environment, access to better data about the client, and better access provided for clients. Even though providing mental health service agencies claim to be "community-based," some end up being their own enclave in a community rather than providing service where it is most needed.

A further problem in community-based services is that mental health problems of the elderly may be undetected by others in the environment, whether they be families, friends, or health professionals. Significant behavior changes will be excused as being part of "old age," physical problems, or "senility." Thus, services for the elderly may not be utilized as effectively as those for other age groups.

Ethnic and racial differences in service utilization can work against minority group elderly. In general, minority group elderly are less likely to use formal services than other elderly. Hispanic elderly may be least likely of all groups to seek help when it is needed, even from families (Weeks & Cuellar, 1981).

Finally, older people are less likely to be a source of "fees for services" than younger persons. Sliding fee scales mean that older persons with limited incomes are seen for a fraction of the cost incurred for professional time. In addition, the special types of mental health services that may be needed are often not reimbursable. Mental health services to the elderly are likely to remain a low priority for the near future.

Types of Services Available
in Community Settings

A vast array of agencies providing mental health services may be available to the elderly in a given community. However, because of logistic, regulatory, and philosophical differences in definition of services, they are not necessarily equally accessible or of uniform quality. The degree to which services are integrated with nonelderly programs is an additional problem in defining or finding programs (Lowy, 1979).

Community Mental Health Centers   Community mental health centers (CMHCs) are agencies set up or designated in specific local geographic areas (catchment areas) to provide five basic mental health services: inpatient, outpatient, emergency, partial hospitalization, and consultation and education. Although centers are currently mandated to serve the elderly, there has been a recent decrease in federal and state support for aging programs and a growing tendency for aging programs to have to compete under block grant funds rather than have funds earmarked for their purposes. Finally, older clients are underrepresented in CMHCs despite the potentially wide range of supportive services such centers could provide (Lowy, 1979).

Adult Day Care and Geriatric Day Hospitals   One of the most rapidly growing services for the elderly is geriatric or adult day care centers. Adult day care centers are settings where a frail older adult can spend several hours or most of the day in a supervised setting. Adult day care settings fall under two general types: a medical-rehabilitative model and a psychosocial model (Weiler & Rathbone-McCuan, 1978). The former emphasizes recovery and rehabilitation from strokes or surgery; the latter emphasizes adaptation and coping with losses, including cognitive impairment.

Many adult day care centers are based in nursing homes or hospitals, which means that resources within the larger setting can be available for day-care clients. However, the day care center is sometimes more an appendage than an integral part of the institution, isolated within its setting.

Adult day care settings vary considerably. They are generally not regulated or reimbursed by third-party payments (including Medicare). Most programs have been developed at a local level, which makes the setting of national standards difficult.

Adult day care settings are potentially excellent sites for observing and treating the older adult and for providing support programs for families and other caregivers (cf. Leonard, 1980; Edinberg, 1982). However, without better linkage between mental health settings such as community mental health centers as well as a stronger financial base for adult day care, mental health services will not meet their full potential in this setting.

Senior Centers   Funded in part by monies arising from Title V of the Older Americans Act and local sources, multipurpose senior centers have sprung up throughout the United States since the 1960s. Senior centers are based on entitlement; that is, anyone, regardless of income or need, can participate. The emphasis is on recreation and leisure activities. Centers vary considerably in their level and pattern or staffing. Some have active and ongoing programs for health, legal or housing benefits, and mental health treatment; others attempt to utilize existing community services, as the center staff may be limited. Similarly, centers are located in a variety of settings, ranging from church basements to newly built senior centers in the middle of town. Along with adult day care, senior centers represent an excellent opportunity for the delivery of mental health services.

Private, Nonprofit Social Service Agencies Arising primarily from social work agencies, mental health and other programs have been developed for the elderly in many communities. Companion programs, home health aide or home-maker programs, outreach, family support groups, counseling, and other types of programs for the elderly are commonly housed in a private nonprofit social service agency. As these agencies operate autonomously in their communities, programs may or may not be coordinated with publicly funded programs.

One final note is that specific agency programs in private nonprofit agencies are often funded for start-up time of three years or less by local, state, or federal programs. There is a serious question as to how many of these programs agencies can support if funding continues to dry up.

Congregate Meal Sites Funded through Title III of the Older Americans Act, meal sites have been established throughout the United States in churches, housing for the elderly, senior centers, and other gathering places for the elderly. Social services and outreach are supposed to be provided in each of these settings, although the meals and transportation are usually a higher priority. However, meal sites are potentially an excellent setting for outreach, support, and direct service.

State and Municipal Programs Several types of state and municipal programs have been developed that provide mental health assistance, at times being the only source of mental health care for an older client. Departments of social welfare, protective services (Connecticut, for example, has legislated ombudsmen for each region of the state), town or city social services, and other types of program have been developed in varying degrees in different states.

Hospitals, Health Clinics, and Visiting Nurse Associations Another poten-tial source of mental health service for the elderly are existing health delivery systems in the community, including hospitals, health clinics and visiting nurse associations (VNAs). However, when mental health care is available in these settings, it may be separate and isolated from health services. Hospitals and health clinics may be free-standing or municipally controlled. Visiting nurse associations are funded through cities or municipal areas and are often an excellent source of home health services. VNAs are also likely to serve the poor and elderly in a com-munity.

FEDERAL FUNDING SOURCES
FOR ELDERLY PROGRAMS

Federal Legislation

There are four major sources of mental health services for the elderly (Lowy, 1979; Gatz, Smyer & Lawton, 1980).

The Mental Health Centers Act of 1963, with subsequent amendments up to and including legislation passed in 1980

The Older Americans Act of 1963, with subsequent amendments
Revenue sharing, in which federal aid to states is redirected to a variety of purposes
Title XX of the Social Security Act, which allows states to obtain needed social services for needy and eligible persons

The programs funded under any of this legislation can change substantially, depending on both federal policy and federal budget allocations in a given year.

Administration on Aging

One federal agency with a specific charge to work for the elderly is the Administration on Aging. It was set up to allocate funds for programs that fall under the Older Americans Act; specifically (as of 1983) Title III, planning social services and meals; Title IV, research training and model projects; and Title V, community service employment. Some adult day care and outreach programs are funded under its auspices.

The Administration on Aging allocates funds for regional, state, and ultimately, local or area agency on aging offices. National contracts are also given to such agencies as the National Council on Aging and the National Council of Senior Citizens. At each level some decisions can be made about priorities and amounts of funds allocated for projects or for groups at lower bureaucratic levels. There is a fairly complicated set of agreements and limits to these decisions, which are guided by plans developed to address needs of the aged. From the perspective of mental health practice, mental health services are at times a secondary concern as opposed to needs for shelter, food, and legal rights.

EXTENSIONS OF TRADITIONAL SERVICES: OUTREACH, PEER COUNSELORS, AND WORK WITH SUPPORT SYSTEMS

Several trends in mental health, health, and social services to the elderly can be considered extensions of traditional direct service. Three such areas are *outreach, peer counseling,* and *working with support systems.* Each area has several characteristics in common: Direct contact with clients is often carried out by nonprofessionals, the services are not reimbursable, and the role of the professional is that of trainer, facilitator, or coach. Services are designed either to handle adaptive problems or to maintain a person with a severe mental health impairment, as opposed to providing curative treatment. Finally, these services have the potential to reach large numbers of people. For all of these reasons, these types of approaches may serve to close some mental health service gaps to the elderly, although, as has been noted, they are neither designed nor are they likely to be effective for all problems and situations.

Outreach Services

Many agencies and organizations offer outreach services for the elderly. Some have been mandated (nutrition sites); others have been developed out of recognition that needy older people are often not included in the existing service delivery system and "reaching out" is necessary to bring them needed human services.

Outreach services are usually considered as having a twofold purpose: to locate older persons and inform them of available services (Harbert & Ginsberg, 1979). Much of the job may be trying to locate and contact uninformed older adults of available services.

The major mental health service offered through outreach is creating a trusting relationship that becomes the basis for other service. While relationships are the basis for all helping services, in outreach the nature of contact may require a diligent and sophisticated approach to establishing trust. With clients who are suspicious of proffered help, there will be a further problem: Once a trusting relationship is established, it may be virtually impossible to transfer the trust to another worker, agency, or an institution. The outreach worker may, by the nature of the role, end up having to be primary provider for certain clients. A high level of skill and knowledge is needed to be successful such circumstances (Rathbone-McCuan & Claymon, 1979).

There are several issues that should be addressed in developing outreach programs with a mental health focus:

The contract, the mutually accepted goals and limits of the service

Limits of outreach workers and how they can—or should—influence case management, given the realities of other services available

Nature of the relationship: problem solving; providing support, information, and referral; or "doing whatever needs to be done"

"Triage and followup": that is, how decisions are made as to client need and who follows the referral process to conclusion.

Peer Counseling

A current trend in service to the elderly is the development and recognition of the value of "peer counselors," that is, older individuals (usually over fifty-five) who are trained by professionals and offer counseling to their peers under the auspices of a service agency (cf. Schwartz, 1980; Waters, Fink, & White, 1976; Becker & Zarit, 1978; Bratter & Tuvman, 1980). The benefits of this approach are its low cost, the fact that a person from the same cohort as the client is doing counseling, and a subsequent nonlabeling of the client as "sick."

Professionals who write about these programs stress three points: selection of counselors, their training, and focus of service rendered.

Selection of Counselors Although the selection of peer counselors is important and difficult, it is often determined by "who volunteers" (Schwartz, 1980).

Ideally, the peer counselor, like the mental health practitioner, should be able to listen, be empathic, be able to put her or his own problems aside when counseling, and be warm—that is, able to develop close relationships with others (Schwartz, 1980). These characteristics are not easy to assess in potential counselors.

Training   Training and supervision will make or break a peer counseling program. Many volunteers, for example, will think that counseling is advice-giving. Others will not know how to express empathy. Even after training, counselors should undergo a test period and supervisory sessions, ideally done with audio-taped review of counseling sessions.

Schwartz (1980) recommends that peer counselor training be task-oriented (concrete) rather than theoretical. He also suggests seven steps: (1) presenting counseling goals, (2) presenting facts on aging, (3) teaching counselors how to appreciate feelings, (4) teaching them how to understand content, (5) developing counseling responses through audio- and video-taped mock interviews, (6) using experiential exercises, and (7) providing follow-up and supervision. Training may take as little as a few hours per week for eight weeks (see Alpaugh & Haney, 1978, for related materials).

Focus of Service   This area is more difficult to define than the other two. Peer counselors are not, by virtue of their limited training, prepared to handle long-term problems or dramatic crises. However, they may be the only ones in a position to do so, and some will do quite well at it. As Rioch (1966) and others have found, uneducated paraprofessionals can be as effective as highly trained clinicians in certain situations.

The type of problems encountered will vary considerably. As a rule of thumb, clients exhibiting disorientation, noticeable changes or signs of physical deterioration, agitation, suicidal content, looseness of association, and/or signs of alcoholism will need other services along with the service rendered by the peer counselor. While it may be difficult to discern if these behaviors are present, the supervising agency should absolutely have medical, psychological, and social service backup and referral available as supports. Otherwise, peer counselors will be in the unenviable situation of knowing that if they are in over their heads, there is no way out for them that is helpful to the client.

Even with these concerns, the concept of peer counseling has proved to add a new "dimension" to mental health services to the elderly.

Working with Support Systems

The "informal support system" usually refers to family, friends, or neighbors who help maintain the older person in his or her home. Although family is usually the focus of most professional interest, a second type of support is older persons themselves, working together as self-help groups. A third type of support is using the older person as a volunteer.

In working with support systems, the mental health practitioner should be aware that there are fundamental differences in the "client," the nature of the contact, and the outcome than with direct mental health services. First, the support system may be healthy and not pathological. Second, the nature of the contact may be practitioner-initiated and is more likely than not to be of an educational or planning nature. Finally, the outcomes and goals of work with support systems may range widely, including improved client functioning, maintaining a client at current level of functioning, improved support system functioning, training support systems in social skills and advocacy, or providing needed services (respite, financial, health) to the support system.

Mental health practitioners can provide support to support systems in five general ways: identifying and linking parts of the system, giving guidance and information to support-system members, providing structural supports such as counseling and respite services, training support system members to be advocates for their elders, and developing and/or helping support groups.

Identifying and Linking Parts of the Support System   Although most older persons use informal supports (Branch & Jette, 1983) informal support systems rarely develop in an organized manner. Rather, one person in a family may take on primary care responsibilities, others may provide financial or emotional support, and friends or neighbors may provide such services as transportation, shopping, or visiting. There may not be significant contact among individuals or subsystems. Also, the support systems of minority group elderly may function differently among minorities and be different than those of non-minorities (Weeks & Cuellar, 1981).

There is potential benefit in having parts of the support system communicate with each other about how they are helping the older person. Care has to be taken not to disturb existing relationships that work by making them too formal. A final caution is that, occasionally, parts of the system (e.g., certain family members) prefer not to be in communication.

Giving Guidance and Information   The mental health practitioner can function as a source of information about the elderly, the specific condition(s) of the older client, and how supports can best function for the older client.

Another way of providing guidance is to reinforce ideas about how to provide care in a way that maximizes independence and self-worth. The previously discussed "MIDMAED" concept (Mastery, Identity, Decision Making, Meaningfulness of Activity and Environment, and Dignity) is a useful tool in this regard. Along with this, reminding caregivers that the quality of the relationships, not just the quantity, is extremely important (Strain & Chappell, 1982).

Structural Supports   Three major structural supports that can be provided to families are inexpensive health or home health services, counseling, and respite services.

Some support systems need trained help in the homes. The mental health practitioner can be an advocate and source for inexpensive services in a community if they are warranted.

Counseling or family therapy may be needed for parts of the caregiving system on a short-term or even long-term basis. The focus of mental health intervention may be specific to the caregiving process, using behavioral-family approaches to teach families how to make specific gains, such as increasing the amount of time a client can be left alone (Haley, 1983a). Or the focus may be on unresolved conflicts triggered by the need to support the older person.

A third approach is to organize structured respite services, in which the family is relieved of care for a period of time (day, weekend, week), and the older client is cared for either at home or in a hospital or institutional setting. Respite beds are slowly being developed in long-term care settings. Care will have to be taken to prepare the older client for this shift in care and to prepare the family and respite caregivers for types of reactions that may occur in respite care. Little is known at this time about the best ways to manage respite care, although the relocation literature suggests that older clients be involved in decisions and be prepared for the transitions.

Support Groups   One trend in helping informal support systems is the establishment of peer support groups. The groups have been started under a variety of auspices. Some have sprung from "You and Your Aging Parents" workshops, others have been started by concerned persons in a community. A national organization, Alzheimer's Disease and Related Disorders Association, Inc. (360 North Avenue, Chicago, Illinois 60601), has been developed to aid family members in developing such groups.

Many groups are self-directed. The members decide when and were to meet; they run their own rap sessions or meetings on a regular basis, providing time to share problems and solutions and giving each other emotional support. Some use outside speakers, and some use professionals as resources or facilitators (Zarit, 1982).

Several reports of successful support groups have been published (Steuer & Clark, 1982; Roozman-Weigensberg & Fox, 1980; Hausman, 1979; Barnes et al., 1981; Hartford & Parsons, 1982). A range of concerns comes up in groups, including:

Knowledge—about the diagnosis, prognosis, and care plans
Support—knowing one is not alone
Problem solving and decision making—including how to include others in caregiving
Advocacy—banding together to air grievances or advocate changes in policies

It is continually stressed that the professional leader's role in support groups is facilitative or consultative, that the format should be flexible and open, and that the group needs to retain as much self-direction as possible.

As leaderless groups, support groups have certain advantages: They are democratic, they provide a forum for peer sharing, and there is a sense of member ownership of the group. There are also some potential problems. One is that a few members can dominate groups, especially in early stages, with irrelevant concerns or with personal problems that are beyond the focus of the group. There is likely to be little screening in the formation of a support group, nor is there likely to be an effective way to get members out or referred to more appropriate services (such as individual counseling) if needed. Many groups will have an informal leader. If that leader moves or leaves the group, it may be difficult for the group to maintain a sense of continuity.

This is not to say that professionals should lead or facilitate support groups. The emergence of support groups is certainly positive; mental health practitioners need to develop effective working relationships with groups to provide support for the problems mentioned above. There will be guesswork as to how much each of these aspects is operating, but, if the practitioner can accurately assess the relative impact of these factors, she or he can also take steps to decrease or eliminate barriers and improve the quality of the group.

SUMMARY AND CONCLUSIONS

The history of mental health care to the aged has been marked by a transition from institutional to community care due to legislation, such as Medicare and the Community Mental Health Centers Act, and availability of medication to control the most dramatic symptoms of mental disorders. However, both long-term care and community services have been ill prepared to handle the problems of older deinstitutionalized mental patients. In addition, decreases in monies earmarked for the elderly (some of which are only available in block grant categories) have led to decreases in services specifically for the aged.

Organizational dynamics, including formal and informal power, staff issues, and professionals' motivations all have impact on mental health services. In institutional settings, staff roles, an implicit norm of "allow no harm," and reaction to likely increases in workload may work against institutional support of mental health treatment. In community settings, fragmentation of service, lack of resources, and underdetection of mental health problems may work against effective mental health care. Yet, effective programs can be implemented in either type of setting, although the mental health practitioner will need to tend to organizational issues to ensure their survival.

Along with the range of interventions discussed in this text, three "nontraditional" approaches that hold promise are outreach, peer counseling, and service to support systems. The mental health delivery system has at best a spotted record in meeting the needs of the elderly. However, the commitment of a growing number of practitioners, demographic changes, and increased appreciation of nontraditional approaches are strong evidence that the professional community may change its focus to better serve our nation's elders.

References

ACKERMAN, N. *The psychodynamics of family life.* New York: Basic Books, 1958.

ACKERMAN, N. *Treating the troubled family.* New York: Basic Books, 1966.

ADAMS, R. D. The morphological aspects of aging in the human nervous system. In J. E. Birren & R. B. Sloane (Eds.), *Handbook of mental health and aging.* Englewood Cliffs, N.J.: Prentice-Hall, 1980.

ADAMS, R. D., FISHER, C. M., HAKIM, S., OJEMANN, R. C., & SWEET, W. H. Symptomatic occult hydrocephalus with "normal" cerebrospinal fluid pressure: A treatable syndrome. *New England Journal of Medicine,* 1965, *273,* 1195-1207.

ALBERTI, R. H., & EMMONS, N. L. *Your perfect right.* San Luis Obispo, Calif.: Impact Books, 1970.

ALEXANDER, F. G. The indication for psychoanalytic therapy. *Bulletin of the New York Academy of Medicine,* 1944, *20,* 319-334.

ALMOND, R. *The healing community.* New York: Jason Aronson, 1974.

ALPAUGH, P., & HANEY, M. *Counseling the older adult—A training manual.* Los Angeles: Andrus center, University of Southern California, 1978.

AMERICAN PSYCHIATRIC ASSOCIATION. *Diagnostic and statistical manual of mental disorders* (3rd ed.). Washington, D.C.: Author, 1980.

ANASTASI, A. *Psychological testing* (14th ed.). New York: MacMillan, 1976.

ATCHLEY, R. C. *The social forces in later life* (3rd ed.). Belmont, Calif.: Wadsworth, 1980.

AVERILL, J. R., & WISOCKI, P. A. Some observations on behavioral approaches to the treatment of grief among the elderly. In H. J. Sobel (Ed.), *Behavior therapy in terminal care: A humanistic approach.* Cambridge, Mass.: Ballinger Publishing Co., 1981.

BAHRICK, H. P., BAHRICK, P. O., & WITTLINGER, R. P. Fifty years of memory for names and faces: A cross sectional approach. *Journal of Experimental Psychology,* 1975, *104,* 54-75.

BALDWIN, D. C. Jr., BALDWIN, M. A., EDINBERG, M. A., & ROWLEY, B. D. A model for recruitment and service—The University of Nevada's summer preceptorships in Indian communities. *Public Health Reports,* 1981, *95*(1), 19-22.

BANDLER, R., & GRINDER, J. *The structure of magic I.* Palo Alto, Calif.: Science and Behavior Books, 1975.

BANDLER, R., & GRINDER, J. *Frogs into princes: Neurolinguistic programming.* Moab, Utah: Real People Press, 1979.

BANDLER, R., GRINDER, J., & SATIR, V. *Changing with families.* Palo Alto, Calif.: Science and Behavior Books, 1976.

BANDURA, A. *Principles of behavior modification.* New York: Holt, Rinehart & Winston, 1969.

BANZIGER, G., & ROUSH, S. Nursing homes for the birds: A control-relevant intervention with bird feeders. *The Gerontologist,* 1983, *23,* 527-531.

BARNES, J. A. Effects of reality orientation classroom on memory loss, confusion, and disorientation in geriatric patients. *The Gerontologist,* 1974, *14,* 138-142.

BARNES, R. R., RASKIND, M. A., SCOTT, M., & MURPHY, C. Problems of families caring for Alzheimer patients: Use of a support group. *Journal of the American Geriatrics Society,* 1981, *29,* 80-85.

BARTON, E. M., BALTES, M. M., & ORZECH, M. J. Etiology of dependency in older nursing home residents during morning care: The role of staff behavior. *Journal of Personality and Social Psychology,* 1980, *38,* 423-431.

BECK, A. T. *Depression: Clinical, experimental, and theoretical aspects.* New York: Harper & Row, 1967.

BECK, A. T. The core problem in depression: The cognitive triad. *Science and Psychoanalysis,* 1970, *17,* 47-55.

BECK, A. T. *Cognitive therapy and emotional disorders.* New York: International Universities Press, 1976.

BECK, C. M., & FERGUSON, D. Aged abuse. *Journal of Gerontological Nursing,* 1981, *7,* 333-336.

BECKER, F., & Zarit, S. Training older adults as peer counselors. *Education Gerontology,* 1978, *3,* 241-250.

BENGTSON, V. L. *The social psychology of aging.* New York: Bobbs-Merrill, 1973.

BENGTSON, V. L., & TREAS, J. The changing family context of mental health and aging. In J. E. Birren & R. B. Sloane, (Eds.), *Handbook of mental health and aging.* Englewood Cliffs, N.J.: Prentice-Hall, 1980.

BENNETT, R., & EISDORFER, C. The institutional environment and behavior change. In S. Sherwood (Ed.), *Long-term care: A handbook for researchers, planners, and providers.* Holliswood, N.Y.: Spectrum Publications, 1975.

BENNIS, W. F., & SHEPPARD, H. A. A theory of group development *Human Relations,* 1956, *9,* 415-437.

BERGER, R. Nutritional needs of the aged. In I. M. Burnside (Ed.), *Nursing and the aged.* New York: McGraw-Hill, 1976.

BERGER, R. M., & ROSE, S. D. Interpersonal training with institutionalized elderly patients. *Journal of Gerontology,* 1977, *32,* 346-353.

BERTALANFFY, L. General systems theory and psychiatry. In S. Ariete (Ed.), *American handbook of psychiatry* (Vol. III). New York: Basic Books, 1966.

BERARDO, F. M.   Survivorship and social isolation: The case of the aged widower. *Family Coordinator,* January 1970, pp. 11-25.

BILLINGSLEY, A.   *Black families in white America.* Englewood Cliffs, N.J.: Prentice-Hall, 1968.

BION, W. R.   *Experiences in groups.* New York: Basic Books, 1961.

BLAKE, R. H., & BICHEKAS, G.   How can I build and maintain helping relations with older persons? In J. E. Myers & M. L. Ganikos (Eds.), *Counseling older persons: Volume II. Basic helping skills for service providers.* Falls Church, Va.: American Personnel and Guidance Association, 1981.

BLAZER, D. G. II.   Family therapy with the depressed older adult. In D. G. Blazer II, *Depression in late life.* St. Louis, C. V. Mosby, 1982.

BLOCK, M. R., DAVIDSON, J. L., GRAMBS, J. D., & SEROCK, K. E.   *Unchartered territory: Issues and concerns of women over 40.* College Park, Md.: University of Maryland, 1978.

BLOCK, M. R. & SINNOTT, J. D.   (1979). *The battered elder syndrome: An exploratory study.* College Park, Md.: Center on Aging, University of Maryland, 1979.

BOTWINICK, J.   *Aging and behavior* (2nd ed.). New York: Springer Publishing Co., 1978.

BOTWINICK, J., & STORANDT, M.   *Memory related functions and age.* Springfield, Ill.: Charles C Thomas, 1974.

BOWEN, M.   The use of family therapy in clinical practice. In J. Haley (Ed.), *Changing families: A family therapy reader.* New York: Grune & Stratton, 1971.

BRADLEY, J. C., & EDINBURG, M. A.   *Communication in the nursing context.* New York: Appleton-Century-Crofts, 1982.

BRAMMER, L. M.   (1979). *The helping relationship: Process and skills* (2nd ed.). Englewood Cliffs, N.J.: Prentice-Hall, 1979.

BRAMMER, L. M.   What is a helping relationship? In J. E. Myers & M. L. Ganikos (Eds.), *Counseling older persons. Vol. II: Basic helping skills for service providers.* Falls Church, Va.: American Personnel and Guidance Association, 1981.

BRANCH, L. G., & JETTE, A. M.   Elders' use of informal long-term care assistance. *The Gerontologist,* 1983, *23,* 51-56.

BRATTER, B., & TUVMAN, E.   A peer counseling program in action. In S. S. Sargent (Ed.), *Nontraditional therapy and counseling with the aging.* Springer series on adulthood and aging. New York: Springer Publishing Co., 1980.

BRICKEL, C. M.   The therapeutic roles of cat mascots with a hospital-based geriatric population: A staff survey. *The Gerontologist,* 1979, *19,* 368-372.

BRICKEL, C. M.   A review of the roles of pet animals in psychotherapy with the elderly. *International Journal of Aging and Human Development,* 1980-1981, *12,* 119-129.

BRIDGE, T. P., CANNON, H. E., & WYATT, R. J.   Burned-out schizophrenia: Evidence for age effects on schizophrenic symptomatology. *Journal of Gerontology,* 1978, *33,* 835-839.

BRINK, T. L.   Geriatric-paranoia: Case report illustrating behavioral management. *Journal of the American Geriatrics Society,* 1980, *28,* 519-522.

BRINK, T. L.   Self-rating of memory versus psychometric ratings of memory and hypochondriasis. *Journal of the American Geriatrics Society,* 1981, *29,* 537-538.

BRINK, T. L., YESAVAGE, J. A., LUM, O., HEERSEMA, P. H., ADEY, M., & ROSE, T. L.   Screening tests for geriatric depression. *Clinical Gerontologist,* 1982, *1,* 37-43.

BRODY, E. M.   The aging family. *The annals of the American Academy of Political and Social Science*, 1978, *438*, 13-27.

BRODY, E. M., & KLEBAN, M. H.   Physical and mental health symptoms of older people: Who do they tell? *Journal of the American Geriatrics Society*, 1981, *29*, 442-449.

BROWN, F. R.   Cardiovascular assessment. In W. J. Phipps, B. C. Long, & N. F. Woods (Eds.), *Medical-surgical nursing: Concepts and clinical practice*. St. Louis: C. V. Mosby., 1979.

BRUDNO, J., & SELTZER, J.   Resocialization therapy through group process with senile patients in a geriatric hospital. *The Gerontologist*, 1968, *8*, 211-214.

BULLOUGH, V., BULLOUGH, B., & MAURO, M.   Age and achievement: A dissenting view. *The Gerontologist*, 1978, *18*, 584-587.

BURNS, D. D.   *Feeling good: The new mood therapy*. New York: Signet Books, 1980.

BURNSIDE, I. M.   The special senses and sensory deprivation. In I. M. Burnside (Ed.), *Nursing and the aged*. New York: McGraw-Hill, 1976.

BURNSIDE, I. M.   Principles from Yalom. In I. M. Burnside (Ed.), *Working with the elderly: Group processes and techniques*. North Scituate, Mass.: Duxbury Press, 1978.

BURNSIDE, I. M.   Symptomatic behaviors in the elderly. In J. E. Birren & R. B. Sloane (Eds.). *Handbook of mental health and aging*. Englewood Cliffs, N.J.: Prentice-Hall, 1980.

BUTLER, R. N.   The life review: An interpretation of reminiscence in the aged. *Psychiatry*, 1963, *26*, 65-76.

BUTLER, R. N.   Age-ism: Another form of bigotry. *The Gerontologist*, 1968, *9*, 243-246.

BUTLER, R. N.   *Why survive? Being old in America*. New York: Harper & Row, 1975.

BUTLER, R. N., & LEWIS, M. I.   *Sex after sixty: A guide for men and women for their later years*. New York: Harper & Row, 1976.

BUTLER, R. N., & LEWIS, M. I.   *Aging and mental health: Positive psychosocial approaches* (3rd ed.). St. Louis: C. V. Mosby, 1982.

CAINE, L.   *Widow*. New York: Morrow, 1974.

CALAHAN, D., CISIN, I. H., & CROSSLEY, H. M.   *American drinking practices*. New Brunswick, N.J.: Rutgers Center of Alcohol Studies, 1969.

CANESTRARI, R. E., Jr.   Paced and self-paced learning in young and elderly adults. *Journal of Gerontology*, 1963, *18*, 165-168.

CAPLOW-LINDNER, E., HARPAZ, L., & SAMBERG, S.   *Therapeutic dance/movement: Expressive activities for older adults*. New York: Human Sciences Press, 1979.

CARKHUFF, R. R.   *Helping and human relations*. New York: Holt, Rinehart & Winston, 1969.

CARP, F. M.   Some components of disengagement. *Journal of Gerontology*, 1968, *23*, 282-286.

CARTER, J. H.   The black aged: Implications for mental health care. *Journal of the American Geriatrics Society*, 1982, *32*, 67-70.

CAUTELA, J.   A classical conditioning approach to the development and modification of behavior in the aged. *The Gerontologist*, 1969, *9*, 109-113.

CHRISTAKIS, G. (Ed.).   Nutritional assessment of the elderly. *American Journal of Public Health*, 1973, Supplement (11), 1-37.

CHUBON, S.   A novel approach to the process of life review. *Jounal of Gerontological Nursing*, 1980, *10*, 543-546.

CITRIN, R., & DIXON, D.   Reality orientation: A milieu therapy used in an instituion for the aged. *The Gerontologist*, 1977, *17*, 39-43.

COBLENTZ, J. N., MATTIS, S., ZINGESSER, L. H., KASOFF, S. S., WISNIEWSKI, H. M., & KATZMAN, R.   Presenile dementia, clinical aspects, and evaluation of cerebrospinal fluid dynamics. *Archives of Neurology*, 1973, *29*, 299-308.

COHEN, F.   Coping with surgery: Information, psychological preparation, and recovery. In L. W. Poon (Ed.), *Aging in the 1980s: Psychological issues*. Washington, D.C.: American Psychological Association, 1980.

COHEN, G.   Prospects for mental health and aging. In J. E. Birren & R. B. Sloane (Eds.), *Handbook of Mental Health and Aging*. Englewood Cliffs, N.J.: Prentice-Hall, 1980.

CONTE, H. R., WEINER, M. B., & PLUTCHIK, R.   Measuring death anxiety: Conceptual, psychometric, and factor-analytic aspects. *Journal of Personality and Social Psychology*, 1982, *43*, 775-785.

COOPER, A. F., & PORTER, R.   Visual activity and ocular pathology in the paranoid and affective psychoses of later life. *Journal of Psychosomatic Research*, 1976, *20*, 107-114.

COOPER, A. F., GARSIDE, R. F., & KAY, D. W. K.   A comparison of deaf and non-deaf patients with paranoid and affective psychoses. *British Journal of Psychiatry*, 1976, *129*, 532-538.

COPELAND, R. R. M., KELLEHER, M. J., KELLETT, J. M., GOURLAY, A. J., COWAN, D. W., BARRON, G., GRUNCH J., GURLAND, B. J., SHARPE, L., SIMON, R., KURIANSKY, J., & STILLER, P.   Cross-national study of diagnosis of mental disorders: A comparison of the diagnoses of elderly psychiatric patients admitted to mental hospitals serving Queens County, New York, and the former borough of Camberwell, London. *British Journal of Psychiatry*, 1975, *126*, 11-20.

Coping with Cancer: A resource for the health professional. (1980). Bethesda, M.D.: U.S. Department of Health and Human Resources, NIH Publication No. 80-2080.

CORBY, N.   Assertive training with aged populations. *Counseling Psychologist*, 1975, *5*, 69-73.

CORBY, N., & SOLNICK, R. L.   Psychosocial and physiological influences on sexuality in the older adult. In J. E. Birren & R. B. Sloane (Eds.), *Handbook of mental health and aging*. Englewood Cliffs, N.J.: Prentice-Hall, 1980.

COREY, G.   *Theory and practice of counseling and psychotherapy* (2nd ed.). Belmont, Calif.: Wadsworth, 1982.

CORSON, S. A., & CORSON, E. O'L.   The role of pet animals as nonverbal communication links in mental health programs. Paper presented at the annual meeting of the American Public Health Association, Washington, D.C., 1982.

CORSON, S. A., CORSON, E. O'L., & GWYNNE, P. H.   Pet-facilitated psychotherapy. In R. S. Anderson (Ed.), *Pet animals and society*. London: Balilliere Tindall, 1975.

CORSON, S. A., CORSON, E. O'L., GWYNNE, P. H., & ARNOLD, L. E.   Pet dogs as nonverbal communication links in hospital psychiatry. *Comprehensive Psychiatry*, 1977, *18*, 61-72.

COSTA, P. T., & MC CRAE, R. R.   Age differences in personality structure revisited: Studies in validity, stability, and change. *International Journal of Aging and Human Development*, 1977, *8*, 261-275.

CRAIGHEAD, W. E., KAZDIN, A. E., & MAHONEY, M. J.   *Behavior modification: Principles, issues, and applications*. Boston: Houghton Mifflin, 1976.

CRAIK, F. M.   Age' differences in human memory. In J. E. Birren & K. W. Shaie (Eds.), *Handbook of the psychology of aging.* New York: Van Nostrand Reinhold, 1977.

CRAIK, F. M. & SIMON, E.   Age differences in memory: The roles of attention and depth of processing. In L. W. Poon, J. L. Fozard, L. S. Cermak, D. Arenberg, & L. W. Thompason (Eds.), *New directions in memory and aging.* Proceedings of the George Tallaud Memorial Conference. Hillsdale, N.J.: Lawrence Erlbaum, 1980.

CRANDALL, R. C.   *Gerontology: A behavioral science approach.* Reading, Mass.: Addison-Wesley, 1980.

CRAPPER, D. R., KRISHNAN, S. S., & DALTON, A. J.   Brain aluminum distribution in Alzheimer's disease and experimental neurofibrillary degeneration. *Science,* 1973, *18,* 511-513.

CROOK, T.   Central-nervous stimulants: Appraisal of use in geropsychiatric patients. *Journal of the American Geriatrics Society,* 1979, *27,* 476-477.

CUMMING, E., & HENRY, W. E.   *Growing old.* New York: Basic Books, 1961.

DAILEY, M.   Sexual expression and aging. In F. J. Berghorn & D. E. Schafer (Eds.), *The dynamics of aging: Original essays on the processes and experiences of growing old.* Boulder, Colo.: Westview Press, 1981.

DAVIES, P.   Studies on the neurochemistry of central cholinergic systems in Alzheimer's disease. In D. Katzman, R. D. Terry & K. L. Dick (Eds.), *Alzheimer's disease: Senile dementia and related disorders.* New York: Raven Press, 1978.

DAVIS, J. M., SEGAL, N. L., & LESSER, J. M.   Use of antipsychotic drugs in the elderly. In C. Eisdorfer & W. E. Fann (Eds.), *Treatment of psychopathology in the aging.* Springer Series on psychiatry, 2. New York: Springer Publishing Co., 1982.

DEBONI, U., & CRAPPER, D. R.   Paired helical filaments of the Alzheimer type in cultured neurons. *Nature,* 1978, *271,* 566-568.

DEBOR, L., GALLAGHER, D., & LESHER, E.   Group counseling with bereaving elderly. *Clinical Gerontologist,* 1983, *1,* 81-89.

DENNIS, H.   Remotivation therapy for the elderly: A suprising outcome. *Journal of Gerontological Nursing,* 1976, *2,* 28-30.

DENNIS, H.   Remotivation therapy groups. In I. M. Burnside (Ed.) *Working with the elderly: Group processes and techniques.* North Scituate, Mass.: Duxbury Press, 1978.

DENNIS, W.   Creative productivity between ages of 20 to 80 years. *Journal of Gerontology,* 1966, *21,* 1-8.

DEWDNEY, I.   An art therapy program for geriatric patients. *American Journal of Art Therapy,* 1973, *12,* 249-254.

DILLON, K.   The need for psychological services for geriatric patients in long-term care facilities. *Long Term Care and Health Administration Quarterly,* 1978, *2,* 29-35.

DOWD, J. D., & BENGTSON, V. L.   Aging in minority populations: An examination of the double jeopardy hypothesis. *Journal of Gerontology,* 1978, *33,* 427-436.

Duke University Center for the Study of Aging and Human Development.   *Multidimensional functional assessment: The OARS methodology.* Durham, N.C.: Duke University, 1978.

DUNNER, D. L.   Lithium treatment of the aged. In C. Eisdorfer & W. E. Fann (Eds.), *Treatment of psychopathology in the aging.* Springer Series on psychiatry 2. New York: Springer Publishing Co., 1982.

DURKHEIM, E.   *Suicide.* New York: Free Press, 1951.

DYCHTWALD, K.   The SAGE project: A new image of age. *Journal of Humanistic Psychology,* 1978, *18* (Spring), 69-74.

DYE, C. J., & ERBER, J. T.   Two group procedures for the treatment of nursing home patients. *The Gerontologist,* 1981, *21,* 539-544.

DYE C. J., & RICHARDS, C. C.   Facilitating the transition to nursing home. In S. S. Sargent (Ed.), *Nontraditional therapy and counseling with the aging.* New York: Springer Publishing Co., 1980.

EBERSOLE, P. P.   A theoretical approach to the use of reminiscence. In I. M. Burnside (Ed.), *Working with the elderly: Group processes and techniques.* North Scituate, Mass.: Duxbury Press, 1978a.

EBERSOLE, P. P.   Establishing reminising groups. In I. M. Burnside, (Ed.), *Working with the elderly: Group processes and techniques.* North Scituate, Mass.: Duxbury Press, 1978b.

EBERT, N. J. (1980a). The nursing process applied to the aged person receiving medication. In A. G. Yurick, S. S. Robb, B. E. Apier, & N. J. Ebert. *The aged person and the nursing process.* New York: Appleton-Century-Crofts, 1980a.

EBERT, N. J.   Nutrition and elimination in the aged and the nursing process. In A. G. Yurik, S. S. Robb, B. E. Apier, & N. J. Ebert. *The aged person and the nursing process.* New York: Appleton-Century-Crofts, 1980b.

EDINBERG, M. A.   Behavioral assessment and assertion training of the elderly. Unpublished doctoral dissertation, University of Cincinnati, 1975.

EDINBERG, M. A.   The family life chronology, an introductory step into a family's part: Developed by Virginia Satir. *Interaction,* 1978, *1,* 36-38.

EDINBERG, M. A.   Day care—Untapped potential? In M. Edinberg (Chair), *Aging and mental health: A continuum of care?* Symposium at annual meeting of American Psychological Association. Washington, D.C., 1982.

EDINBERG, M. A., KAROLY, P., & GLESER, G. C.   Assessing assertion in the elderly: An application of the behavioral-analytic model of competence. *Journal of Clinical Psychology,* 1977, *33,* 869-874.

EGAN, G.   *The skilled helper,* Monterey, Calif.: Brooks/Cole.

EISDORFER, C., NOROLIN, J., & WILKIE, F.   Improvement of learning in the aged by modification of the autonomic nervous system. *Science,* 1970, *170,* 1327-1329.

EISDORFER, C., & WILKIE, F.   Stress, disease, aging, and behavior. In J. E. Birren and K. W. Schaie (Eds.) *Handbook of the psychology of aging.* New York: Van Nostrand Reinhold, 1977.

ELLIS, A.   *Reason and emotion in psychotherapy.* New York/ Lyle Stuart, 1962.

ELLIS, A.   *Rational-emotive therapy and cognitive behavior therapy.* New York: Springer Publishing Co., 1981a.

ELLIS, A.   The rational-emotive approach to thanatology. In H. J. Sobel (Ed.), *Behavior therapy in terminal care: A humanistic approach.* Cambridge, Mass.: Ballinger, 1981b.

ELLIS, A., & HARPER, R. A.   *A guide to rational living.* Hollywood, Wilshire Books, 1973.

ELLISON, K. B.   Working with the elderly in a life review group. *Journal of Gerontological Nursing,* 1981, *7,* 537-541.

EPSTEIN, C.   *Nursing the dying patient.* Reston, Va.: Reston, 1975.

EPSTEIN, L. J.   Depression in the elderly. *Journal of Gerontology,* 1976, *31,* 278-282.

EPSTEIN, L. J., & SIMON, J.   Organic brain syndrome in the elderly. *Geriatrics,* 1967, *22,* 145-150.

ERIKSON, E. H. *Childhood and society* (2nd ed.), New York: W. W. Norton & Co., 1963.

ESTES, C. L. *The aging enterprise.* San Francisco: Jossey-Bass, 1979.

FAGAN, J., & SHEPHERD, I. (Eds.), *Gestalt therapy now.* New York: Harper & Row, 1970.

FALCIONI, D. Assessing the abused elderly. *Journal of Gerontological Nursing,* 1982, *8,* 208-212.

FEIL, N. W. Group therapy in a home for the aged. *The Gerontologist,* 1967, *7,* 192-195.

FILLENBAUM, G. G., & SMYER, M. A. The development, validity, and reliability of the OARS multidimensional functional assessment questionnaire. *Journal of Gerontology,* 1981, *36,* 428-434.

FINE, R. *The healing of the mind.* New York: D. McKay, 1971.

FISKE, M. Tasks and crisis of the second half of life: The interrelationship of commitment, coping, and adaptation. In J. E. Birren & R. B. Sloane (Eds.), *Handbook of Mental Health and Aging.* Englewood Cliffs, N.J.: Prentice-Hall, 1980.

FOLSOM, J. C. Reality orientation for the elderly mental patient. *Journal of Geriatric Psychiatry,* 1968, *1,* 291-307.

FONER, A., & SCHWAB, K. *Aging and retirement.* Monterey, Calif.: Brooks/Cole, 1981.

FORD, C. V., & WINTER, J. W. Computerized axial tomograms and dementia in elderly patients. *Journal of Gerontology,* 1981, *36,* 164-169.

FRANK, J. D. Psychotherapy of bodily disease: An overview. *Psychotherapy and Psychosomatics,* 1975, *26,* 192-202.

FRY, P. S. Structured and unstructured reminiscence training and depression among the elderly. *Clinical Gerontologist,* 1983, *1,* 15-35.

FULTON, R. Death, grief, and social recuperation. *Omega,* 1970, *1,* 22-28.

FULTON, R. *Death and identity.* Bowie, Md.: Charles Press Publishers, 1976.

GAITZ, C. M. Identifying and treating depression in an older patient. *Geriatrics,* 1983, *38*(2), 42-46.

GALLAGHER, D. E., & THOMPSON, L. W. Effectiveness of psychotherapy for both endogenous and nonendogenous depression in older adult outpatients. *Journal of Gerontology,* 1983, *38,* 707-712.

GARCIA, C. A., REDING, M. S., & BLASS, J. P. Overdiagnosis of dementia. *Journal of the American Geriatrics Society,* 1981, *29,* 407-410.

GARDNER, E. A., BAHN, A. K., & MACK, M. Suicide and psychiatric care in the aging. *Archives of General Psychiatry,* 1981, *10,* 547-553.

GATZ, M., SMYER, M. A., & LAWTON, M. P. The mental health system and the older adult. In L. W. Poon (Ed.), *Aging in the 1980s: Psychological issues.* Washington, D.C.: American Psychological Association, 1980.

GETZEL, J. Resident councils and social action. *Journal of Gerontological Social Work,* 1982, *5,* 179-185.

GIAMBRA, L. M., & ARENBERG, D. Problem solving, concept learning, and aging. In L. W. Poon (Ed.), *Aging in the 1980s: Psychological issues.* Washington, D.C.: American Psychological Association, 1980.

GLAMSER, F. D. The impact of preretirement programs on the retirement experience. Journal of Gerontology, 1981, 36, 244-250.

GLASSCOTE, R. M., GUDEMAN, J. E., & MILES, D. G. *Creative mental health services for the elderly.* Washington, D.C.: Joint Information Service, 1978.

GLICK, I. O., WEISS, R. S., & PARKES, C. M. *The first year of bereavement.* New York: John Wiley, 1974.

GODBOLE, A., & VERINIS, J. S. Brief psychotherapy in the treatment of emotional disorders in physically ill geriatric patients. *The Gerontologist,* 1974, *14,* 143-148.

GOFFMAN, E.   *Asylums.* New York: Anchor Books, 1961.

GOLDFARB, A. I., & TURNER, H.   Psychotherapy of aged persons. *American Journal of Psychiatry,* 1953, *109,* 916-921.

GONZALEZ DEL VALLE, A., & USHER, M.   Group therapy with aged Latino women: A pilot project and study. *Clinical Gerontologist,* 1982, *1,* 51-57.

GORDON, T.   *Parent effectiveness training.* New York: Peter Wyden, 1970.

GÖTESTAM, K. G.   Training in reality orientation of patients with senile dementia. In L. Levi (Ed.), *Society, stress, and disease: Aging and old age.* London: Oxford University Press, 1979.

GÖTESTAM, K. G.   Behavior and dynamic psychotherapy with the elderly. In J. E. Birren & R. B. Sloane (Eds.), *Handbook of Mental Health and Aging.* Englewood Cliffs, N.J.: Prentice-Hall, 1980.

GRANGER, C. V., SHERWOOD, C. C., & GREER, D. S.   Functonal status measures in a comprehensive stroke care program. *Archives of Physical Medicine and Rehabilitation,* 1977, *58,* 555-561.

GREENBLATT, D. J., & DIVOLL, M.   Benzodiazepines in the elderly. In C. Eisdorfer & W. E. Fann (Eds.), *Treatment of psychopathology in the aging.* Springer Series on psychiatry, 2, New York: Springer Publishing Co., 1982.

GREENE, R. R.   Life review: A technique for clarifying family roles in adulthood. *Clinical Gerontologist,* 1982, *1,* 59-67.

GREENE, V. L., & MONAHAN, D. J.   The impact of visitation on patient well-being in nursing homes. *The Gerontologist,* 1982, *22,* 418-423.

GRINDER, J., & BANDLER, R.   *The structure of magic II.* Palo Alto, Calif.: Science and Behavior Books, 1976.

GROB, D.   Common disorders of muscles in the aged. In A. B. Chinn (Ed.), *Working with older people: A guide to practice.* Vol. IV: *Clinical aspects of aging,* Washington, U. S. Public Health Service Publication 1459, 1971, 156-162.

Guide for Reality Orientation. Veteran's Administration Hospital. Tuscaloosa, Ala.: Nursing Service, 1974.

GURLAND, B.   The assessment of the mental health status of older adults. In J. B. Birren & R. B. Sloane (Eds.), *Handbook of mental health and aging.* Englewood Cliffs, N.J.: Prentice-Hall, 1980.

GURLAND, B., KURIANSKY, J., SHARPE, L., SIMON, R., STILLER, P., & BIRKETT, P.   The comprehensive assessment and referral evaluation (CARE) Rationale, development and reliability: Part II. A factor analysis. *International Journal of Aging and Human Development,* 1977, *8,* 9-42.

HALE, W. E., MARKS, R. G., & STEWART, R. B.   Drug use in a geriatric population. *Journal of the American Geriatrics Society,* 1979, *27,* 374-377.

HALEY, J.   *Strategies of psychotherapy.* New York: Grune & Stratton, 1963.

HALEY, W. E.   A family behavioral approach to the treatment of the cognitively impaired elderly. *The Gerontologist,* 1983a, *23,* 18-20.

HALEY, W. E.   Behavioral self-management: Application to a case of agitation in an elderly chronic psychiatric patient. *Clinical Gerontologist,* 1983b, *3*(1), 45-52.

HAMILL, C. M., & OLIVER, R. C.   *Therapeutic activities for the handicapped elderly.* Rockville, Md.: Aspen Systems Corporation, 1980.

HARBERT, A. S., & GINSBERG, L. H.   *Human services for older adults: Concepts and skills.* Belmont, Calif.: Wadsworth, 1979.

HARBIN, H. T., & MADDEN, D. J.   Battered parents: A new syndrome. *American Journal of Psychiatry,* 1979, *136,* 1288-1291.

HARRIS, C. S. *Fact book on aging: A profile of America's older population.* Washington, D.C.: National Council on the Aging, 1978.

HARRIS, L., & ASSOCIATES *The myth and reality of aging in America.* Washington: National Council on Aging, 1975.

HARRIS, R. Special features of heart disease in elderly patients. In A. B. Chinn (Ed.), *Working with older people: A guide to practice.* Volume IV: *Clinical aspects of aging.* Washington, D.C.: U.S. Department of Health, Education, and Welfare, 1971.

HARRIS, R. Cardiopathy on aging: Are the changes related to congestive heart failure? *Geriatrics,* 1977, *32* (Feb.), 42-46.

HARTFORD, M. E. The use of group methods for work with the aged. In J. E. Birren & R. B. Sloane (Eds.), *Handbook of mental health and aging.* Englewood Cliffs, N.J.: Prentice-Hall, 1980.

HARTFORD, M. E., & PARSONS, R. Groups with relatives of dependent older adults. *The Gerontologist,* 1982, *22,* 394-398.

HATTON, J. Aging and the glare problem. *Journal of Gerontological Nursing,* 1977, *3,* 38-44.

HAUSMAN, C. P. Short-term counseling groups for people with elderly parents. *The Gerontologist,* 1979, *19,* 102-107.

HAVIGHURST, R. J., & ALBRECHT, R. *Older people.* New York: D. McKay, 1953.

HAYTER, J. Helping families of patients with Alzheimer's disease. *Journal of Gerontological Nursing,* 1982, *8,* 81-86.

HEADLEY, L. *Adults and their parents in family therapy: A new direction in treatment.* New York: Plenum Press, 1977.

HEAMAN, D. & MOORE, J. A pet show for remotivation. *Geriatric Nursing,* March-April, 108-110, 1982.

Help Begins at Home. International Center for the Disabled. New York, undated.

HENNESSEY, M. J. Music and music therapy groups. In I. M. Burnside (Ed.), *Working with the elderly: Group processes and techniques.* North Scituate, Mass.: Duxbury Press, 1978.

HERR, J. J., & WEAKLAND, J. H. *Counseling elders and their families: Practical techniques for applied gerontology.* New York: Springer Publishing Co., 1979.

HILL, R. A demographic profile of the black aged. *Aging,* 1978, *287-288,* 2-9.

HILL, R., FOOTE, N., ALDOUS, J., CARLSON, R., and MACDONALD, R. *Family development in three generations.* Cambridge: Schenkman, 1970.

HINTON, J. Speaking of death with the dying. In *Dying.* New York: Penguin Books, 1967. (Reprinted in E. S. Schneidman, Ed., *Death: Current perspectives.* Palo Alto, Calif.: Mayfield Publishing Company, 1976.)

HOGAN, R. Neoplasia. In W. J. Phipps, B. C. Long, N. F. Woods, *Medical-surgical nursing.* St. Louis: C. V. Mosby, 1979.

HOLMES, M., STEINFELD, E., SCHIAFFINO, K., & SILVERSTEIN, M. Volume III: Guidelines for the development of services and appropriate architectural design features in public housing for the elderly. New York: Community Research Applications, Inc., 1979.

HOLMES, T., & RAHE, R. H. The social readjustment scale. *Journal of Psychosomatic Research,* 1967, *11,* 213-217.

HOYER, W. J., KAFER, R. A., SIMPSON, S. C., & HOYER, F. W. Reinstatement of verbal behavior in elderly mental patients using operant procedures. *The Gerontologist,* 1974, *14,* 149-152.

HUBER, C. H., & WOLFF, A. R. Know thyself. Unit III in J. E. Myers & M. L. Ganikos (Eds.), *Counseling older persons Vol II: Basic helping skills for service providers*. Falls Church, Va.: American Personnel and Guidance Association, 1981.

HUSSIAN, R. A.   *Geriatric Psychology: A behavioral perspective*. New York: Van Nostrand Reinhold, 1981.

HUYCK, M. H., & HOYER, W. J.   *Adult development and aging*. Belmont, Calif.: Wadsworth, 1982.

HYATT, L. S.   Environment and the aged. Workshop presented at Bentley Gardens extended care facility. West Haven, Conn., October, 1982.

HYER, L., COLLINS, J., & BLAZER, DAN II.   Community adjustment of older schizophrenics. *Journal of Clinical Psychology*, 1983, *39*, 160-164.

INGERSOLL, B., & SILVERMAN, A.   Comparative group psychotherapy for the aged. *The Gerontologist*, 1978, *18*, 201-206.

INGERSOLL, B., & GOODMAN, L.   History comes alive: Facilitating reminiscence in a group of institutionalized elderly. *Journal of Gerontological Social Work*, 1980, *2*, 305-319.

IVEY, A., & AUTHIER, J.   *Microcounseling: Innovations in interviewing, counseling, psychotherapy, and psychoeducation* (2nd ed.), Springfield, Ill.: Charles C. Thomas, 1978.

JACKSON, J. J.   *Minorities and aging*. Belmont, Calif.: Wadsworth, 1980.

JACOBSON, E.   *Progressive relaxation*. Chicago: University of Chicago Press, 1938.

JARVIK, L. F.   Diagnosis of dementia in the elderly: A 1980 perspective. In C. Eisdorfer, (Ed.), *Annual Review of Gerontology and Geriatrics*, 1980, *1*, 180-203.

JARVIK, L. F., MINTZ, J., STEUER, J., & GERNER, R.   Treating geriatric depression: A 26-week interim analysis. *Journal of the American Geriatric Society*, 1982, *30*, 713-717.

JARVIK, L. F., & RUSSELL, D.   Anxiety, aging, and the third emergency reaction. *Journal of Gerontology* 1979, *34*, 197-200.

JENIKE, M. A.   Electroconvulsive therapy: What are the facts? *Geriatrics*, 1983, *38*(4), 33-38.

JESSE, E. M.   Pet therapy for the elderly. *Aging*, September-October, 1982, pp. 26-28.

JOHNSON, D. W., & JOHNSON, F. P.   *Joining together: Group therapy and group skills* (2nd Ed.). Englewood Cliffs, N.J.: Prentice-Hall, 1982.

JONES, M.   *The therapeutic community*. New York: Basic Books, 1953.

JONES, S. L.   *Family therapy:A comparison of approaches*. Bowie, Md.: Robert J. Brady Co., 1980.

JOURARD, S.   *The transparent self*. New York: Van Nostrand Reinhold, 1971.

KAHN, R. L.   The mental health system and the future aged. *The Gerontologist*, 1975, *15*, 24-31.

KAHN, R. L., GOLDFARB, A. I., POLLACK, M., & PECK, A.   Brief objective measures for the determination of mental status of the aged. *American Journal of Psychiatry*, 1960, *117*, 326-328.

KAHN, R. L., & MILLER, N. E.   Assessment of altered brain function in the aged. In M. Storandt, I. C. Siegler, & M. F. Elias, (Eds.) *The Clinical Psychology of Aging*, New York, Plenum, 1978.

KALISH, R. A.   Death and dying in a social context. In R. Binstock & E. Shanas (Eds.), *Handbook of aging and social sciences*. New York: Behavioral Publications, 1976.

KAMINSKY, M.   Pictures from the past: The use of reminiscence in casework with the elderly. *Journal of Gerontological Social Work*, 1978, *1*, 19-31.

KANE, R. A., & KANE, R. L. *Assessing the elderly: A practical guide to measurement.* Lexington, Mass.: Lexington Books, 1981.

KANFER, F. H., & PHILLIPS, J. S. *Learning foundations of behavior therapy.* New York: John Wiley, 1970.

KANFER, F. H., & SASLOW, G. Behavioral analysis: An alternative to diagnostic classification. *Archives of General Psychiatry,* 1965, *12,* 529-538.

KANFER, F. H., & SALSLOW, G. Behavioral diagnosis. In C. Franks (Ed.), *Assessment and status of the behavior therapies and associated developments.* New York: McGraw-Hill, 1969.

KARASU, T. B., & KATZMAN, R. Organic brain syndromes. In L. Bellak & T. B. Karasu (Eds.). *Geriatric psychiatry: A handbook for psychiatrists and primary care physicians.* New York: Grune & Stratton, 1976.

KART, C. S. *The realities of aging: An introduction to gerontology.* Boston: Allyn & Bacon, 1981.

KART, C. S., METRESS, E. S., & METRESS, J. F. *Aging and health: Biologic and social perspectives.* Reading, Mass.: Addison-Wesley, 1978.

KASTENBAUM, R. The realm of death: An emerging area in psychological research. *Journal of Human Relations,* 1965, *13,* 538-552.

KASTENBAUM, R. *Death, society, and human experience* (2nd ed.). St. Louis: C. V. Mosby, 1981.

KASTENBAUM, R., & AISENBERG, R. *The psychology of death.* New York: Springer Publishing Co., 1972.

KASTENBAUM, R., & CANDY, S. The 4 percent fallacy: A methodological and empirical critique of extended care facility population statistics. *International Journal of Human Development,* 1973, *4,* 15-31.

KATCHNER, A. H. Are companion animals good for your health? *Aging,* September-October 1982, pp. 2-8.

KATZ, D., & KAHN, R. L. *The social psychology of organizations.* New York: John Wiley, 1966.

KATZ, S., FORD, A. B., MOSKOWITZ, R. W., JACKSON, B. A., & JAFFEE, M. W. Studies in illness in the aged. The index of ADL: A standardized measure of biological and social function. *Journal of the American Medical Association,* 1963, *185,* 914-919.

KATZMAN, R. The prevalence and malignancy of Alzheimer's disease. *Archives of Neurology,* 1976, *33,* 217-218.

KAY, D. W. K., & ROTH, D. Environmental and hereditary factors in the schizophrenias of old age ("late paraphrenia") and their bearing on the general problem of causation in schizophrenia. *Journal of Mental Science,* 1961, *107,* 649-686.

KELLER, J. F., CROAKE, J. W., & BROOKING, J. Y. Effects of a program in rational thinking on anxieties in older persons. *Journal of Counseling Psychology,* 1975, *22,* 54-57.

KELLY, J. The aging male homosexual: Myth and reality. *The Gerontologist,* 1977, *17,* 328-332.

KEMPLER, W. Gestalt therapy. In L. Corsini (Ed.), *Current psychotherapies.* Ithica, Ill.: F. E. Peacock, 1973.

KENT, S. Preventing senile dementia: Hope for the future. *Geriatrics,* 1981, *36*(9), 130-136.

KIMMEL, D. C. *Adulthood and aging* (2nd ed), New York: John Wiley, 1980.

KITANO, H. H. L. *Race relations.* Englewood Cliffs, N.J.: Prentice-Hall, 1974.

KNIGHT, R. G. "There is no continuum of care." Discussant's remarks. In M. Edinberg (Chair) *Aging and mental health: A continuum of care?* Symposium presented at annual meeting of the American Psychological Association, Washington, D.C., August, 1982.

KOBATA, F. S., LOCKERY, S. A., & MORIWAKI, S. Y.   Minority issues in mental health and aging. In J. E. Birren & R. B. Sloane (Eds.). *Handbook of Mental Health and Aging.* Englewood Cliffs, N.J.: Prentice-Hall, 1980.

KOFF, T. H.   Death, dying, and survivorship. In M. Ganikos (Ed.), *Counseling the aged: A training syllabus for educators.* Falls Church, Va.: American Personnel and Guidance Association, 1978.

KOUZES, J. M., & MICO, P. R.   Domain theory: An introduction to organizational behavior in human service organizations. *Journal of Applied Behavioral Science,* 1979, *15,* 449-469.

KRAMER, M., TAUBE, C. A., & REDICK, R. W.   Patterns of use of psychiatric facilities by the aged: Past, present, and future. In C. Eisdorfer & M. P. Lawton (Eds.), *Psychology of adult development and aging.* Washington, D. C.: American Psychological Association, 1973.

KUBEY, R. W.   Television and aging: Past, present, and future. *The Gerontologist,* 1980, *20,* 16-35.

KÜBLER-ROSS, E.   *On death and dying.* New York: Macmillan, 1969.

KUYPERS, J. A., & BENGTSON, V. L.   Competence and social breakdown: A social-psychological view of aging. *Human Development,* 1973, *16,* 37-49.

LAGO, D., KNIGHT, B., & CONNELL, C.   PACT: A pet placement organization for the elderly living at home. *Aging,* September-October, 1982, pp. 19-25.

LAING, R. D.   *The politics of experience.* New York: Ballantine Books, 1968.

LAMM, L. B., & FOLSOM, J. C.   Attitude therapy and the team approach. *Mental Hospitals,* 1965, *16,* 307-320.

LANGER, E., & RODIN, J.   The effects of choice and enhanced personal responsibility for the aged: A field experiment in an institutional setting. *Journal of Personality and Social Psychology,* 1976, *34,* 191-198.

LAWRENCE, P.   Applying skills with special populations. In J. E. Myers & M. L. Ganikos (Eds.), *Counseling older persons. Volume II: Basic helping skills for service providers.* Falls Church, Va.: American Personnel and Guidance Association, 1981.

LAWTON, M. P., & BRODY, E.   Assessment of older people: Self maintaining and instrumental activities of daily living. *The Gerontologist,* 1969, *9,* 179-186.

LAWTON. M. P., & NAHEMOW, L.   Ecology and the aging process. In C. Eisdorfer & M. P. Lawton (Eds.), *Psychology of adult development and aging.* Washington, D.C.: American Psychological Association, 1973.

LAWTON, M. P., WHELIHAN, W. M., & BELSKY, J. K.   Personality tests and their uses with older adults. In J. E. Birren & R. B. Sloane (Eds.), *Handbook of Mental Health and Aging.* Englewood Cliffs, N. J.: Prentice-Hall, 1980.

LAZARUS, L. W., GUTMANN, D., GRUNES, J., RIPECKYJ, A., GROVES, L., NEWTON, N., FRANKEL, R., & HAVASY-GALLOWAY, S.   Process and outcome of brief psychotherapy with the elderly. Presented at annual meeting of the Gerontological Society, Boston, November, 1982.

LAZARUS, L. W., STAFFORD, F., COOPER, D., COHLER, B., & DYSKEN, M.   A pilot study of an Alzheimer patients' relatives discussion group. *The Gerontologist,* 1981, *21,* 353-358.

LEECH, S., & WITTE, K. L.   Paired associate learning in elderly adults as related to pacing and incentive condition. *Developmental Psychology,* 1974, *5,* 180.

LEERING, C.   A structural model of functional capacity in the aged. *Journal of the American Geriatrics Society,* 1979, *27,* 314-316.

LEHMAN, H. The influence of longevity upon curves showing man's creative production rate at successive age levels. *Journal of Gerontology,* 1958, *13,* 187-191.

LEONARD, L. Adult day care centers: A potent force for individual and family change. In S. S. Sargent (Ed.), *Nontraditional therapy and counseling with the aged.* New York: Springer Publishing Co., 1980.

LERNER, M. "When, why, and where people die." In O. G. Brim, Jr., H. E. Freeman, S. Levine, & N. A. Scotch, (Eds.), *The dying patient.* New York: Russell Sage Foundation, 1970.

LESSER, J., LAZARUS, L. W., FRANKEL, R., & HAVASY, A. Reminiscence group therapy with psychotic geriatric inpatients. *The Gerontologist,* 1981, *21,* 291-296.

LEVENKRON, J. C., COHEN, J. D., FISHER, B. B., & MUELLER, H. S. Modifying the type A coronary-prone behavior pattern. *Journal of Consulting and Clinical Psychology,* 1983, *51,* 192-194.

LEVINE, N. B., DASTOOR, D. P., & GENDRON, M. A. Coping with dementia: A pilot study. *Journal of the American Geriatrics Society,* 1983, *31,* 12-18.

LEVINSON, D. J. *The seasons of a man's life* (with N. Darrow, E. B. Klein, H. Levison & B. McKee). New York: Knopf, 1978.

LEVITSKY, A., & PERLS, F. The rules and games of Gestalt therapy. In J. Fagan & I. Shepherd (Eds.), *Gestalt therapy now.* New York: Harper & Row, 1970.

LEVY, R. Choline in Alzheimer's disease. *Lancet,* 1978, *2,* 944-945.

LEWINSOHN, P. M., BIGLAN, A., & ZEISS, A. M. Behavioral treatment of depression. In P. O. Davidson (Ed.), *The behavioral management of anxiety, depression, and pain.* New York: Brunner/Mazel, 1976.

LEWINSOHN, P. M., MUNOZ, R. F., YOUNGREN, M. A., & ZEISS, A. M. *Control your depression.* Englewood Cliffs, N. J.: Prentice-Hall, 1978.

LEWIS, M. I., & BUTLER, R. N. Life review therapy: Putting memories to work in individual and group psychotherapy. *Geriatrics,* 1974, *29,* 165-169; 172-173.

LIBB, J. W., & CLEMENTS, C. B. Token reinforcement in an exercise program for geriatric patients. *Perceptual and Motor Skills,* 1969, *28,* 957-958.

LIBOW, L. S. Senile dementia and "pseudosenility." In C. Eisdorfer & R. O. Friedel (Eds.), *Cognitive and emotional disturbance in the elderly: Clinical issues.* Chicago: Year Book Medical Publishers, 1977.

LIEBERMAN, M. A. Group methods. In F. Kanfer & A. Goldstein (Eds.), *Helping people change.* New York: Pergamon Press, 1980.

LIEBERMAN, M. A., & GOURASH, N. Evaluation the effects of change groups on the elderly. *International Journal of Group Psychotherapy,* 1979, *29,* 283-304.

LIEBERMAN, M. A., YALOM, I. D., & MILES, M. B. *Encounter groups: First facts.* New York: Basic Books, 1973.

LINDEMANN, E. Symptomatology and management of acute grief. *American Journal of Psychiatry,* 1944, *101,* 141-148.

LINDEN, M. E. Group psychotherapy with institutionalized senile women: Study in gerontologic human relations. *International Journal of Group Psychotherapy,* 1953, *3,* 150-170.

LINDEN, M. E. The significance of dual leadership in gerontologic group psychotherapy: Studies in gerontologic human relations. *International Journal of Group Psychotherapy,* 1954, *4,* 262-273.

LINDEN, M. E. Transference in gerontologic group psychotherapy: Studies in gerontologic human relations IV. *International Journal of Group Psychotherapy,* 1955, *5,* 61-79.

LIPOWSKI, Z. J.   Differentiating delirium from dementia in the elderly. *Clinical Gerontologist,* 1982, *1,* 3-10.

LOPATA, H.   *Women as widows: Support systems.* New York: Elsevier North Holland, 1979.

LOPATA, H. Z.   *Widowhood in an American city.* Cambridge, Mass.: Schenkman, 1973.

LOPEZ, M., HOYER, W. J., GOLDSTEIN, A. P., GERSHAW, N. J., & SPRAFKIN, R. P.   Effects of overlearning and incentive on the acquisition and transfer of interpersonal skills with institutionalized elderly. *Journal of Gerontology,* 1980, *35,* 403-408.

LOPICCOLO, J., & LOPICCOLO, L.   (Eds.), *Handbook of sex therapy.* New York: Plenum, 1978.

LOWENTHAL, M F.   The relationship between social factors and mental health in the aged. Psychiatric research report 23. American Psychiatric Association, February 1968.

LOWENTHAL, M. F.   Psychosocial variation across the adult life course: Frontiers for research and policy. *The Gerontologist,* 1975, *15,* 6-15.

LOWENTHAL, M. F., & HAVEN, C.   Interaction and adaptation: Intimacy as a critical variable. *American Sociological Review,* 1968, *33,* 414-420.

LOWY, L.   *Social work with the aging: The challenge and promise of the later years.* New York: Harper & Row, 1979.

LUCE, G. G.   *Your second life.* Lawrence, N.Y.: Delacorte Press/Seymour, 1979.

LUDEMAN, K.   The sexuality of the older person: Review of the literature. *The Gerontologist,* 1981, *21,* 203-208.

MACDONALD, M. L.   Teaching assertion: A paradigm for therapeutic intervention. *Psychotherapy: Theory, Research and Practice,* 1975, *12,* 60-67.

MACDONALD, M. L., & BUTLER, A. K.   Reversal of helplessness: Producing walking behavior in nursing home wheelchair residents using behavior modification procedures. *Journal of Gerontology,* 1974. *29,* 97-101.

MACDONALD, M. L., & SETTIN, J. M.   Reality orientation versus sheltered workshops as treatment for the institutionalized aging. *Journal of Gerontology,* 1978, *33,* 416-421.

MACE, N. L., & RABINS, P. V.   *The 36-hour day.* Baltimore: The Johns Hopkins University Press, 1981.

MADDOX, G. L.   Disengagement theory: A critical evaluation. *The Gerontologist,* 1964, *4,* 80-82.

MAGNUSSEN, M. H.   Body protection in the aged and the nursing process. In A. G. Yurik, S. S. Robb, B. E. Spier, & N. J. Ebert. *The aged person and the nursing process.* New York: Appleton-Century-Crofts, 1980.

MAHONEY, F. I., & BARTHEL, D. W.   Functional evaluation: The Barthel index. *Rehabilitation,* 1965, *14,* 61-65.

MAHONEY, M. J.   *Cognition and behavior modification.* Cambridge, Mass.: Ballinger, 1974.

MARMOR, J.   Psychiatrists and their patients: A national study of private practice psychiatrists. Washington, D.C.: American Psychiatric Association, 1975.

MARSHALL, J. R.   The geriatric patient's fears about death. *Postgraduate Medicine,* 1971, *57,* 144-149.

MASLOW, A.   *Toward a psychology of being.* Princeton, N.J.: Van Nostrand, 1968.

MASLOW, A.   *Motivation and personality* (Rev. ed.), New York: Harper & Row, 1970.

MASTERS, W. H., & JOHNSON, V. E.   *Human sexual response.* Boston: Little, Brown, 1966.

MASTERS, W. H. & JOHNSON, V. E. *Human sexual inadequacy.* Boston: Little, Brown, 1970.

MASTERS, W. H. & JOHNSON, V. E. Sex and the aging process. *Journal of the American Geriatrics Society,* 1981, *29,* 385-390.

MAXEY, L. B. Therapeutic interaction with families of th confused elderly. In M. O. Wolanin, & L. R. Phillips, *Confusion: Prevention and care.* St. Louis: C. V. Mosby, 1981.

MAY, E. E., WAGGONER, N. R., & HOTTE, E. B. *Independent living of the handicapped elderly.* Boston: Houghton Mifflin, 1974.

MAY, R. *Man's search for himself.* New York: Dell Pub. Co., 1953.

MEICHENBAUM, D. *Cognitive-behavior modification.* New York: Plenum, 1977.

MERRIAM, S. The concept and function of reminiscence: Review of the research. *The Gerontologist,* 1980, *20,* 604-608.

MERSKEY, H. The nature of pain. In W. L. Smith, H. Merskey, & S. C. Gross (Eds.), *Pain: Meaning and management.* New York: Spectrum Pubications, 1980.

MILLER, E. Cognitive assessment of the older adult. In J. E. Birren & R. B. Sloane (Eds.), *Handbook of mental health and aging.* Englewood Cliffs, N.J.: Prentice-Hall, 1980.

MINUCHIN, S. *Families and family therapy.* Cambridge, Mass.: Harvard University Press, 1974.

MISHARA, B. L. Environment and face-hand test performance in the institutionalized elderly. *Journal of Gerontology,* 1979, *34,* 692-696.

MISHARA, B. L., & KASTENBAUM, R. *Alcohol and old age.* New York: Grune & Stratton, 1980.

MITFORD, J. *The American way of death.* New York: Simon & Schuster, 1963.

MONGE, R. H., & HULTSCH, D. Paired-associate learning as a function of adult age and the length of the anticipation and inspection intervals. *Journal of Gerontology,* 1971, *26,* 157-162.

MOODY, R. A. *Life after life.* Atlanta, Ga.: Mockingbird Press, 1975.

MOORE, E. C. Using music with groups of geriatric patients. In I. M. Burnside (Ed.), *Working with the elderly: Group process and techniques.* North Scituate, Mass.: Duxbury Press, 1978.

MOOS, R. H. *The human context: Environmental determinants of behavior.* New York: John Wiley, 1976.

MUGFORD, R. A., & M'COMISKY, J. G. Some recent work on the psychotherapeutic value of cage birds with old people. In R. S. Anderson (Ed.), *Pet animals and society.* London: Balilliere Tindall, 1975.

MURRAY, J. Family structure in the preretirement years. *Retirement history study report No. 4.* U.S. Department of Health, Education, and Welfare, 1973.

NEEDLER, W., & BAER, M. A. Movement, music, and remotivation with the regressed elderly. *Journal of Gerontological Nursing,* 1982, *8,* 497-502.

NELSON, F. L., & FARBEROW, N. L. Indirect self-destructive behavior in the elderly nursing home patient. *Journal of Gerontology,* 1980, *35,* 949-957.

NEUGARTEN, B. L. Personality and aging. In J. E. Birren, and K. W. Schaie (Eds.), *Handbook of the psychology of aging.* New York: Van Nostrand Reinhold, 1977.

NEWCOMER, R. J., & CAGGIANO, M. A. Environment and the aged person. In I. M. Burnside (Ed.). *Nursing and the aged.* New York: McGraw-Hill, 1976.

NICHOLS, R., & NICHOLS, J. Funerals: A time for grief and growth. In E. Kübler-Ross (Ed.), *Death: The final stage of growth.* Englewood Cliffs, N.J.: Prentice-Hall, 1975.

NUNNALLY, J. C. *Psychometric theory.* New York: McGraw-Hill, 1967.

NUSSMAN, J., & BURT, M. No room for pets. *Aging,* September-October 1982, pp. 15-18.

OBERLEDER, M. Restoring the mentally ill through reality orientation. In L. P. Stephens (Ed.), *Reality orientation.* Washington, D.C.: American Psychiatric Association, 1969.

O'BRIEN, J. E., & WAGNER, D. L. Help seeking by the frail elderly: Problems in network analysis. *The Gerontologist,* 1980, *20,* 78-83.

O'FARRELL, T. J., KEUTHERN, N. J., CONNORS, G. J., & UPPER, D. Age-related differences among psychiatric inpatients. *International Journal of Behavioral Geriatrics,* 1983, *2,* 29-37.

OKUN, B. F. *Effective helping, interviewing, and counseling techniques* (2nd ed.), Monterey, Calif.: Brooks-Cole, 1982.

OLSON, J. K., & CAHN, B. W. Helping families cope with elderly parents. *Journal of Gerontological Nursing,* 1980, *6,* 152-154.

OSTERWEIS, M., & SZMUSZKOVICZ-CHAMPAGNE, D. The U.S. hospice movement: Issues in development. *American Journal of Public Health,* 1979, *69,* 492-496.

PAGE, J. D. *Psychopathology: The science of understanding deviance.* New York: Aldine, 1971.

PALMORE, E. B. Facts on aging: A short quiz. *The Gerontologist,* 1977, *17,* 315-320.

PALMORE, E. B. The facts on aging quiz: Part two. *The Gerontologist,* 1981, *21,* 431-437.

PALMORE, E. B., CLEVELAND, W. P., NOWLIN, J. B., RAMM, D., & SIEGLER, I. C. Stress and adaptation in later life. *Journal of Gerontology,* 1979, *34,* 841-851.

PARKES, C. M. *Bereavement: Studies of grief in adult life.* New York: International Universities Press, 1972.

PAUL, G. L., & BERNSTEIN, D. A. Anxiety and clinical problems: Systematic desensitization and related techniques. In J. T. Spence, R. C. Carson, & J. W. Thibaut (Eds.), *Behavioral approaches to therapy.* Morristown, N.J.: General Learning Press, 1976.

PECK, R. C. Psychological developments in the second half of life. In J. E. Anderson (Ed.), *Psychological aspects of aging,* Proceedings of a conference in planning research, Bethesda, Md. Washington, D.C.: American Psychological Association, April 1955.

PEGELS, C. C. *Health care and the elderly.* Rockville, Md.: Aspen, Systems Corporation, 1980.

PERLS, F. *Gestalt therapy verbatim.* Moab, Utah: Real People Press, 1969a.

PERLS, F. *In and out of the garbage pail.* Moab, Utah: Real People Press, 1969b.

PERLS, F. Four lectures. In J. Fagan & I. Shepherd (Eds.), *Gestalt therapy now.* New York: Harper & Row, 1970.

PFEIFFER, E. A short portable mental status questionnaire for the assessment of organic brain deficit in elderly patients. *Journal of the American Geriatrics Society,* 1975, *23,* 433-441.

PFEIFFER, E. Psychopathology and social pathology. In J. E. Birren & K. W. Schaie (Eds.), *Handbook of psychology and aging.* New York: Van Nostrand Reinhold, 1977.

PFEIFFER, E., & BUSSE, E. W. Mental disorders in later life-affective disorders: Paranoid, neurotic, and situational reactions. In E. W. Busse & E. Pfeiffer (Eds.), *Mental illness in later life.* Washington, D.C.: American Psychiatric Association, 1973.

PFEIFFER, E., JOHNSON, T. M., & CHIOFOLO, R. C. "Functional assessment of elderly subjects in four service settings." Paper presented at the annual scientific meeting of the Gerontological Society of America, San Diego, Calif., 1980.

PHILLIPS, L. R. F. Care of the client with sensoriperceptual problems. In M. O. Wolanin, & L. R. Phillips, *Confusion: Prevention and Care*. St. Louis: C. V. Mosby, 1981.

POLSTER, E., & POLSTER, M. *Gestalt therapy integrated: Contours of theory and practice*. New York: Brunner/Mazel, 1973.

POST, F. Paranoid, schizophrenia-like, and schizophrenia states in the aged. In J. E. Birren & R. B. Sloane (Eds.), *Handbook of mental health and aging*. Englewood Cliffs, N.J.: Prentice-Hall, 1980.

PUDER, R. S., LACKS, P., BERTELSON, A., & STORANDT, M. Short-term stimulus control treatment of insomnia in older adults. Paper presented at the meeting of the Gerontology Society of America, Boston, 1982.

PUTERSKI, D. The role of the community mental health center: A case study. In M. Edinberg, (Chair) *Aging and mental health: A Continuum of care?* Symposium at annual meeting of the American Psychological Association. Washington, D.C., August 1982.

RAGAN, P. K., & SIMONIN, M. M. *Social and cultural contexts of aging: Community survey report*. Los Angeles: Andrus Gerontology Center, University of Southern California, 1977.

RATHBONE-McCUAN, E. Elderly victims of family violence and neglect. *Social Casework*, 1980, *61* (day), 296-304.

RATHBONE-McCUAN, E., & CLAYMON, C. Counseling the isolated elderly. *Journal of the American Geriatrics Society*, 1979, *27*, 355-358.

REDDY, W. B. Screening and selection of participants. In L. N. Solomon, & B. Berzon, (Eds.), *New perspectives on encounter groups*. San Francisco: Jossey Bass, 1972.

REDDY, W. B., & LIPPERT, K. M. The processes and dynamics within experimental groups. In P. Smith (Ed.), *Small groups and personal change*. London: Methuen, 1980.

REDICK, R. W., & TAUBE, C. A. Demography and mental health care of the aged. In J. E. Birren & R. B. Sloane (Eds.), *Handbook of mental health and aging*. Englewood Cliffs, N.J.: Prentice-Hall, 1980.

REIDEL, R. G. Experimental analysis as applied to adulthood and old age: A review. Paper presented at American Psychological Association meeting, New Orleans, 1974.

REIFLER, B. V., & EISDORFER, C. A clinic for impaired elderly and their families. *American Journal of Psychiatry*, 1980, *137*, 1399-1403.

REINHART, R. A, & SARGENT, S. S. The humanistic approach: The Ventura County creative aging workshops. In S. S. Sargent (Ed.), *Nontraditional therapy and counseling with the aged*. New York: Springer Publishing Co., 1980.

RELF, P. D. Horticulture as a recreational activity. *American Health Care Association Journal*, September 1978, *4*, 68-70.

RESNIK, H. L., & CANTOR, J. M. Suicide and aging. *Journal of the American Geriatrics Society*, 1970, *18*, 152-158.

RICHMAN, S. A couples therapy group on a geriatric service. Presented at annual meeting of the Gerontological Society, Dallas, November 1978.

RIMM, D. C., & MASTERS, J. C. *Behavior therapy: Techniques and empirical findings*. New York: Academic Press, 1974.

RIOCH, M. J. Changing concepts in the training of therapists. *Journal of Consulting Psychology*, 1966, *30*, 290-292.

ROBB, S. S.   The elderly in the United State: Numbers, proportions, health status, and use of health services. In A. G. Yurick, S. S. Robb, B. E. Apier, & N. J. Ebert. *The aged person and the nursing process.* New York: Appleton-Century-Crofts, 1980.

ROBINSON, A. M.   *Remotivation techniques: A manual for use in nursing homes.* American Psychiatric Association and Smith Kline and French Laboratories Remotivation Project, Philadelphia.

RODIN, J., & LANGER, E.   Long-term effects of a control-relevant intervention with the institutionalized aged. *Journal of Personality and Social Psychology,* 1977, *35,* 897-902.

ROGERS, C. R.   *Counseling and psychotherapy.* Boston: Houghton Mifflin, 1942.

ROGERS, C. R.   *Client-centered therapy.* Boston: Houghton Mifflin, 1951.

ROGERS, C. R.   *On becoming a person.* Boston: Houghton Mifflin, 1961.

ROGERS, C. R.   *Carl Rogers on personal power.* New York: Delacorte Press, 1977.

ROOZMAN-WEIGENSBERG, C., & FOX, M.   A group work approach with adult children of institutionalized elderly: An investment in the future. *Journal of Gerontological Social Work,* 1980, *2,* 355-362.

ROSS, M. & BURDICK, D.   *Sensory integration.* Thorofare, N.J.: Charles B. Slack, 1981.

ROTH, M., TOMLINSON, B. E., & BLESSED, G.   The relationship between quantitative measures of dementia and of degenerative changes in cerebral gray matter of elderly subjects. *Proceedings of the Royal Society of Medicine,* 1967, *60,* 254-259.

RYDEN, M.   Nursing intervention in support of reminiscence. *Journal of Gerontological Nursing,* 1981, *1,* 461-463.

SANDEL, S. L.   Integrating dance therapy into treatment. *Hospital and Community Psychiatry,* 1975, *26,* 439-441.

SANDEL, S. L.   Movement therapy with geriatric patients in a convalescent home. *Hospital and Community Psychiatry,* 1978a, *29,* 738-741.

SANDEL, S. L.   Reminscence in movement therapy with the aged. *Art Psychotherapy,* 1978b, *5,* 217-221.

SARASON, S. B.   *Work, aging, and social change.* New York: Free Press, 1977.

SARASON, S. B., & LORENTZ, E.   *The challenges of the resources exchange network.* San Francisco: Jossey-Bass, 1979.

SARGENT, S. S., (Ed.).   *Nontraditional therapy and counseling with the aging.* Volume 7 in the Springer series on adulthood and aging. New York: Springer Publishing Co., 1980.

SATIR, V.   *Peoplemaking.* Palo Alto, Calif.: Science and Behavior Books, 1972.

SAUNDERS, C.   Dying they live: St. Christopher's hospice. In J. S. Quadagno (Ed.), *Aging: The individual and society: Readings in social gerontology.* New York: St. Martin's Press, 1980. Originally printed in H. Feitel, (Ed.), *New meanings of death.* New York: McGraw-Hill, 1971.

SAUNDERS, C.   St. Christopher's hospice. In E. S. Schneidman, (Ed.), *Death: Current perspectives.* Palo Alto: Mayfield Publishing Company, 1976. (Reprinted from St. Christopher's Hospice Annual Report, 1971-72.)

SCHACT, T., & NATHAN, P.   But is it good for psychologists? Appraisal and status of DSM-III. *American Psychologist,* 1977, *32,* 1017-1025.

SCHELL, M. A. Sr.,   *Conversion handbook for remotivation in health care centers.* Wilton, Conn.: School Sisters of Notre Dame, 1975.

SCHNEIDMAN, E. S.   *Death: current perspectives.* Palto Alto, Calif.: Mayfield Publishing Co., 1976.

SCHONFIELD, A. E. D. Learning, memory, and aging. In J. E. Birren, & R. B. Sloane (Eds.), *Handbook of mental health and aging*. Englewood Cliffs, N.J.: Prentice-Hall, 1980.

SCHUCKIT, M. A. Geriatric alcoholism and drug abuse. *The Gerontologist*, 1977, *17*, 168-174.

SCHULZ, R. The effects of control and predictability on the psychological and physical well-being of the institutionalized aged. *Journal of Personality and Social Psychology*, 1976, *33*, 563-573.

SCHULZ, R. *The psychology of death, dying, and bereavement*. Reading, Mass.: Addison-Wesley, 1978.

SCHULZ, R., & BRENNER, G. Relocation of the aged: A review and theoretical analysis. *Journal of Gerontology*, 1977, *32*, 323-333.

SCHULZ, R., & HANUSA, B. H. Long-term effects of control and predictability-enhancing interventions: Findings and ethical issues. *Journal of Personality and Social Psycology*, 1978, *36*, 1194-1201.

SCHWARTZ, A. N. Training of peer counselors. In S. S. Sargent (Ed.), *Nontraditional therapy and counseling with the aging*. Springer series on adulthood and aging. New York: Springer Publishing Co., 1980.

SCHWARTZ, A. N., & PETERSON, J. A. *Introduction to gerontology*. New York: Holt, Rinehart & Winston, 1979.

SCOVERN, A. W., & KILMANN, P. R. Status of ECT: A review of the outcome literature. *Psychological Bulletin*, 1980, *87*, 260-303.

SEIXAS, F. A. Drug/alcohol interactions—Avert potential dangers. *Geriatrics*, 1979, *34*(10), 89-102.

SELYE, H. *Stress without distress*. Philadelphia: Lippincott, 1974.

SETTIN, J. M. Overcoming ageism in long-term care: A solution in group therapy. *Journal of Gerontological Nursing*, 1982, *8*, 565-567.

SHADER, R. I., HARMATZ, J. S., & SALZMAN, C. A. A new scale for clinical assessment in geriatric populations: Sandoz clinical assessment geriatric (SCAG). *Journal of the American Geriatrics Society*, 1974, *22*, 107-113.

SHAFFER, J. *Humanistic psychology*. Englewood Cliffs, N.J.: Prentice-Hall, 1978.

SHANAS, E. The family as a social support system in old age. *The Gerontologist*, 1979, *19*, 169-174.

SHERMAN, E. A cognitive approach to direct practice with the aging. *Journal of Gerontological Social Work*, 1979, *2*, 43-53.

SIMON, A. The neuroses, personality disorders, alcoholism, drug use and misuse, and crime in the aged. In J. E. Birren & R. B. Sloane (Eds.), *Handbook of mental health and aging*. Englewood Cliffs, N.J.: Prentice-Hall, 1980.

SIMONTON, O. C., MATTHEWS-SIMONTON, S., & CREIGHTON, J. *Getting well again*. Los Angeles: J. P. Tarcher, 1978.

SIMONTON, O. C., & SIMONTON, S. S. Belief systems and management of the emotional aspects of malignancy. *Journal of Transpersonal Psychology*, 1975, *7*(1), 29-47.

SIMPSON, M. "Brought in dead." *Omega*, 1976, *7*(3), 243-248.

SKLAR, M. Gastrointestinal diseases in the aged. In A. B. Chinn (Ed.), *Working with older people: A guide to practice*, Vol. 4, *Clinical aspects of aging*. Washington, D.C.: U.S. Public Health Service Publication 1459, 1971, 124-130.

SLATER, E., & ROTH, M. *Clinical psychiatry* (3rd ed.), Baltimore: Williams & Wilkins, 1977.

SLOANE, R. B. Organic brain syndrome. In J. E. Birren & R. B. Sloane (Eds.),

Handbook of mental health and aging. Englewood Cliffs, N.J.: Prentice-Hall, 1980.

SMITH, E.   Are you really communicating? *American Journal of Nursing,* 1977, *77,* 1966-1968.

SMITH, D. W., & GERMAIN, C. P. H.   *Care of the adult patient* (4th ed.), New York: J. B. Lippincott, 1975.

SMITH, K. F., & BENGTSON, V. L.   Positive consequences of institutionalization: Solidarity between elderly parents and their middle-aged children. *The Gerontologist,* 1979, *19,* 438-447.

SMITH, W. L., MERSKEY, D. M., & GROSS, S. L. (Eds.).   *Pain: Meaning and management.* New York: Spectrum Publications, 1980.

SMYER, M. A.   The differential usage of services by impaired elderly. *Journal of Gerontology,* 1980, *35,* 249-255.

SMYER, M. A., & GATZ, M.   Aging and mental health: Business as usual? *American Psychologist,* 1979, *34,* 240-246.

SNYDER, L. H., PYREK, J., & SMITH, K. C.   Vision and mental function of the elderly. *The Gerontologist,* 1976, *16,* 491-495.

SOBEL, W. K.   Behavioral treatment of depression in the dying patient. In H. J. Sobel (Ed.), *Behavior therapy in terminal care: A humanistic approach.* Cambridge, Mass.: Ballinger, 1981.

SOLOMON, C.   Elderly non-whites: Unique situations and concerns. In M. L. Ganikos (Ed.), *Counseling the aged:A training syllabus for educators.* Falls Church, Va.: American Personnel and Guidance Association, 1979.

SOLOMON, R.   Serving families of the institutionalized aged: The four crises. *Journal of Gerontological Social Work,* 1982, *5,* 83-96.

SOMER, R.   Small group ecology in institutions for the elderly. In L. A. Pastalan & D. H. Carson (Eds.), *Spatial behavior of older people.* Ann Arbor: University of Michigan Press, 1970.

SPARACINO, J.   The type A (coronary-prone) behavior pattern, aging, and mortality. *Journal of the American Geriatrics Society,* 1979, *27,* 251-257.

Statistical Abstract of the United States, 1982-1983. National data book and guide to sources. 103rd edition. Washington, U.S. Government Printing Office.

STAUFFER, S. B.   Pet programs for the elderly: Rewards and responsibilities. *Aging,* September-October 1982, 9-14.

STEELE, F.   Physical settings and organization development. Reading, Mass.: Addison-Wesley, 1973.

STENBACK, A.   Depression and suicidal behavior in old age. In J. E. Birren & R. B. Sloane (Eds.), *Handbook of mental health and aging.* Englewood Cliffs, N.J.: Prentice-Hall, 1980.

STENGEL, E.   Psychopathology of dementia. *Proceedings of the Royal Society of Medicine,* 1964, *57,* 911-914.

STEUER, J.   Psychotherapy for depressed elders. In D. G. Blazer II (Ed.), *Depression in late life.* St. Louis: C. V. Mosby, 1982.

STEUER, J., & AUSTIN, E.   Family abuse of the elderly. *Journal of the American Geriatrics Society,* 1980, *28,* 372-376.

STEUER, J., & CLARK, E. O.   Family support groups within a research project on dementia. *Clinical Gerontologist,* 1982, *1,* 87-95.

STINNETT, N., COLLINS, J., & MONTGOMERY, J.   Martial need satisfaction of older husbands and wives. *Journal of Marriage and the Family,* 1970, *32,* 428-434.

STORANDT, M.   *Counseling and therapy with older adults.* Boston: Little, Brown, 1983.

STRAIN, L. A., & CHAPPELL, N. L. Confidants: Do they make a difference in quality of life? *Research on Aging*, 1982, *4*, 479-502.

STREIB, G. F., & SCHNEIDER, C. J. *Retirement in American society: Impact and process*. Ithaca, N.Y.: Cornell University Press, 1971.

SUDNOW, D. *Passing on*. Englewood Cliffs, N.J.: Prentice-Hall, 1967.

SUE, S. Psychological theory and implications for Asian Americans. *Personnel and Guidance Journal*, 1977, *55*, 381-389.

SUINN, R. M. Intervention with type A behaviors. *Journal of Consulting and Clinical Psychology*, 1982, *50*, 933-949.

SZAPOCZNIK, J., SANTISTENBAN, D., HERUIS, O., SPENCER, F., & KURTINES, W. M. Treatment of depression among Cuban American Elders: Some validation evidence for a life enhancement counseling approach. *Journal of Consulting and Clinical Psychology*, 1981, *49*, 752-754.

TANNA, V. Paranoid states, a selected review. *Comprehensive Psychiatry*, 1974, *15*, 453-470.

TATE, J. W. The need for personal space in institutions for the elderly. *Journal of Gerontological Nursing*, 1980, *6*, 439-449.

TAULBEE, L. R. *The ABCs of reality orientation: An instruction manual*. Lucille R. Taulbee (Publisher), 1976.

TAULBEE, L. R. Reality orientation: A therapeutic group activity for elderly persons. In I. M. Burnside (Ed.), *Working with the elderly: Group processes and techniques*. North Scituate, Mass.: Duxbury Press, 1978.

TAULBEE, L. R., & FOLSOM, J. C. Reality orientation for geriatric patients. *Hospital and Community Psychiatry*, 1966, *17*, 133-135.

TERRY, R. D. Dementia: A brief and selective review. *Archives of Neurology*, 1976, *33*, 1-4.

TERRY, R. D. & WISNIEWSKI, H. M. Structural and chemical changes of the aged human brain. In S. Gershin & A. Raskin (Eds.), *Aging: Vol. 2. Genesis and treatment of psychologic disorder in the elderly*. New York: Raven Press, 1975.

TINDALL, J. P. Geriatric dermatology. In A. B. Chinn (Ed.), *Working with older people: A guide to practice*. Vol. 4. *Clinical aspects of aging*. Washington, D.C.: U.S. Public Health Service Publication 1459, 1971, 3-27.

TOBIN, S. S., & LIEBERMAN, M. A. *Last home for the aged: Critical implications for institutionalization*. San Francisco: Jossey-Bass, 1976.

TOBIN, S. S., & NEUGARTEN, B. L. Life satisfaction and social interaction in the aging. *Journal of Gerontology*, 1961, *16*, 344-346.

TOMLINSON, B. E., & HENDERSON, G. Some qualitative findings in normal and demented old people. In R. D. Terry & S. Gershin (Eds.), *Neurobiology of aging*. New York: Raven Press, 1976.

TRAUB, R., GAJDUSEK, N. C., & GIBBS, C. J. Transmissible viris dementia: The relation of transmissible spongiform encephalopathy to Creutz-Feldt-Jacob disease. In W. L. Smith & M. Kinsbourne (Eds.), *Aging and dementia*. New York: Spectrum Publications, 1977.

TREAS, J. Aging and the family. In D. S. Woodruff & J. E. Birren (Eds.), *Aging: Scientific perspectives and social issues*. New York: Van Nostrand Reinhold, 1975.

TREAS, J., & VAN HILST, A. Marriage and remarriage rates among older Americans. *The Gerontologist*, 1976, *16*, 132-136.

TUCKMAN, B. W. Developmental sequence in small groups. *Psychological Bulletin*, 1965, *3*, 384-399.

TURK, D. C., & RENNERT, K. Pain and the terminally ill cancer patient: A cognitive-social learning perspective. In H. J. Sobel (Ed.), *Behavior therapy in terminal care: A humanistic approach.* Cambridge, Mass.: Ballinger, 1981.

U.S. Bureau of the Census (1983). Current population reports, series P-23, #128, America in Transition: An Aging Society. Washington: U.S. Government Printing Office.

VANDEN BOS, G. R., STAPP, J., & KILBURG, R. R.   Health service providers in psychology: Results of the APA human resources survey. *American Psychologist,* 1981, *36,* 1395-1418.

VEITH, R. C.   Depression in the elderly: Pharmacologic considerations in treatment. *Journal of the American Geriatrics Society,* 1981, *30,* 581-586.

VERWOERDT, A.   *Clinical geropsychiatry.* Baltimore: Williams & Wilkins, 1976.

VOELKEL, D.   A study of reality orientation and resocialization groups with confused elderly. *Journal of Gerontological Nursing,* 1978, *4,* 3-18.

WAGNER, D. L., & KEAST, F.   Informal groups and the elderly. *Research in Aging,* 1981, *3,* 325-331.

WATERS, E., FINK, S., & WHITE, B.   Peer group counseling for older people. *Educational Gerontology,* 1976, *1,* 157-170.

WATSON, W.   *Aging and behavior: An introduction to social gerontology.,* Scituate, Mass.: Duxbury Press, 1982.

WAUGH, N. C., & NORMAN, D. A.   Primary memory. *Psychological Bulletin,* 1965, *72,* 89-104.

WEED, L.   *Medical records, medical education, and patient care: The problem oriented record as a basic tool.* Cleveland: Press of Case Western University, 1969.

WEEKS, J. R., & CUELLAR, J. B.   The role of family members in the helping networks of older people. *The Gerontologist,* 1981, *21,* 388-394.

WEILER, P. G, & RATHBONE-MCCUAN, E.   *Adult day care: Community work with the elderly.* New York: Springer Publishing Co., 1978.

WEINER, R. D.   The role of electroconvulsive therapy in the treatment of depression in the elderly. *Journal of the American Geriatrics Society,* 1982, *30,* 710-712.

WEISMAN, A. D.   Common fallacies about dying patients. From: *On dying and denying: A psychiatric study of terminality.* New York: Behavioral Publications, Inc. 1972a. (Reprinted in E. S. Schneidman (Ed.), *Death: Current perspectives.* Palo Alto, Calif.: Mayfield Publishing Company 1976.)

WEISMAN, A. D.   *On Dying and Denying: A psychiatric study of terminality.* New York: Behavioral Publications, 1972b.

WEISMAN, A. D.   *The realization of death.* New York: Jason Aronson, 1974.

WEISMAN, A. D., & KASTENBAUM, R.   The psychological autopsy: a study of the terminal phase of life. *Community Mental Health Journal* Memograph No. 4, 1968.

WELLS, C. E.   *Dementia* (2nd ed.). Philadelphia: F. A. Davis, 1977.

WESTIN, A.   *Privacy and freedom.* New York: Atheneum Press, 1970.

WHEELER, E.   Assertive training groups for the aging. In S. S Sargent (Ed.), *Nontraditional therapy and counseling with the aging.* New York: Springer Publishing Co., 1980.

WHITAKER, D. S., & LIEBERMAN, M. A.   *Psychotherapy through the group process.* Chicago: Aldine, 1964.

WILLINGTON, F. L.   Incontinence—5: Training and retraining for continence. *Nursing Times,* 1975, *71* (March 27), 500-503.

WILLINGTON, F. L. (Ed.).   *Incontinence in the elderly.* New York: Academic Press, 1976.

WILLIS, S. L., & BALTES, P. B.   Intelligence in adulthood and aging: Contemporary issues. In L. W. Poon (Ed.), *Aging in the 1980s: Psychological issues.* Washington, D.C.: American Psychological Association, 1980.

WINDLEY, P. G., & SCHEIDT, R. J.   Person-environment dialectics: Implications for competent functioning in old age. In L. W. Poon (Ed.), *Aging in the 1980s: Psychological issues.* Washington, D.C.: American Psychological Association, 1980.

WISOCKI, P. A., & MOSHER, P.   Peer-facilitated sign language training for a geriatric stroke victim with chronic brain damage. *Journal of geriatric psychiatry,* 1980, *13,* 89-102.

WOLANIN, M. O., & PHILLIPS, L. R. F., (Eds.),   *Confusion prevention, and care.* St. Louis: C. V. Mosby, 1981.

WOLCOTT, A. B.   Art therapy: An experimental group. In I. M. Burnside (Ed.), *Working with the elderly: Group processes and techniques.* North Scituate, Mass.: Duxbury Press, 1978.

WOLF, R. S., STRUGNELL, C. P., & GODKIN, M. A.   Preliminary findings from three model projects on elderly abuse. Worcester, Mass.: University of Massachusettes Medical Center, 1982.

WOLFF, A. R., & MEYER, G. W.   Counseling older adults: Suggested approaches. In M. L. Ganikos (Ed.), *Counseling the aged: A training syllabus for educators.* Falls Church, Va.: American Personnel and Guidance Association, 1979.

WOLFF, K.   Comparison of group and individual psychotherapy with geriatric patients. *Diseases of the Nervous System,* 1967, *28,* 384-386.

WOLPE, J.   *Psychotherapy by reciprocal inhibition.* Stanford, Calif.: Stanford University Press, 1958.

WOLPE, J., & LAZARUS, A.   *Behavior therapy techniques: A guide to the treatment of neuroses.* Oxford: Pergamon Press, 1966.

WORTMAN, C. B., & DUNKEL-SCHETTER, C.   Interpersonal relationships and cancer: A theroretical analysis. *Journal of Social Issues,* 1979, *35,* 120-155.

YALOM, I. D.   *The theory and practice of group psychotherapy.* New York: Basic Books, 1970.

YEATES, A.   *Behavior therapy.* New York: John Wiley, 1970.

YEATES, W. K.   Normal and abnormal bladder function in incontinence of urine. In F. L. Willington (Ed.), *Incontinence in the elderly.* New York: Academic Press, 1976.

YESAVAGE, J. A., ADEY, M., & WERNER, P. D.   Development of a geriatric behavioral self-assessment scale. *Journal of the American Geriatrics Society,* 1981, *29,* 285-288.

YESAVAGE, J. A., & BERENS, E. S.   Multiple monitored electroconvulsive therapy in the elderly. *Journal of the American Geriatrics Society,* 1980, *28,* 206-209.

YURICK, A. G., ROBB, S. S., SPIER, B. E., & EBERT, N. J.   *The aged person and the nursing process.* New York: Appleton-Century-Crofts, 1980.

ZARIT, J. M.   *Familial role, social supports, and their relation to caregiver's burden.* Presented at an annual meeting of the Western Psychological Association. Sacramento, Calif., 1982.

ZARIT, S. H.   *Aging and mental disorders.* New York: Free Press, 1980.

ZARIT, S. H., GALLAGHER, D., & KRAMER, N.   Memory training in the community aged: Effects on depression, memory, complaint, and memory performance. *Educational Gerontology,* 1981, *6,* 11-27.

ZARIT, S. H., & KAHN, R. L.   Aging and adaptation to illness. *Journal of Gerontology,* 1975, *30,* 67-72.

ZARIT, S. H., MILLER, N. E., & KAHN, R. L.   Brain function, intellectual impairment, and education in the aged. *Journal of the American Geriatrics Society,* 1978, *26,* 58-67.

ZEMORE, R., & EAMES, N.   Psychic and somatic symptoms of depression among young adults, institutionalized aged, and noninstitutionalized aged. *Journal of Gerontology,* 1979, *34,* 716-722.

ZEPELIN, H., WOLFE, R., & NORRIS, A.   Evaluation of a year-long reality orientation program. *Journal of Gerontology,* 1981, *36,* 70-77.

ZIEGER, B. L.   Life review in art therapy with the aged. *American Journal of Art Therapy,* 1976, *15,* 47-50.

ZIMBERG, S.   The elderly alcoholic. *The Gerontologist,* 1974, *14,* 221-224.

ZUNG, W. W. K.   A self-rating depression scale. *Archives of General Psychiatry,* 1965, *12,* 63-70.

ZUNG, W. W. K.   Depression in the normal aged. *Psychosomatics,* 1967, *8,* 287-292.

Index

Ross, M., 217
Roth, M., 112, 117
Roush, S., 3
Rowley, B.D., 47
Ryden, M., 165

SAGE Project, 200-201
Salzman, C.A., 135
Samberg, S., 203, 204
Sandel, S., 203-5
Sandoz Clinical Assessment, 135
Sarason, S.B., 259, 261, 262
Sargent, S.S., 13, 142, 200, 201
Saslow, G., 137, 169
Satir, V., 193, 230, 236
Saunders, C., 67, 68
Schact, T., 77
Scheidt, R.J., 247, 252, 255
Schell, M.A., Sr., 218
Schiaffino, K., 250-51, 253
Schizophrenialike illnesses, 82-83
Schizophrenic disorders, 79-84
Schneider, C.J., 50
Schneidman, E.S., 65, 69
Schonfield, A.E.D., 180
Schovern, A.W., 89
Schuckit, M.A., 97
Schulz, R., 59, 60, 63-65, 68, 241, 245, 246, 265
Schwab, K., 50
Schwartz, A.N., 45, 273, 274
Scott, M., 276
Screening, group, 211, 213
Secondary memory, 18
Segal, N.L., 80-81, 83
Seixas, F.A., 97
Selection of peer counselors, 273-74
Selective abstraction, 186
Self
  -actualization, 192
  -awareness, 70, 193
  -care, widowhood and, 54-55
  -confidence, 12
  -disclosure, 145, 194, 221
  groups focusing on development of, 220-22
  -image, internalizing, 12
  -reliance, 12
  sense of, 193
Self-assessment Scale-Geriatric, 135
Seltzer, J., 218

Selye, H., 33
Senile brain disease, 111-15, 119-20
Senile macular degeneration, 30
Senile plaques, 112
Senile pruritus, 26
Senility, myth of, 3
Senior Actualization and Growth Experience (SAGE) project, 200-201
Senior centers, 270
Senior's Assertion Manual, The (Edinberg), 181
Sense of self, 193
Sense organs, changes in, 30-31
Sensory awareness, 217
Sensory stimulation, environmental, 248-50
Sensuality, 21
Services
  coordination, 121
  delivery of, 257-77
    in community settings, 268-71
    extensions of traditional, 272-77
    federal funding sources for programs, 271-72
    in institutions, 262-68
    nature of system, 258-59
    observations about, 260-62
  need for nontraditional, 142-43
Sessions, 143, 212-13
Settin, J.M., 180, 210
Setting
  appropriate, 145
  community, 121, 268-71
  institutional, 262-68
  integration of group into, 214-15
Sexuality, aging and, 3-4, 20-25
Shader, R.I., 135
Shaffer, J., 191
Shanas, E., 42, 263
Sharpe, L., 104, 111, 137
Shepherd, I., 192, 196
Sheppard, H.A., 208
Sherwood, C.C., 127
Shifts, issues between staff, 266-67
Shock therapy, electroconvulsive, 88-89
Short Portable MSQ (SPMSQ), 132-33
"Sick role," acceptance of, 175-76
Siegler, I.C., 33
Significant others, involvement of, 175
Silverman, A., 217
Silverstein, M., 250-51, 253